Sociology for Nurses

Third Edition

Edited by Elaine Denny, Sarah Earle and Alistair Hewison

polity

Copyright © Polity Press 2016

The right of Elaine Denny, Sarah Earle and Alistair Hewison to be identified as Authors of this Work has been asserted in accordance with the UK Copyright, Designs and Patents Act 1988.

First published in 2016 by Polity Press

Polity Press
65 Bridge Street
Cambridge CB2 1UR, UK

Polity Press
350 Main Street
Malden, MA 02148, USA

ISBN-13: 978-1-5095-0540-1
ISBN-13: 978-1-5095-0541-8(pb)

A catalogue record for this book is available from the British Library.

Library of Congress Cataloging-in-Publication Data

Names: Denny, Elaine, editor. | Earle, Sarah, editor. | Hewison, Alistair, editor.
Title: Sociology for nurses / [edited by] Elaine Denny, Sarah Earle, Alistair
    Hewison.
Description: Third edition. | Cambridge, UK ; Malden, MA : Polity Press,
    2016. | Includes bibliographical references and index.
Identifiers: LCCN 2015038012| ISBN 9781509505401 (hardcover : alk. paper) |
    ISBN 1509505407 (hardcover : alk. paper) | ISBN 9781509505418 (pbk. : alk.
    paper) | ISBN 1509505415 (pbk. : alk. paper)
Subjects: | MESH: Nursing Care--psychology. | Sociology--Nurses' Instruction.
Classification: LCC RT86.5 | NLM WY 87 | DDC 610.73--dc23 LC record
available at http://lccn.loc.gov/2015038012

Typeset in 10.5 on 13pt Minion Pro by Servis Filmsetting Ltd, Stockport, Cheshire
Printed and bound in Italy by Rotolito Lombarda

For further information on Polity, visit our website: politybooks.com

Contents

Boxes, Figures and Tables

Figures

Tables

Contributors

Elaine Denny is emeritus professor of health sociology at Birmingham City University. Her research interests focus around women as recipients and providers of health care, in particular reproductive health, and she has published work on women's experience of IVF, the experience of endometriosis, and the occupation of nursing. She has conducted qualitative research within Health Technology Assessment funded randomized controlled trials on a variety of women's health topics. With Sarah Earle, she co-edited the previous two editions of *Sociology for Nurses*, and with Ruth Deery and Gayle Letherby she co-edited *Sociology for Midwives* (Polity, 2015). She is currently on the editorial board of *BJOG An International Journal of Obstetrics and Gynaecology*.

Sarah Earle is associate dean for research in the Faculty of Health & Social Care at the Open University. Her research interests include reproductive and sexual health and the role of sociology within health-care education and practice. She has published widely in these fields and is the co-editor of *Understanding Reproductive Loss: Perspectives on Life, Death and Fertility* (Ashgate, 2012), with Carol Komaromy and Linda Layne, and sub-editor of the international journal *Human Fertility*. With Elaine Denny she co-edited the first two editions of *Sociology for Nurses*.

Alistair Hewison is senior lecturer and research lead for Nursing in the School of Nursing at the University of Birmingham. His current research and teaching activities are centred on the management and organization of care. He has served as principal investigator for several studies, including a large-scale National Institute of Health Research funded examination of service re-design in three acute NHS Trusts, and a number investigating the organization of end-of-life care services. He has an honorary contract with Birmingham St Mary's Hospice, where he is responsible for research development. With colleagues at the Health Services Management Centre at the University of Birmingham he is investigating the organizational factors which contribute to failures in nursing care, and was recently appointed to the advisory board of the prestigious Langston Center for Quality, Safety and Innovation in Richmond, Virginia, USA. He has written widely on health-care management and policy issues in papers published in scholarly journals and chapters in edited collections.

Carol Komaromy is a medical sociologist who has worked as a full-time academic at the Open University since 1994 and is now a visiting research associate. Prior to this, she worked in health care, midwifery and counselling. Since moving from practice to academia, Carol has been involved in research and teaching in end-of-life and palliative care. She has also worked as media fellow and is currently co-editor of the international journal, *Mortality*, and vice president of the Association of Death and Society. She is committed to the belief that sociological research should make a difference to the experience of service users and providers. With Jenny Hockey and Kate Woodthorpe, she is co-editor of *The Matter of Death: Space, Place and Materiality* (Palgrave, 2010), and, with Sarah Earle and Linda Layne, she co-edited *Understanding Reproductive Los*s (Ashgate, 2012).

Sue Ledger is a researcher with the Faculty of Health & Social Care at the Open University. Her interests include life-story methods, consent, inclusive research, health-care improvement and the involvement of people with high support needs in research. Sue published, peer-reviewed and presented with people with learning disabilities on a range of issues. Most recently she has co-edited a book entitled *Sexuality and Relationships in the Lives of People with Intellectual Disabilities: Standing in My Shoes* (Jessica Kingsley Publishers, 2015).

Gayle Letherby is honorary professor of sociology at Plymouth University and combines freelance academic activities with work as a civil celebrant (<http://www.arwenack.co.uk/p/home.html>). Academic research and writing interests embrace all things methodological (including feminist, auto/biographical and creative approaches); reproductive and non/parental identities; gender, health and wellbeing; loss and bereavement; travel and transport mobility and working and learning in higher education. Most recent publications include *An Introduction to Gender: Social Science Perspectives* (revised 2nd edn, Routledge, 2014), with Jennifer Marchbank, and 'Gendered Methodology', in *Introducing Gender and Women's Studies* (4th edn, Palgrave, 2015), edited by Victoria Robinson and Diane Richardson.

Paula McGee is emeritus professor of nursing in the Faculty of Health, Education and Life Sciences at Birmingham City University. Her main interests are in nursing practice and in the impact of race, culture and diversity on care. She has published widely on both subjects. In 2005 she was awarded the title of Transcultural Nursing Scholar in recognition of her work, the first nurse in the UK to receive this award. She has launched and edited several international professional journals, including *British Journal of Nursing* and *Diversity and Equality in Health and Care*, and has acted as guest editor for other publications. She is currently associate editor of the *Journal of Transcultural Nursing*.

Catherine Needham is a reader in public policy and public management at the Health Services Management Centre, University of Birmingham. Her areas of special interest include: reform of public services through co-production and personalization; public-sector workforce change; and individualized budgets within public services. Her most recent book was published by the Policy Press in 2014, entitled *Debates in Personalization*.

Lindy Shufflebotham has worked for the past twenty-five years in both statutory and voluntary sectors, in the provision of support to people with learning disabilities. Particular areas of interest include: access to ordinary housing, user involvement in organizational strategy and governance arrangements and the role and contribution of community organizations in enabling improved health care.

Kate Thomson has been teaching health policy and sociology at Birmingham City University since 2004, where she has gained substantial experience in curriculum development and in teaching health practitioners at undergraduate and postgraduate levels. She is currently director of postgraduate research degrees in health. Her research interests centre on health and social policy, with a particular focus on international and cross-cultural comparisons (particularly in relation to Russia and Eastern Europe), and on the wider politics of health.

Jan Walmsley is an independent researcher and teacher with honorary chairs at both the Open University and London South Bank University. She is a fellow of the National Institute of Health Research's School of Social Care Research, and on the editorial board of two leading disability journals, *Disability and Society* and the *British Journal of Learning Disabilities*. She has practised and written extensively about 'inclusive research', working and publishing alongside intellectually disabled researchers.

Acknowledgements

The editors would like to acknowledge the contribution of the following people to the first edition of *Sociology for Nurses*:
Keith Sharp (Chapter 1)
Barbara Green (Chapter 2)
Corinne Wilson and Geraldine Brown (Chapter 7)
Pat Chambers (Chapter 8)
Terry O'Donnell (Chapter 11)

Figure 8.3 contains public-sector information licensed under the Open Government Licence v3.0.

We are grateful to the Lambeth Learning Disability Forum and Jane Abraham for permission to use their photograph (Figure 10.4).

Figure 14.1 contains public-sector information licensed under the Open Government Licence v3.0.

Illustration Credits

The publisher would like to acknowledge permission to reproduce the following images:

Chapter 1:
Figure 1.1 © Monkeybusinessimages/iStock
Figure 1.2 © Jacky Fleming (www.jackyfleming.co.uk)
Figure 1.3 © Jean Schweitzer/iStock

Chapter 2:
Figure 2.1 © Roman Milert/iStock
Figure 2.2 © Chris Schmidt/iStock
Figure 2.3 © Steve Vidler/Alamy Stock Photo

Chapter 3:
Figure 3.1 © Maria Perry
Figure 3.2 © Keith Brofsky/Getty
Figure 3.4 © Fertnig/iStock

Chapter 4:
Figure 4.2 © Steve Debenport/iStock
Figure 4.3 © Annett Vauteck/iStock
Figure 4.4 © Darren Baker/iStock

Chapter 5:
Figure 5.1 © Shaith/iStock
Figure 5.2 © Photofusion/ Getty
Figure 5.3 © Carolyn Jenkins/Alamy Stock Photo

Chapter 6:
Figure 6.1 © David Monniaux/Wikimedia Commons;
Figure 6.2 © Alex Belomlinsky/iStock
Figure 6.3 © ACORN 1/Alamy Stock Photo
Figure 6.4 © Tim Hales – The FA/Getty

Chapter 7:
Figure 7.1 © Yuri_Arcurs/iStock
Figure 7.2 © duncan1890/iStock
Figure 7.3 © Susan Chang/iStock
Figure 7.4 Adapted from O'Keefe et al., 2007

Chapter 8:
Figure 8.1 © Jui Chen/iStock
Figure 8.2 © DurdenImages/iStock
Figure 8.3 Adapted from National Statistics online
Figure 8.4 © Sturti/iStock

Chapter 9:
Figure 9.1 © snapphoto/iStock

Figure 9.2 © vandervelden/iStock
Figure 9.3 © NoDerog/iStock
Chapter 10:
Figure 10.1 © herjua/iStock
Figure 10.2 © UPPA/Photoshot
Figure 10.3 © abalcazar/iStock
Figure 10.4 © Jane Abraham
Chapter 11:
Figure 11.1 Adapted from Health Survey England, 2013
Figure 11.2 © Christopher Futcher/iStock
Figure 11.3 Adapted from Dahlgren and Whitehead, 1991
Figure 11.4 ©Photofusion Picture Library/Alamy Stock Photo
Chapter 12:
Figure 12.1 © Cathy Yeulet/iStock
Figure 12.2 © PYMCA/Getty
Figure 12.3 © Photofusion/Getty
Chapter 13:
Figure 13.1 © Cameron Spencer/Getty
Figure 13.3 © danhughes/iStock
Figure 13.4 © OLI SCARFF/Getty
Chapter 14:
Figure 14.2 © choja/iStock
Figure 14.3 Adapted from Schein, 1985
Figure 14.4 © Janine Wiedel Photolibrary/Alamy Stock Photo
Chapter 15:
Figure 15.1 © David Callan/iStock
Figure 15.2 Adapted from SCIE's *Personalization: A Rough Guide*, 2013
Figure 15.3 © Alex Raths/iStock
Chapter 16:
Figure 16.1 © Jaymast/iStock
Figure 16.2 Adapted from WHO, 2009
Figure 16.3 © relax360/iStock
Figure 16.4 © Jonathan Torgovnik/Getty

Introduction

Sarah Earle, Elaine Denny and Alistair Hewison

The Nursing and Midwifery Council (NMC 2010) requires nurses across the UK to respond to changing needs, developments and priorities within health and health care, and to possess the knowledge, skills and behaviours that will enable them to do so effectively. The standards for competence (NMC 2010) that all student nurses must achieve ensure that nurses are able to meet future challenges, drive up standards and improve the population's health and well-being. In order to achieve these competencies, nurses are expected to consider up-to-date evidence and are required to draw on knowledge from a range of disciplines, including the social sciences.

Nursing is no longer (if it ever was) the sum of its tasks – or what nurses 'do' – but has become a complex set of relationships. Society has changed since the inception of the NHS, deference towards health professionals has lessened and individuals are more willing to challenge 'experts'. Professional boundaries are becoming less rigid and many client groups are demanding a more active part in decision-making. The NHS itself has seen many reorganizations, and nurses, along with other health-care workers, have had to adapt to changing structures and ideologies of health care.

The impact of these changes has been immense, and many nurses have found themselves at a loss to know how to prepare themselves for the new demands made of them. There are probably few nurses who would turn to sociology to provide answers, as it is a discipline frequently perceived to be not of direct relevance to nursing work. This book has, therefore, deliberately set out to demonstrate the usefulness of sociology by relating the concepts and theories of sociology and health policy to nursing practice, with examples from all four branches of nursing. The aim of the book is to provide an accessible sociological textbook on health, illness and health care, based on the needs of pre-registration nursing courses. It is also of relevance to post-registration students on 'top-up' degree programmes, particularly those who are new to the study of sociology.

The book is divided into three parts and each part enables you to draw on sociology to help you meet the requirements of *The Code* for nurses and midwives in the UK (NMC 2015).

Part I considers the contribution that sociological knowledge and research methods can make to the delivery of nursing care. *The Code* for nurses and midwives requires you to think about your own professional development and to practise effectively, using the best evidence available and best practice. Part I starts by introducing the key sociological theories and approaches that underpin many of the concepts discussed later in the book. It then turns to the frequently raised question of why nurses need to study sociology, and how knowledge of these theories may make a difference to nursing practice. One of the tasks of sociology is to encourage us to apply a 'sociological imagination' to things we may take for granted; the concepts of 'health' and 'nursing' are explored here using just such an approach. Part I also introduces you to sociological research methods and encourages you to think about how best to use research and evidence.

Part II explores diversity and inequality in health and health care, demonstrating the link between client groups and the structures of society. These structures will advantage some groups and disadvantage others, resulting in wide variations in the incidence and experience of morbidity and mortality. A continuing theme here will be the role of nurses in challenging inequality and becoming advocates for patients and clients. *The Code* for nurses and midwives requires nurses to prioritize people and recognize diversity, and to ensure that discriminatory attitudes and behaviours are challenged. Engaging with the issues raised in this section may result in confronting and questioning your own beliefs and values.

Nurses are required to be models of integrity and leadership for others to aspire to, and they must work within the law and other relevant policies and guidance (NMC 2015). Reflective practice requires a broader understanding of the context of how and why policies are made and the extent to which these change and aid, or constrain, practice. Part III of the book moves on to explore some of the wider influences on health and health care, and considers the relevance of policy and management issues to nurses at all levels, not just those in senior roles, and the opportunity for nurses to engage in policy debate. The book finishes by moving outside of the NHS and direct patient/client care to think about health within a global context and the implications of this for nurses.

The chapters are similarly structured and designed to enable you to reflect on the sociological issues raised and to relate them to nursing practice:

- Each chapter begins with the key issues, giving you signposts on what to expect.

- Learning outcomes enable you to assess whether you have understood and learnt from what you have read.
- Key terms are explained in the glossary boxes in the margins, to aid understanding at a glance.
- There are activities to carry out with colleagues from your own, or different, branches of nursing, enabling reflection and encouraging you to relate theory to practice.
- At the end of each chapter there are summary points.
- To expand your knowledge, annotated further reading and questions for discussion are included at the end of the chapter.
- There is also a website accompanying this volume, providing further reading, questions for discussion, and links to Internet resources.

Once you have read this book and engaged with the activities and discussion questions, we hope that you will feel equipped to use a sociological approach as one of your tools for formulating and delivering optimum nursing care. You may also wish to enter into the debates about the future of nursing and its place in determining health policy. Most of all, you should be able to look beyond the simple explanations of everyday issues and problems to gain a deeper, more meaningful understanding.

References

NMC 2015 *The Code: Professional Standards of Practice and Behaviour for Nurses and Midwives*. Available at: <http://www.nmc.org.uk/globalassets/ sitedocuments/nmc-publications/revised-new-nmc-code.pdf>.

NMC 2010 *Standards for Pre-registration Nursing Education*. Available at: <http://www.nmc.org.uk/globalassets/sitedocuments/nmc-publications/ standards-for-pre-registration-nursing-education-16082010.pdf>.

Part I
Nursing and the Sociology of Health and Health Care

Sociology is exciting and can transform the way you think about the world, but is not always easy to understand – even for sociology students – and its relevance to nursing, and nurses, is not readily apparent. There is considerable controversy regarding whether nurses should study sociology and we have attempted to reflect this within Part I of this book. Some commentators have suggested that sociology should not be included in the nursing curriculum, arguing that it can add no value to nurse education and training. Others have suggested that sociology is vital to nurse education and to the future of nursing as a profession!

Student nurses often ask: 'Why do we have to do sociology?' It is as a response to this question that we have written this book and, more specifically, chosen to include the chapters in this section. Each of these chapters examines key concepts and debates in relation to nursing, and the sociology of health and health care.

The first chapter, 'What is Sociology?', introduces you to key sociological approaches, concepts and theories. With this in mind, some of you may find it useful to start with this chapter, whereas others of you may wish to come back to it after reading the later chapters within this section. This first chapter begins by outlining the distinction between sociological knowledge and other forms of knowledge, and considers the role of sociology within society. Sociology is often criticized as just 'common sense' and this chapter addresses this distinction. The chapter then moves on to examine the distinction between social 'structure' and social 'action', outlining key sociological theories and their relevance to our understanding of health and health care. The chapter concludes by encouraging you to think about how sociologists might theorize mental health.

The second chapter specifically addresses the question of 'Why Should Nurses Study Sociology?', and explores the role of sociological knowledge within nursing practice. Following on from the discussion begun in Chapter 1, this chapter examines how, far from being just 'common sense', sociology can help to develop a range of thinking skills which are vital to contemporary nursing. This chapter highlights the problem of the 'theory–practice gap' and focuses on the sociology of nursing as well as the role of sociology in nursing. By drawing on a variety of empirical studies, this chapter explores the value of sociological knowledge to nurses. The chapter also explores the importance of sociological research methods as both a tool for carrying out research and as a resource for evaluating published research. At the end of the chapter there is a special focus on why sociology is relevant to experiences of diabetes.

Nurses are involved in caring for people who are ill or dying, as well as promoting health and well-being. Whichever is the case, understanding what being 'healthy' means is important – although it is a challenging task, to say the least. In Chapter 3, 'What is Health?', we consider the range of ways that health has been defined, looking at 'official' definitions of health, as well as the distinction between professional and lay definitions. Models of health are also explored and, here, we contrast the biomedical model, which has been influential within medicine and health care, with the social model, which focuses on the social causes of disease. In this chapter we also consider the social construction of health and illness, examining how normal healthy processes become medicalized, and discuss the iatrogenic effects of medicalization on individuals and on society. Here we focus on obesity and the sociological debates on the medicalization of fatness. This chapter also considers a more holistic approach to care within nursing and offers some sociological reflections on this.

Chapter 4, 'Nursing as an Occupation', provides a brief historical overview of nursing, mapping the development of nursing and nurse registration from the nineteenth century and beyond. Just as other chapters within this section consider issues of definition, this chapter explores the debates which attempt to define what nursing is – is it an art or a science? In this chapter we consider the process of becoming a nurse and the socialization of students into nursing. Following on from the debate identified in Chapter 3, this chapter further highlights the tension of the 'theory–practice gap' within the socialization of student nurses. The gendered nature of nursing is also considered, and the role and status of men within nursing. Power relations are explored, and elitism within nursing and the relationships between nurses and other health-care workers are considered. Drawing on the concept of emotion work, relationships between nurses and patients are also discussed and the challenge of dementia for nursing as an occupation is considered.

In the final chapter of Part I, methodological approaches and some of the research methods commonly used by sociologists to explore health and illness are explored. In particular, the chapter focuses on the distinction between quantitative and qualitative methods, exploring when and why different research methods would be used. The chapter encourages critical reflection on the use of different research methods, outlining the key strengths and limitations of different methods of data collection. At the end of the chapter, the principles of research discussed are applied to the case of coronary heart disease.

What is Sociology?

Sarah Earle

KEY ISSUES IN THIS CHAPTER:

▶ The nature of sociological inquiry.
▶ Sociology, 'common sense' and lay reasoning.
▶ The role of sociology in society and in nursing.
▶ An introduction to sociological theory.
▶ Theorizing mental health and illness.

BY THE END OF THIS CHAPTER YOU SHOULD BE ABLE TO:

▶ Understand the nature of sociological inquiry.
▶ Recognize the distinction between sociology, 'common sense' and lay reasoning.
▶ Engage in some of the debates concerning the role of sociology within society and nursing.
▶ Discuss different sociological theories.
▶ Apply sociological theories to the issue of mental health and illness.

1 Introduction

Sociology is concerned, in the broadest sense, with the study of human society. As this implies, its scope is almost limitless: it is possible, in principle, to have a sociology of any activity in which human beings engage. Inevitably the sorts of activities that have concerned sociologists have changed somewhat over time. The principal concerns of sociologists writing in the nineteenth century, when sociology was just beginning as an academic discipline, were the major social, political and economic changes which had taken place across Europe since the late Middle Ages. Early sociological writing was dominated, for example, by attempts to chart and explain the rise of industrial capitalism and

modernity:
a focus on achieving progress, synonymous with industrialization

the changing nature and role of religion in society, and to understand the new forms which social and political institutions had taken since the Industrial Revolution (Giddens 2001); this period of time is known as **modernity**. Today, the changed concerns of sociologists largely reflect the changing nature of society. A shift in sexual attitudes and behaviours, gender relations, globalization and new communications technologies, as well as changing patterns of criminality and social aspects of health and illness – the subject of this book – have all loomed large in recent sociological literature (see, for example, Letherby et al. 2008; Earle and Sharp 2007; Sassen 2007; and Nettleton 2006). Most recently, attention has turned to the subject of happiness. For instance, some of the debates have focused on the individual and social benefits of being happy, such as improved mental health and well-being, as well as on the more controversial economic and political benefits for society generally (such as increased productivity and less frequent use of health services).

Activity 1.1 The benefits of happiness

David Cameron's 2006 speech to Google Zeitgeist can be found at: <http://www.guardian.co.uk/politics/2006/may/22/conservatives.davidcameron.co.uk/ politics/2006/may/22/conservatives.davidcameron>. When you have read this, answer the questions below.

(a) What is happiness? Can you define it?
(b) Can you make patients happy? If so, how?
(c) Is happiness important in nursing?
(d) Why do you think happiness is a sociological concern?

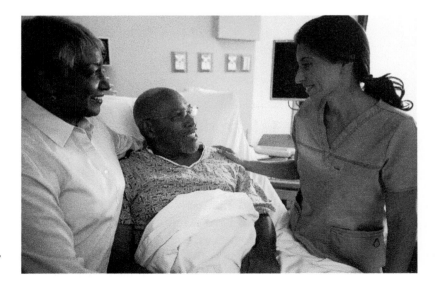

Figure 1.1 'It's time we admitted that there's more to life than money and it's time we focused not just on GDP but on GWB – general well-being.' David Cameron, British Prime Minister

There are a number of key questions and issues which lie at the heart of sociological inquiry, whatever the specific topic to which it is directed. The aim of this chapter is to introduce the most important of these. Before doing so, it is important to make a few general points about the nature of sociological inquiry and how it may differ from other disciplines. The remainder of this chapter is devoted to a discussion of the main theoretical debates in sociology.

In particular, the chapter will consider the main competing theoretical positions adopted by sociologists, and illustrate the implications of these different positions for the ways in which sociology can shed light on the nature of society and its institutions. An appreciation of these debates will be helpful in understanding many of the chapters that follow and in evaluating the contribution that sociology can make to nursing practice.

2 The nature of sociological inquiry

The first thing to note about the discipline of sociology is that it is characterized by diversity. While in any discipline we will find a certain amount of disagreement between practitioners, this is especially marked in the case of sociology. Unlike disciplines such as chemistry or biology, sociologists disagree even about the most fundamental principles of their methods of working. Some of these disagreements will be examined later in this chapter. What this means is that sociology cannot, in general, be used to 'solve' technical problems in the way that knowledge from other 'scientific' disciplines may be able to.

Sociology and other disciplines

A second point worth noting about sociology is that many of the topics with which it is concerned are also of interest to researchers from other disciplines. It is therefore prone to 'boundary disputes'. A good example of this is the relationship between sociology and psychology. In broad terms it is possible to say that while sociology is concerned with understanding societies, psychology is concerned with understanding individuals. But very quickly the value of this distinction starts to break down. Rather obviously, societies are made up of individuals, so cannot be understood entirely without reference to individuals. Let us take a concrete example. Sociologists often like to use the term **socialization**. However, it seems clear that the processes by which individuals are socialized fall within the domain of psychology, and the whole subfield of learning has a great deal to say about this. Unfortunately, sociologists rarely seem to take much notice of the wealth of psychological literature which details the complexity of the socialization process; similarly, psychologists are often accused of failing to give proper attention to the insights of sociologists on the complex effects of wider social processes on individual learning.

socialization: processes by which individuals acquire the roles, norms and cultures of society

The role of sociology within society

Finally, it is worth noting that sociology must confront a particularly wide range of ethical issues. Not only must sociologists deal with the sorts of issues around the avoidance of individual harm in the course of conducting their research, which any human scientist must confront (and this is discussed in Chapter 5), but there is also a wider set of ethical concerns about the role of sociology in society. Is it the role of sociology, for example, to make recommendations about the kinds of social arrangements that are most desirable? Or should it, as the sociologist Max Weber argued, avoid such essentially political questions and focus instead on developing a neutral understanding of the social world, leaving questions of how society should be organized to politicians? As you will see from Part II of this book, sociology has been particularly influential in identifying social inequalities in health. Is it the role of sociology to comment on the extent to which such inequalities should be eradicated (bearing in mind that even beginning to do so would entail massive costs which would have to be funded somehow), or should sociologists be content merely to describe and explain the extent of the inequality that exists? Some sociologists argue that sociology should offer solutions to social problems. For instance, Widdance Twine (2011), who writes about gestational surrogacy, argues that sociology has always been dedicated to analysing social problems, offering diagnoses as well as solutions. Others, such as Bruce (2000), are quite against this idea, suggesting that sociologists should focus on issues that are sociologically interesting, rather than issues that might be socially problematic. In doing so, Bruce argues, sociologists can discover some quite interesting and unexpected findings.

Sociology versus 'common sense'

An often voiced criticism of sociology is that it is just 'common sense', and that sociologists do little more than state the obvious. So it is important to explain why sociology is, and must be, more than just common sense (see also Chapter 2). The first point to make about this is that there is often more than one 'common-sense' view on any given issue. One viewpoint is that it is just 'common sense' that people are poor because they are lazy, stupid and work-shy. From another perspective, it is just common sense that poverty results from historical inequalities in society, and hence has nothing to do with individual attributes. Clearly both views cannot be correct, and so little will be gained in this case by relying on common sense. In fact, the explanation of poverty is a highly complex example, which requires sophisticated sociological research and analysis (see Chapter 11).

Similarly, 'common sense' often conceals positions of self-interest – or **partisanship**. It might be common sense for the rich to regard the

partisanship: bias or allegiance to the view of a particular social group

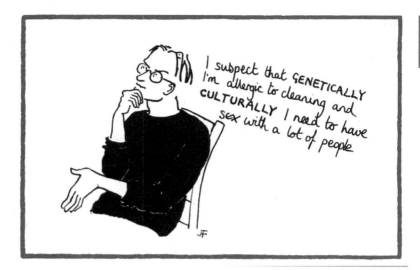

Figure 1.2
Genetically

poor as lazy, stupid and work-shy, but it seems most unlikely that such a view would be regarded as common sense by someone in poverty. In other words, it can be tempting, when adopting a common-sense view, to regard one's own views and ideas as correct, and the views of others as incorrect, or merely ideology. However, the role of sociology is to challenge the obvious, and to assess the evidence and arguments for and against any particular position that is advanced.

Another important distinction to be made between sociology and common sense is that any good scientific theory – whether sociological or not – must be internally consistent. It is this fact that distinguishes theory from common sense or what might otherwise be known as **lay reasoning**. Writing specifically about this, the sociologist Steve Bruce (2000: 1) writes:

lay reasoning:
everyday thinking about the world that is neither consistent nor scientifically rigorous

> My mother contradicted herself more often than not. That something she said one moment was incompatible with her next pronouncement hardly ever troubled her. She once criticized a roadside café by asserting that the food was vile and the portions were too small!

As you will read in more detail in the chapter on research methods (Chapter 5), sociologists draw on rigorous evidence to make claims about the world and how it works. Sociologists also engage in the open exchange of ideas and seek evidence that refutes their ideas, rather than just looking for evidence that supports what they want to argue. In other words, sociology is different from common sense or 'lay reasoning' because a traditional scientific approach is followed, meaning that sociological theories are internally consistent and rigorously applied.

3 Classical theoretical debates in sociology

structure:
organized patterns of social behaviour and the social institutions within society

The aim of this section is not to provide you with a comprehensive summary of debates in sociological theory, but rather to highlight some of the most important and to sketch out their implications for how sociologists concerned with health and illness go about their work. The distinction between **structure**, on the one hand, and **action**, on the other, is fundamental to theoretical debates within sociology, and these are discussed below.

action:
purposeful and conscious behaviour

Structural theories

A question often posed by sociologists is: what is society? Although this may appear rather simple at first sight, we can quickly see that it does in fact raise a number of different possibilities. One general view of society can be called structural. This view tends to see societies as systems of interconnected parts, which influence each other in a variety of complex ways. The focus is less on the specific actions of individuals, than on the roles they occupy and the ways in which these roles relate to each other. Structural theories are also sometimes referred to as macro-sociological theories.

Let us consider the example of a hospital. A structural view of a hospital might focus, first of all, on how power and authority are distributed throughout the organization. At the top of the hospital (or in modern Britain the Trust) might be a Chief Executive who has ultimate responsibility for the operational and strategic management of the hospital. The hospital's administration might be organized into a number of departments – human resources, finance, estates, etc. – each of which has a head, who is accountable to the Chief Executive and to whom staff of the department are responsible. The various clinical services provided by the Trust will similarly be organized into units, with heads, each of whom will be responsible to the Chief Executive for the effective and efficient delivery of their own particular service.

role:
expected behaviour of holders of particular positions within society

Within these structures individuals occupy a particular **role**. Notice that in talking about roles, we are not talking about the individuals who occupy them. Take, as an example, the role of a consultant surgeon employed by an NHS Trust in a large metropolitan hospital. To a very significant extent, the behaviour and performance of any consultant surgeon employed in such a context will be substantially the same. The same job needs to be done, the same standard of professional performance is expected, and even similar codes of dress and personal demeanour are expected (and usually found) amongst the individuals who occupy these roles. Plainly these similarities do not derive from essentially similar personalities just happening to find themselves in the same job; rather, they derive from the expectations associated with the role in question.

culture:
the ways of life of members of any given society

Sociologists distinguish between the concepts of society and **culture**. Society is the system that connects individuals to one another, whereas culture refers to the way of life of those individuals. A variety of social mechanisms tend to ensure that individuals conform to the expectations of the roles they occupy. Hospitals, like any other institution, have a particular culture that reinforces ways of thinking and doing. The Francis Report (2013), for example, which reported on the failings of the Mid Staffordshire NHS Foundation Trust, noted that there was an institutional culture that failed patients (see Box 1.1).

> **Box 1.1 The warning signs of a failing culture at Mid Staffordshire NHS Foundation Trust**
>
> * A culture focused on doing the system's business – not that of the patients.
> * An institutional culture which ascribed more weight to positive information about the service than to information capable of implying cause for concern.
> * Standards and methods of measuring compliance which did not focus on the effect of a service on patients.
> * Too great a degree of tolerance of poor standards and of risk to patients.
> * A failure of communication between the many agencies to share their knowledge of concerns.
> * Assumptions that monitoring, performance management or intervention was the responsibility of someone else.
> * A failure to tackle challenges to the building up of a positive culture, in nursing in particular but also within the medical profession.
> * A failure to appreciate until recently the risk of disruptive loss of corporate memory and focus resulting from repeated, multi-level reorganization.
>
> *Francis (2013)*

norms:
rules of behaviour that reinforce the culture of society

Cultures are reinforced by **norms**. Norms are fundamental because they provide the rules for social behaviour that reinforce a culture's values. Some of these norms are very formal. For example, it is a (not unreasonable) expectation that anyone occupying the role of consultant surgeon will take all reasonable steps to ensure that their patients are operated on in a safe and competent manner. If in a particular case a surgeon does not do this, then there exist various formal and legal sanctions which either ensure future conformity to this aspect of the role, or remove the individual from that role altogether. Others are much more informal. For example, a surgeon who reports to work unshaven, unwashed and dressed in a dirty tracksuit will probably suffer the disapproval of his colleagues and superiors, which may or may not be enough to cause a change in behaviour before more formal sanctions are invoked.

The concepts of culture, role and norms allow sociologists to think about societies and organizations within societies as having a life independent of the individuals who make them up. In a very real sense, then, individual people, their hearts, minds and personalities, do not really figure in the sort of sociology that emphasizes structure. Hospitals, governments, prisons, families and other groups operate in the way they do, with the consequences they have, not because of anything to do with the individuals who make them up, but because of the structures, cultures and roles which define them.

'Structural' sociologists share a common view of how we should conceptualize society. While at one level this is true, it is important to point out that there are various types of approaches and these exhibit some quite fundamental differences that fall under the general umbrella of structural sociology. We shall now consider two of these: functionalism and Marxism.

Functionalism

The origins of sociology lie in the nineteenth century, and no one was more significant in its development than the Frenchman Émile Durkheim. Although the term 'sociology' had been coined by the French philosopher Auguste Comte, it was Durkheim who established it as a serious academic discipline. It was, moreover, Durkheim who established the principles of the theoretical approach known as functionalism.

The starting point for Durkheim, and for functionalist sociology in general, is the idea that societies are complete systems and that their component parts cannot be viewed in isolation from each other. Sometimes an analogy with a living organism is used. Consider a dog. It is composed of various limbs, organs, connective tissues, and so on. In itself, each of these constitutive parts does very little; it is only when they are all connected together to form an actual living dog that we can appreciate the functions of each part and, crucially, how each part contributes to the overall functioning and performance of the dog. For functionalists like Durkheim, this is how we should view societies. We cannot take each part in isolation but rather need to consider each element of a society in relation to the whole.

Durkheim was fond of illustrating this point with seemingly unpromising examples. For example, in his classic text *The Rules of Sociological Method* (1964), he sought to illustrate that even crime – something we are accustomed to regarding as a social problem – makes a positive contribution to the overall functioning of society. Durkheim makes two important points about crime: first, that without crime (that is, the breaking of legally sanctioned social norms) there would be no innovation and societies would stagnate; second, that crime (and, importantly, its punishment) serves to heighten society's collective commitment to certain core values without which no society could exist. In other words, by punishing law-breakers, societies reinforce the boundaries of acceptable conduct and the commitment of their members to upholding these.

Although Durkheim had little to say about health care (he was, after all, writing at the turn of the twentieth century), later 'functionalist' sociologists have applied the idea of 'function' to various aspects of health and its management. Most famous perhaps was the work of Talcott Parsons on the 'sick role'. This is explored in more detail in Chapter 3, but in essence Parsons argued that there was a socially defined 'role' which, in modern societies, individuals adopt when they become sick. The sick role has both rights and obligations attached to it: the sick individual has the right to refrain from work and other normal social duties, but also the obligation to seek appropriate medical advice and seek a speedy return to full health. For Parsons, this role – and note, it is the role to which Parsons refers, rather than the individuals who occupy that role – that ensures the smooth functioning of society. Disease and ill health are potentially disruptive to society, and so the existence of the sick role ensures that this disruption is kept to a minimum.

While there is something very appealing about the functionalist view of the world, it is not without criticisms. First of all, by concentrating almost exclusively on the positive social functions of institutions and roles, functionalists like Parsons have been accused of ignoring their negative or harmful consequences. For example, we might criticize the sick role by pointing out that in cases of chronic illness and disability, the adoption of this role discourages full participation in society and encourages dependency (see Chapters 9 and 10).

Similarly, the prestige and independence accorded to the medical profession might encourage the abuse of medical power and the exploitation of patients for personal gain. Functionalism tends to ignore conflict at all levels. Second, functionalism – like other structural theories – can be accused of playing down the degree of independence which social actors actually possess. They tend to be treated as 'pawns' in a larger game, and are assumed to be unable to alter social institutions or roles as a result of their own independent actions.

Marxism

means of production:
the means by which surpluses are extracted

bourgeoisie:
those who own the means of production

proletariat:
those who sell their labour

A second structural theory within sociology is Marxism – named after its founder, Karl Marx (1818–83). If functionalism can be accused of understating the degree of conflict in society, the same cannot be said of Marxism. For Marx, the starting point for social analysis was the inherent conflicts – economic in origin – that exist between social classes. For Marx, a social class is a group of people who share a common economic position. In all forms of pre-socialist society, Marx claimed, there were essentially two classes: those who owned the **means of production** and those who did not. Much of Marx's analysis concentrated on capitalist society. Under capitalism, the two classes for Marx are the **bourgeoisie** and the **proletariat**.

Marx claimed that the relationship between the two classes was inevitably exploitative. Wage labourers (the proletariat) generate more wealth for their employers than they are allowed to keep: in short, the rich get richer at the expense of the poor. For Marx, this relationship (part of the economic infrastructure) was fundamental to explaining the nature of society. For him, and his followers, the nature of the institutions and roles that make up a society can be explained with reference to these fundamental inequalities, and their inherently volatile nature. Let us take the example of religion. For Marx, religious beliefs were **ideologies** and form part of the superstructure of society. Religion under capitalism (at least the sort of nineteenth-century industrial capitalism about which Marx wrote) stressed that social inequalities were just and, indeed, ordained by God. Just think of the words of the hymn 'All Things Bright and Beautiful': 'The rich man in his castle, The poor man at his gate, God made them, high or lowly, And ordered their estate.' These words epitomize the ideological function of religion: it encourages the poor to accept their condition and to tolerate, graciously, the superior economic position of the bourgeoisie.

There have been many attempts to apply Marxist thought to the study of health and illness; for example, the theory of **commodification**. One such account is offered by McKinlay (1985), who suggests that, under modern capitalism, medicine, like any other good or service, has become commodified. In other words, medicine has become just another product which is bought and sold, and out of which significant profits are generated for those who own the means of production. Although McKinlay's analysis focuses on the United States, where health care is explicitly provided primarily by the private sector, it may still have resonance in countries like the UK where health care is provided principally by the state. One illustration of this is the way in which medical practice is influenced by the activities of the large pharmaceutical companies. It could well be argued that drugs are developed and marketed to medical practitioners not out of a sense of social responsibility, but primarily as a means of making profits – and pretty huge ones at that. Thus, the motivating factor for the development of a drug therapy is not need (or, arguably, far more research would have been done to develop drugs to combat diseases of the developing world), but the potential to generate profit. There is simply more money to be made from treating 'diseases' of the rich, than diseases of the poor (see, for example, Williams, Gabe and Davis 2009; Law 2006).

ideologies: system of ideas underlying social action

commodification: when economic value is given to something previously without economic value

---

Activity 1.2 The commodification of health

Read the case study below and then answer the questions.

Alison is a student nurse in her second year. She is currently on placement and has just finished a morning shift. Although she's exhausted she decides to pop in to her local health club for a swim before heading off home (she gets a specially discounted rate). After her swim, Alison remembers that there is almost nothing in the fridge so she drives to the nearest supermarket to get some food. It's difficult to know what to buy; there are lots of offers. She buys – amongst other things – some yoghurts and margarine which promise to 'lower cholesterol', some cereal bars packed with 'all 9 essential amino acids', and some bread which claims to be 'medium GI' and 'low in fat'. She also buys a newspaper and a women's magazine. She sets off home and does some work on her next assignment, before preparing something to eat. Later that evening, she switches on the television to wind down and watches a programme on celebrity diets. She picks up the magazine that she bought earlier that day and skims through it; there are lots of adverts for teeth whitening, eye laser treatment and cosmetic surgery. Eventually the programme ends, Alison puts down her magazine and goes up to bed.

(a) Drawing on the case study, make a list of the different ways in which health can be described as commodified.
(b) Do you agree that health and medicine have been commodified?
(c) Who benefits from the commodification of health?

Action theories

Both of the approaches considered above have in common the idea that wider social forces exert powerful influences on individual behaviour. Although there are stronger and weaker formulations of the idea, the essential assumption shared by structural approaches is that they seek to explain patterns of individual behaviour in terms of the location of individuals within wider social structures. It is perhaps not surprising, therefore, that some sociologists have criticized these approaches for underestimating the role of individual action in society. Action theories are also sometimes referred to as micro-sociological theories.

One of the first sociologists to develop a critique of what he saw as the overemphasis on structural determinants of action was Max Weber. Weber's sociology is rich and complex and encompasses a recognition that human beings do not act merely in response to wider social forces, but rather for conscious reasons and towards certain purposes. At its simplest it was not enough, for Weber, to say that events occur because social structures ordain them; instead, he was concerned to understand how individuals come to see the world in such a way that they voluntarily choose a particular course of action. To capture the importance of this dimension, Weber used the German term *verstehen*, which translates, approximately, as 'empathetic understanding'. This means, in essence, that to gain a full understanding of an individual's action, we must look at the world from their point of view and, as it were, step into their shoes. This approach is evident in Weber's analysis of the origins of capitalism (Weber 1958). Unlike Marx, who saw capitalism as the inevitable outcome of an economically driven process, Weber insisted that it was essential to put oneself in the shoes of the early capitalist entrepreneurs and to try to understand how their view of the world differed from those which had gone before. By doing this, Weber develops a theory of how a particular interpretation of the world – that of the early Calvinist Protestants – led to patterns of behaviour which resulted, eventually, in the emergence of capitalism as an economic system.

Symbolic interactionism

While Weber was responsible for sensitizing sociologists to the need to account for social action from the point of view of the actor, it was a group of philosophers and sociologists from the University of Chicago who developed a major theory of social action which became known as symbolic interactionism. Undoubtedly the most significant figure in the development of this approach was George Herbert Mead.

The starting point for Mead's analysis was his recognition that human beings are fundamentally different from animals, not only because their behaviour is more complex, but because it is of a fundamentally different kind. Take a simple example. If a man kicks a dog, the response of the dog is predictable. It may be that the dog's previous experiences will influence its response, and that, because of this, all dogs will not react in exactly the same way. Nevertheless, the essential feature of its response is that it is predictable and, in a genuine sense, automatic. Now imagine that you are standing at a bus stop and someone walks up to you and kicks you. How will you react? Your immediate reaction might be to say you would kick them back, but a moment's reflection will reveal that the situation is more complicated than this. In fact your reaction will be influenced by a wide range of factors. Who kicked you? If it was your best friend, you might assume either that it was intended as a prank, or perhaps that you had upset them and the kick was intended maliciously. Which you choose will depend on a further set of factors: what is the expression on their face, was the kick accompanied by any words, are there any background circumstances which might explain their anger with you, and so on? If the kick was from a stranger, then a whole new set of factors will need to be considered before you can decide how to react. The point is that, unlike the dog – who reacts automatically – a human being can, and indeed must, choose how to react. And, in making that choice, they must place themselves in the position of the kicker and interrogate their motives. We ask the question: why did that person kick me? Only when we have done that do we select a course of action and, as this example illustrates, that could vary from laughter if we decide it was a prank by a friend, to extreme fear and panic if we decide it was an assault by a malicious stranger. This contrasts very sharply with the reaction of the dog, which is completely oblivious to the point of view of its attacker.

Mead (1934) describes this process as taking the role of the other. Human beings do not merely react to situations in automatic and predictable ways (as both functionalists and Marxists might be accused of assuming), but rather interpret situations and select courses of action according to this interpretation. For Mead, this is because we

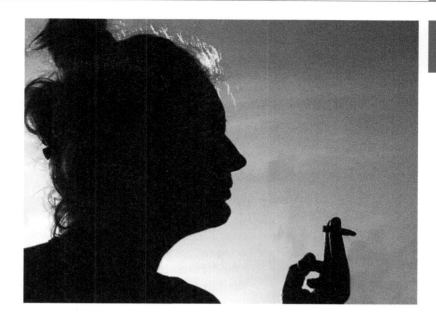

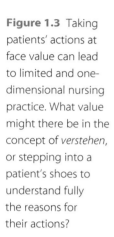

Figure 1.3 Taking patients' actions at face value can lead to limited and one-dimensional nursing practice. What value might there be in the concept of *verstehen*, or stepping into a patient's shoes to understand fully the reasons for their actions?

possess a social self. Mead's concept of self has two parts: the I and the Me. Although this idea appears rather abstract, in essence it is quite simple. Think of the Me as the public part of yourself, which you place on display to others, and the I as the private part, which is accessible only to yourself. Now think about how you choose a course of action: what you are going to wear to an interview, for instance. You imagine yourself in your pinstripe suit, or your floral dress, and imagine how others will react to you. In other words, your Me has a 'conversation' with your I and, on the basis of taking the role of the other, you choose a course of action which suits your goals.

Activity 1.3 Taking the role of the other

(a) Describe what is meant by 'taking the role of the other'.
(b) Is taking the role of the other important to the provision of good nursing practice? What role does it play in developing reflective practice?
(c) How easy is it to take the role of the other when nursing children, people with mental health problems or people with learning disabilities?

What all of this means is that symbolic interactionists tend to reject theories which see human beings as passive pawns in the play of wider social forces. Rather, they are concerned with understanding how people interpret situations and how these interpretations influence their future conduct. It should be obvious that this approachintroducesa significant element of uncertainty in our understanding of human action: indeed, for interactionists, human conduct is to a large extent unpredictable.

4 Contemporary theoretical debates in sociology

Contemporary approaches to social theory have sought to bridge the gap between structure and action. This section introduces you to two of these contemporary sociological perspectives.

Structuration theory

This theory was proposed by the well-known sociologist Anthony Giddens (1984). Giddens argued against the separation of structure from action within sociological theory, suggesting that this distinction no longer applies within modern social life – which he refers to as **late modernity**. Instead, Giddens argues that structure and action are interrelated and that it is the repeated actions of individuals which reproduce the structures of society. In other words, structure and agency are two sides of the same coin. Within this theoretical perspective, individuals have considerable power to act in their own interests.

late modernity: continuation of modern societies in a highly connected and globalized world

Giddens's theory of structuration has been criticized by other sociologists, who suggest that he does not fully explain and consider the role and power of social structures. One such sociologist is Greener (2008), who has argued that Giddens's structuration theory has been extremely influential within health policy, especially in relation to the UK government's approach to the 'expert patient' and the management of long-term conditions, but that it is of concern too. Criticizing the notion of the 'expert patient' – which encourages patients to take responsibility for their health and treatment – Greener argues:

> The long term ill start with the disadvantage of having to manage a condition that may involve use of medication in imprecise circumstances and frequent consultation with the medical profession. Those who suffer from physical or psychological disabilities are often not in the best position to negotiate their care. For the government to pretend that these inequalities do not exist is hugely problematic, and perhaps even dangerous.

While structuration theory is not unproblematic, it is helpful when thinking about the way in which individuals live within, and influence, social structures.

Post-modern perspectives

These are not one single theory but rather a number of different perspectives which share both similarities and differences with Giddens's theory of structuration. They are similar insofar as they reject the distinction between structure and action. However, they differ in that post-modernity does not propose a single **grand narrative** (such

grand narrative: an overarching single theory of society and social change

as those proposed by Marx, Weber, Durkheim and even Giddens), but rather consists of a number of theories of society. Post-modern perspectives also differ from structuration theory in that Giddens views society as late modern – a continuation of modernity – and post-modern thinkers view society as **post-modern**.

post-modern:
the view that society is chaotic and in flux

Whereas modern societies are characterized by the pursuit of progress, post-modernists would suggest that post-modern societies are characterized by change, ambivalence and insecurity. In contrast with the perspective put forward by a sociologist such as Marx – in which individuals are primarily defined by the class structure – post-modern thinkers would suggest that individuals are now more able to define themselves. While this freedom from social order and tradition provides opportunities for action, this freedom can also create insecurity because individuals have to work out who they are and where they fit in society. Additionally, post-modernists would argue that experiences are fragmented. So, for example, while Marx would have argued that experiences of health and illness are determined by class, post-modernists would point out that individuals are defined by much more than class and that other differences – such as gender, age and ethnicity – are also important.

The work of the social theorist Michel Foucault (1974) is really important because he highlighted the importance of power. While power is generally an important sociological concept, Foucault argued that the use of language was a really important form of power because it influences the way people think. Language is therefore a **discourse** that can determine how a phenomenon is understood. For example, if you think about the way language is used in the media to describe obesity you can see how it might influence the way you think about the issues (see Box 1.2).

discourse:
a way of thinking through language

Box 1.2 Talking about obesity in the media

Child obesity: Why do parents let their kids get fat? (*BBC News Magazine*, 26 September 2012). Available at: <http://www.bbc.co.uk/news/magazine-19661085>

Britain's obesity epidemic worse than feared (the *Telegraph*, 13 January 2014). Available at: <http://www.telegraph.co.uk/news/10566705/Britains-obesity-epidemic-worse-than-feared.html>,

'Babies getting fat in the WOMB is to blame for obesity spiralling out of control, warns top child doctor' (Harriet Crawford for the *Daily Mail*, 26 May 2015). Available at: <www.dailymail.co.uk/news/article-3096796/obesity-warning-UK-s-senior-children-s-doctor-says-babies-getting-fat-mothers-wombs-html>.

The benefits couple who are too FAT to work (*Mail Online*, 5 January 2015). Available at: <http://www.dailymail.co.uk/news/article-2897024/Couple-weigh-54-stone-claim-2-000-month-benefits-fat-work-use-pay-3-000-dream-wedding.html>.

Table 1.1 Sociological theories	
Focus on social structure	**Focus on social action**
Classical sociological theories	
Functionalism focuses on the maintenance of order and cohesion and views society as a number of interdependent parts	*Symbolic interactionism* focuses on the process of symbolic interaction and the symbolic meanings that people develop
Marxism focuses on conflict (rather than cohesion) and views society as fragmented, emphasizing the role of coercion in producing social order	
Contemporary sociological theories	
Structuration theory seeks to bridge the distinction between structure and action and views society as late modern	
Post-modern perspectives views society as post-modern rather than modern and is a collection of theories that rejects the distinction between structure and action	

There is some debate as to how far post-modern perspectives have influenced thinking within the sociology of health and illness (for example, see Cockerham 2009). However, it has been influential within some areas, such as the sociology of the body and identity and the sociology of disability.

The final section of this chapter encourages you to apply your understanding of different sociological theories to the important subject of mental health and illness. Before you move on to this section, try to summarize your knowledge, using Table 1.1.

5 Theorizing mental health and illness

Mental health and illness is an interesting subject to study from a sociological perspective, and many sociologists have explored this subject in different ways, depending upon their theoretical persuasion. There is no commonly accepted definition of the term 'mental illness'. Many different words can be used to describe mental illness and these are often derogatory, for example, 'crazy', 'loony', 'nutter' and 'mad'. Medicine and psychiatry have a long history in trying to define behaviour that is different, believing that they do so in a way that is rigorous and scientific. For instance, behaviour that is melancholy would be described as depression, and nervous behaviour described as anxiety. However, sociologists would suggest that medical professionals still draw on value judgements to ascribe certain behaviours to these rigid categories (Szasz 1961).

Sociologists such as Durkheim – a functionalist – would argue that definitions of what is normal and abnormal (or pathological) serve to strengthen social cohesion and perform a necessary function. Additionally, they would claim that what is defined as normal and abnormal depends upon the values of the social group that is doing the defining. Over time there have been many different explanations for abnormal behaviour. For example, in the fifteenth century, strange behaviour was thought to be caused by witchcraft. In the nineteenth century, some believed that abnormal behaviour had biological causes, whereas others, such as Sigmund Freud, believed in psychological explanations (Rosenhan and Seligman 1989). Sociologists show that certain behaviours are labelled as deviant and also that what is labelled as abnormal changes over time.

Conflict perspectives in the sociology of mental illness are also useful because they demonstrate how mental health and illness are socially patterned. In particular, they highlight that experiences of mental health are gendered; women are more likely to be diagnosed with depression than men. Mental health issues also increase with decreasing socioeconomic status (those who are poorest are most likely to experience mental illness). Sociologists have also pointed out that mental health is racially patterned. The Count Me In censuses, which were published annually up to 2011 by the Care Quality Commission, have consistently shown that rates of admission and detentions for black people are higher than for the rest of the population (Health and Social Care Information Centre 2013).

Activity 1.4 Discrimination and mental illness

In a blog posted on the mental health charity MIND's website, Louise describes her experience of discrimination and mental illness.

I've always been what some may call neurotic. I'm uptight, nervous and sensitive . . .

I've suffered from depression, anxiety and borderline Obsessive-Compulsive Disorder (OCD) for around ten years now, and I do a damn good job of coping with it, even when the conditions conspire to bring me to my lowest ebb . . .

I always disclose to my immediate family any health issues I'm having, including mental health. I'd been struggling with anxiety since the death of a very close loved one and depression was clouding my mind, making me tearful and not as robust as I usually am. I'd been to my GP and was on appropriate medication, and simply taking each day as I found it. I always believed my immediate family loved me unconditionally, regardless of my 'flaws' or my mental health. But it turns out, for one non-blood relative, they were simply masking how they truly perceived me.

'She's an attention seeker; she just wants all the focus on her. She's a weak person. She needs to grow a spine. Everyone thinks she's a hypochondriac.'

I was aghast, my mouth wide open in shock, when these words reached me from another room. I sat there, numb, tears in my eyes, wondering what I'd done to bring about such a character assassination . . . I thought families were supposed to be caring, accepting, a safe haven from the other people who used stigma and discrimination.

(Louise, 'Stigma in my family', MIND (<www.mind.org.uk>))

(a) You will no doubt have some experience of mental illness; either your own, that of a family member or a friend, or you may have cared for someone with mental illness. Have you ever come across the sort of discrimination described by Louise? Think about this and reflect on your own attitude to mental illness.

(b) Consider the fact that Foucault describes language as discourse. Read Louise's account of stigma and mental illness again and think about the importance of how we talk about things and how this might influence the way we think about them.

In summary, sociology is often described as multi-paradigmatic; this means that there are many different competing sociological explanations. Sociological theories are generally divided into theories of social structure, such as functionalism, or theories of social action, such as symbolic interactionism. More contemporary social theories seek to consider structure and action together. The following chapters within this book will introduce you to some other important sociological theories, and it is worth remembering that all theories are concerned with the relationship between structure and action. For example, see Chapters 6 and 7 for a fuller discussion of feminist theories, Chapter 8 for theories of ageing, Chapter 9, which focuses on theories of chronic illness, and Chapter 12, in which you will find a theoretical discussion of 'race' and 'ethnicity'.

Activity 1.5 Nursing: menial and mundane?

If nursing involves anything more complex than the most menial of tasks, and if nurses enjoy any sort of decision-making capacities independent of medicine, then they require . . . knowledge on which to base their decisions about what sort of actions they should be taking, and when they should be taking them. In other words, nurses require a theoretical grounding for their actions. This, of course, says nothing about the sort of theory that should underpin nursing practice, specifically whether or not sociology is an appropriate theoretical source . . .

The point to be made at this stage of the argument is that, given that nurses deal with a myriad of different people and a multiplicity of problems, using various, often complex, methods, it is inconceivable that they would be capable of making informed decisions about care if they were not in possession of some sort of overarching model of their professional activity. In short, given the nature of their job, it is axiomatic that nurses require theoretical knowledge of some sort . . .

The deprecation of nursing as mundane work is often articulated by identifying it as 'women's work' . . . nothing more than a public extension of private domestic labour, which in itself is seen as requiring little thought or skill. (Porter 1995: 1131)

(a) Do you agree with the position expressed by Porter?

(b) Should nurses just know how to do things or should they also understand the theory behind what they are doing?

(c) Do you think that sociology can provide nurses with the theoretical underpinnings for practice?

Summary and Resources

1

Summary

▶ Sociology is concerned with the study of human societies.

▶ Sociology is distinct from 'common sense' because it challenges the obvious and assesses evidence for and against any position taken.

▶ There can be a sociology of virtually anything as long as the theory is internally consistent.

▶ There is debate concerning the role of sociology within society. That is, should sociologists simply report what they see or should they be concerned with changing the social world around them?

▶ There are two major types of classical sociological theory and they can be categorized according to whether they focus on 'structures' or 'action'.

▶ Contemporary sociological theories often seek to bridge the gap between structure and action approaches.

Questions for Discussion

1 Should sociologists develop neutral understandings of the social world or should they seek to influence change?

2 Next time you are on placement, ask yourself, 'What is going on here?' Describe what you are doing, or seeing, and then try to explain it.

3 Is it useful to think of the world in terms of 'structure' and 'action'?

Glossary

action: an important sociological term that refers to purposeful and conscious behaviour initiated by individuals in society

bourgeoisie: those who own the means of production; the capitalist class that owns most of society's wealth

commodification: assigning an economic value to something that does not generally possess one; judging something solely on this economic value; a market in health care, where investigations and treatment are provided according to ability to pay, is an example of commodification

culture: the ways of life of members of any given society or part of society that influence ways

	of thinking, behaving and being in the social world
discourse:	within sociology, discourse means more than just discussion or verbal communication, and refers to how power relations are expressed through language; for example, if a patient is in hospital when they do not need to be there, 'bed blocker' implies a failing by the patient, whereas 'delayed discharge' is a problem of the health system; the use of different terminology may influence how the individual is perceived and treated
grand narrative:	a comprehensive theory that explains historical meaning, experience or knowledge; sometimes called meta-narrative, which means that the overarching narrative (or story) explains the smaller narratives contained within it
ideologies:	systems of beliefs, attitudes and opinions for explaining the social world, such as Marxism, fascism, liberalism; they are often associated with political views, and governments may develop policy based on ideology, but also encompass religion and philosophy
late modernity:	sociologist Anthony Giddens argues that society is developing in a way that he refers to as late modernity; by this he means that the social forces that structured modernity are being developed and extended, rather than being superseded by post-modernity
lay reasoning:	describes everyday thinking about the world that is neither consistent nor rigorous insofar as it is not located within any particular set of scientific beliefs
means of production:	the means by which all physical surpluses (for example, machines, tools and supplies) are extracted to produce goods and services in a society
modernity:	modernity developed from pre-modern societies which existed before the late sixteenth century and refers to a focus on achieving progress; it is synonymous with industrialization and stretches into the late twentieth century
norms:	rules of behaviour that serve to reinforce the culture of society; some sociologists believe that both the following and breaking of social norms serves to reinforce culture

partisanship:	bias or allegiance to the view of a particular social group, political party or cause
post-modern:	a move against the fixed condition of universality characterizing the period of modernity; it encompasses a scepticism towards social structures of society, an acceptance of a range of philosophical and ideological positions, and a fluidity of traditional boundaries
proletariat:	those who sell their labour to the capitalist class; the working classes who do not control capital or own wealth or property
role:	refers to the part that someone plays within society or some other group, which then determines the expected behaviours of those people depending on the role(s) they perform
socialization:	processes by which individuals acquire the roles, norms and cultures of society, thus enabling them to participate in society; socialization regulates behaviour and brings about conformity
structure:	an important sociological term that refers to the organized patterns of social behaviour and the social institutions within society

Further Reading

S. Bruce: *Sociology: A Very Short Introduction*. Oxford University Press: Oxford, 2000.
Written in an accessible style, this book really does what it says on the tin! It will give you a very short introduction to sociology in just over 100 pages.

S. Earle and G. Letherby (eds): *The Sociology of Healthcare: A Reader for Health Professionals*. Basingstoke: Palgrave, 2008.
This is an excellent collection of readings exploring many aspects of the sociology of health care, including: sociological theory; sociological research; inequalities and diversity; the body and the mind; and power and professional practice.

A. Giddens and P. W. Sutton: *Sociology*. 7th edn, Cambridge: Polity, 2013.
This is a comprehensive sociological text written by an influential and well-known sociologist and social theorist. The book explores a wide range of useful topics. It is well illustrated and easy to read.

References

Allan, H. T. 2006 Using participant observation to immerse oneself in the field. The relevance and importance of ethnography for illuminating the role of emotions in nursing. *Journal of Research in Nursing* 11/5: 397–407.

Blaxter, M. 1990 *Health and Lifestyles*. London: Tavistock.

Bruce, S. 2000 *Sociology: A Very Short Introduction*. Oxford: Oxford University Press.

Cockerham, W. C. 2009 Deflecting a postmodernist critique. *Social Theory & Health* 7: 74–7.

Department of Health 2005 *Research Governance Framework for Health and Social Care*, 2nd edn. London: Department of Health.

Durkheim, E. 1964 *The Rules of Sociological Method*. New York: Free Press.

Earle, S. and Sharp K. 2007 *Sex in Cyberspace: Men who Pay for Sex*. Aldershot: Ashgate.

Foucault, M. 1974 *The Archaeology of Knowledge*. Tavistock: London.

Francis, R. 2013 *Report of the Mid Staffordshire NHS Foundation Trust Public Inquiry*. London: The Stationery Office. At: <http://www.midstaffspublicinquiry.com/report>.

Giddens, A. 1984 *The Constitution of Society*. Cambridge: Polity.

Giddens, A. 2001 [1971] *Capitalism and Modern Social Theory*. Cambridge: Cambridge University Press.

Greener, I. 2008 Expert patients and human agency: Long-term conditions and Giddens' Structuration Theory. *Social Theory & Health* 6: 273–90.

Health & Social Care Information Centre 2013 *Mental Health Bulletin: Annual Report from MHMDS Returns – England 2012/13*.

Healthcare Commission, 2004 *Patient Survey Report, 2004: Young Patients*. London: Healthcare Commission. At: <http://www.nhssurveys.org/Filestore/CQC/YP_KF_2004.pdf>.

Hine, C. 2005 *Virtual Methods: Issues in Social Research on the Internet*. Oxford: Berg Publishers.

Hutchinson, A. M. and Johnston, L. 2008 An observational study of health professionals' use of evidence to inform the development of clinical management tools. *Journal of Clinical Nursing* 17/6: 2203–211.

Law, J. 2006 *Big Pharma*. London: Robinson Publishing.

Lehna, C. and McNeil, J. 2008 Mixed-methods exploration of parents' health information understanding. *Clinical Nursing Research* 17/2: 133–44.

Letherby, G., Williams, K., Birch, P. and Cain, M. (eds) 2008 *Sex as Crime?* Devon: Willan.

McKinlay, J. B. (ed.) 1985 *Issues in the Political Economy of Healthcare*. London: Tavistock Press.

Mead, G. H. 1934 *Mind, Self, and Society: From the Standpoint of a Social Behaviourist*. London: University of Chicago Press.

Nettleton, S. 2006 *The Sociology of Health and Illness*, 2nd edn. Cambridge: Polity.

O'Baugh, J., Wilkes, L. M., Luke, S. and George, A. 2008 Positive attitude in cancer: The nurses' perspective. *International Journal of Nursing Practice* 14/2: 109–14.

Porter, S. 1995 Sociology and the nursing curriculum: a defence. *Journal of Advanced Nursing* 21/6: 1130–5.

Rosenhan, D. and Seligman, M. 1989 *Abnormal Psychology*. New York: W.W. Norton.

Sassen, S. 2007 *A Sociology of Globalization*. London: W. W. Norton and Co.

Szasz, T. 1961 *The Myth of Mental Illness*. London: Paladin.

Weber, M. 1958 *The Protestant Ethic and the Spirit of Capitalism*. New York: Charles Scribner's Sons.

Widdance Twine, F. 2011 *Outsourcing the Womb: Race, Class and Gestational Surrogacy in a Global Market*. Abingdon: Routledge.

Williams, S., Gabe, J. and Davis, P. 2009 *Pharmaceuticals and Society: Critical Discourses and Debates*. Oxford: Wiley-Blackwell.

Why Should Nurses Study Sociology?

Sarah Earle

KEY ISSUES IN THIS CHAPTER:

▶ The difference between sociology in nursing and sociology of nursing.
▶ The value of developing sociological skills.
▶ Using sociological skills in nursing practice.
▶ The contribution of sociology to nursing knowledge.
▶ The sociology of diabetes.

BY THE END OF THIS CHAPTER YOU SHOULD BE ABLE TO:

▶ Discuss the reasons why nurses should study sociology.
▶ Understand the distinction between sociology of nursing and sociology in nursing.
▶ Understand the value of sociological skills.
▶ Discuss the role of sociological knowledge within nursing practice.
▶ Think about diabetes sociologically.

1 Introduction

As your experience in clinical practice develops you will come across patients with a wide range of concerns and from a diversity of social backgrounds. The main aim of this chapter is to demonstrate the practical relevance of sociology to nursing, and to explore how sociology may provide you with exciting new ways with which to understand the needs of your patients.

The second section of this chapter discusses conceptual differences between sociology in nursing and sociology of nursing. Section 3 focuses on the **cognitive** skills that an appreciation of sociology may encourage, enabling you to positively shape and influence practice.

cognitive:
relating to thinking
processes

2

Section 4 draws on empirical studies to demonstrate the role of sociology in exploring social issues in health and the social worlds of patients, nurses and other health-care workers. Finally, Section 6 addresses the role of sociological knowledge in relation to diabetes, a serious public-health problem globally.

2 Sociology in nursing and sociology of nursing

There are two main types of sociological knowledge relevant to nurses: one is identified as sociology *in* nursing and the other as the sociology *of* nursing. Each type of knowledge has the scope to enable the 'ordinary' day-to-day work of nurses to be seen in a different light; it is this alternative perspective which is characteristic of sociology. Sociology encourages us to view everyday **phenomena** in a different way. It is like being given a new pair of glasses. This is sometimes referred to as **problematizing**; that is, what at first sight might seem unremarkable becomes problematic. More will be said about this later, but first let us turn to the distinction between sociology in and of nursing.

Sociology can be defined most simply as the scientific study of 'human life' (Giddens 2009: 6) (also see Chapter 1 for a further discussion of defining sociology). A sociological approach to nursing locates the work of individual nurses squarely within a social context, rather than considering it in isolation. In general terms, when a sociological analysis is applied to the essence of individual health-care experience, whether it be that of patients or health-care workers, this is termed 'sociology in nursing'. 'The sociology of nursing' usually refers to issues affecting the profession as a whole, such as its occupational status, or recruitment and attrition problems (see Chapter 5 for further discussion of nursing as an occupation). The role of sociology in relation to nursing is continuously debated within the literature. However, as Pinikahana (2003) has argued, the most important thing to remember is that sociology is only relevant to nurses if it is *applied* to nursing.

phenomena:
states or processes that can be observed

problematizing:
looking beyond the obvious to seek an explanation

3 Sociology: helping develop skills

Is sociology just 'common sense'?

It is important to clarify exactly how a knowledge of sociology can be of value to practising nurses. As explored in Chapter 1, can sociology be described as 'just common sense'? Let us consider what sociology does have to offer nursing practice.

In her treatment of the question, Hannah Cooke (1993: 215) describes sociology as an 'emancipatory discipline'. By this she means that nurses need to be self-critical and to question the long-held assumptions of the profession. This may seem difficult in the light of your limited practical experiences, or an unfamiliarity with academic study. Although 'training' still has a valuable part to play in nurse education, for example in the learning of practical skills such as aseptic or injection techniques, it is important to distinguish between this and the acquisition of a higher education, of which the study of sociology is an example. It is argued by Ross (1981), for example, that the concept of learning in education, as opposed to training, is characterized by discovery and transformation of thought, which suggests personal growth and a radical shift in previously held beliefs and values. Ellis (1992) describes this as a 'personal education'. Arguably, any academic discipline in its authentic form is a valuable experience for students on vocational courses, but classical authors of sociology, notably Wright Mills (1959) and Berger (1963), would argue that the subject holds a unique fascination and distinctiveness.

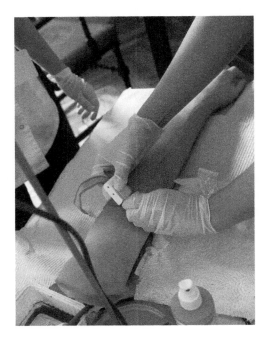

Figure 2.1 Learning practical skills such as taking blood are central to becoming a nurse – but is this the limit of nursing?

Wright Mills (1959: 7) coined the term 'sociological imagination' to describe his particular view of the sociological enterprise in his classic work of the same name. What he meant by this is the ability to shift one's thinking from one perspective to another, or possession of a certain quality of mind, open to different interpretations of phenomena. This can also be applied to the difference between education and training. As previously stated, we do need elements of training in nurse education, but there is an often quoted saying that 'dogs can be trained to jump through hoops', referring to the fact that people can be trained to do tasks without really having to think very much about them. The consequences of this in nursing can be, and have been, disastrous.

2

Activity 2.1 Sociology in nursing or sociology of nursing?

Read Items A and B and answer the questions below. Item A is an extract from a study that explores patients' experiences of day surgery using a sociological framework of analysis. Item B is an extract from a study exploring the theoretical literature on the body and its relevance to nursing practice.

Item A

Innovations such as day surgery may not be in accord with patient and caregiver expectations. Shorter hospital stays, minimal interaction with medical staff and greater responsibility placed on patients and families for self-care all reduce the traditional markers and rituals of being accepted into the traditional sick role.

For many of the patients, families and employers the term 'same day surgery' was synonymous with 'same day recovery'. Confusion surrounding the sick role appears to be aggravated by social expectations that serious illness is equated with in-patient hospital treatment lasting days or weeks. Consequently, only individuals who undergo longer hospital stays are allowed the privileges of the sick role. . . The perceived expectations which meet day surgery patients are considerably different from those which meet inpatients. The former are expected to be 'street ready' within a few hours, and can only relinquish their social roles for a few hours at most. Even though they are advised to give themselves appropriate time for recovery, in many cases this is no time at all. (Mottram 2010: 145–6)

Item B

An example of nursing's turn away from embodied practice and towards technology is evidenced in the simple case study of blood-pressure measurement. In hospitals in the western hemisphere, blood-pressure measurement is now largely undertaken using the electronic sphygmomanometer. The cuff is placed on the arm of the patient and, with a press of a button, the cuff is electronically inflated and the patient's blood pressure automatically displayed on a screen. Prior to the widespread adoption of this electronic device, nurses learnt to measure a patient's blood pressure in a very different way; through a rich, embodied encounter of touch, sight and sound, using her own body as an instrument through which to read that of her patient's. The heightened skills of touch (sensing the delicate cessation and subsequent re-emergence of the brachial pulse) and sound (listening for the disappearance and reappearance of the 'lub dub' sounds associated with the pulse) are powerful examples of the embodied nature of much of nursing's work. With the routine use of technology such as this we risk losing our mastery of these and other embodied encounters, with significant implications for subsequent generations of nurses.

Greater focus on embodied practice should assist us to attend more insightfully to the lived health and illness experiences of our patients and our own embodied skills as nurses. (Draper 2014: 2236–9)

(a) Identify whether items A and B portray sociology in nursing or sociology of nursing and explain why.

(b) What type of sociology most interests you and why?

Conversely, the possession of this difference in quality of mind and approach to practice, when transferred into appropriate action by nurses, will arguably ensure the evidence base for practice required by the profession. But, more than this, it represents an approach to practice underpinned by critical thinking, analytic and questioning skills, which is crucial to achieve the 'new futures for nursing' envisioned by Cooke (1993: 215).

So, what are these new futures likely to be? Why do nurses always seem to come 'back to basics'? What are the essentials of nursing care and do you need a degree to give a bedpan? The following subsection will demonstrate how knowledge of sociology can help you in addressing such questions.

Activity 2.2 Sociology and 'common sense'

(a) Explain your understanding of the term 'common sense'. Do you think that sociology is 'just common sense'? How useful is this term when talking to patients?

(b) Imagine a patient experiencing quite severe wound pain two days post-operatively following a cholecystectomy (gall bladder removal). Leaving aside the intervention of prescribed analgesia, what kind of social influences do you think might affect this person's reaction to pain?

(c) 'It is the capacity of sociology to take nurses temporarily "out of nursing" that represents one of its strongest attributes' (Mulholland 1997: 850). What do you think that Mulholland means by this statement?

---

4 Nursing skills and reflective practice

With Project 2000 (P2K), nursing moved from an apprentice to an education-based model within universities (you can read more about this in Chapter 5). More recently, in 2013, the goalposts have shifted again and all new nurses must be degree educated. Commenting on this shift, the Nursing and Midwifery Council's then chief executive Dickson Weir-Hughes said that 'Raising the minimum level of education programmes to degree is essential in ensuring that future nursing students are fully prepared to undertake the new roles and responsibilities that will be expected of them' (reported in the *Guardian* (Bowcott 2009)). These new roles and responsibilities include advanced-level practice, which the Department of Health defines as:

Advanced level practice encompasses aspects of education, research and management but is firmly grounded in direct care provision or clinical work with patients, families and populations. Nurses working at an advanced level promote public health and well-being. They understand the implications of the social, economic and political context of healthcare. Their expertise, experience and professional and clinical judgement are demonstrated in the expert nature of their practice and the depth of their knowledge. Patients, clients

2

and other professionals acknowledge their highly developed and extensive knowledge in areas such as diagnostics, therapeutics, the biological, social and epidemiological sciences and pharmacology, and their enhanced skills in areas such as consultation and clinical decision-making. Nurses working at an advanced level use complex reasoning, critical thinking, reflection and analysis to inform their assessments, clinical judgements and decisions. They are able to apply knowledge and skills to a range of clinically and professionally challenging and complex situations. (Department of Health 2010: 7)

However, not everybody agrees with the shift to degree-level education. For example, the Patients' Association argued:

The basics of nursing care are dignity, compassion and, above all, safety. The academic must be secondary to the practical. Only then will patients get the nurses they want and trust ... It must never become more important to write about care than to give it. If our nurses do not have the basics of training, the costs of care will soar because of infection rates and overblown bureaucracy. (Reported in the *Guardian* (Bowcott 2009))

In 2012, the Department of Health published the strategy document *Compassion in Practice*. This document sets out to build a culture of compassionate care in all nursing, midwifery and caregiving settings throughout the NHS and social care in England and Wales. The strategy also sets out six key values for nursing and midwifery – these values are known as the six Cs (see Box 2.1).

Box 2.1 Compassion in nursing and the six Cs

Care is our core business and that of our organizations, and the care we deliver helps the individual person and improves the health of the whole community. Caring defines us and our work. People receiving care expect it to be right for them, consistently, throughout every stage of their life.

Compassion is how care is given through relationships based on empathy, respect and dignity – it can also be described as intelligent kindness, and is central to how people perceive their care.

Competence means all those in caring roles must have the ability to understand an individual's health and social needs and the expertise, clinical and technical knowledge to deliver effective care and treatments based on research and evidence.

Communication is central to successful caring relationships and to effective teamworking. Listening is as important as what we say and do and essential for 'no decision about me without me'. Communication is the key to a good workplace with benefits for those in our care and staff alike.

Courage enables us to do the right thing for the people we care for, to speak up when we have concerns and to have the personal strength and vision to innovate and to embrace new ways of working.

> **Commitment** to our patients and populations is a cornerstone of what we do. We need to build on our commitment to improve the care and experience of our patients, to take action to make this vision and strategy a reality for all and meet the health, care and support challenges ahead.

Activity 2.3 The 'stark reality' of care?

Few care processes are more complex than terminal care of the distressed, incontinent elderly patient. When I and my loved ones are sick or dying, I want our nurses to be caring, patient and tolerant – and well-educated into the bargain. But perhaps most policy makers have not experienced such situations and cannot imagine why a trained intellect is crucial, even when wiping a bottom. (Salvage 2001: 21)

(a) Can you think of other examples of what Salvage describes as the 'stark reality' of hands-on care?
(b) Why do you think that Salvage uses this term?
(c) Do you agree that a trained intellect is crucial, even when wiping a bottom?

It is widely recognized that reflective practice can play a key role in the development of the skills and competencies required to work as a nurse. The development of reflective practice can bridge the theory–practice gap and there is a wealth of literature suggesting that sociology can play an important role in the development of reflective skills within nursing (see, for example, Aranda and Law 2007). The problem of theory–practice integration in the nursing curriculum is particularly pertinent in relation to sociology. One reason for this is that sociology is concerned with the exposure of key issues such as health inequalities. Not only do these have a detrimental effect on individual health care, but they may be constructed and maintained at an institutional level and subject to covert structural processes of which individual practitioners may be unaware. It is useful here to return to Wright Mills (1959), who argued that the sociological imagination is at its most effective in making the distinction between personal troubles and public issues, the idea that what may appear to be an individual phenomenon is actually highly determined by social structures. Consequently, it can be argued that the crux of the sociological enterprise for nursing should be a focused concern with the concept of power and power relations at all levels of health-care practice, an area where nurses have traditionally been invisible.

All this implies that in order for nurses to use sociological knowledge effectively both *in* nursing and at the broader policy level, a more overtly political focus and agenda to the inclusion of sociology in the nursing curriculum is required. It is possible that this may be immediately problematic to some students in terms of their own current values and beliefs about educational requirements for nursing, and it is worth thinking at this stage how comfortably (or not) these ideas about sociology sit with your own views as novice practitioners. Clifford (2000),

2

in her discussion of international politics and nurse education, suggests that although issues of politics, power and control have been of concern to nurses, there has, to date, not been a framework in place to integrate one with the other. Writing specifically about the theory–practice gap, Thompson and Pascal (2015) suggest that reflective practice is, ironically, relatively under-theorized. Drawing broadly on sociological theories of learning, they attempt to broaden the theory base and, as part of this, suggest that it is important not to neglect the emotional dimensions of learning. For example, they suggest that many forms of professional practice can be emotionally demanding. They also argue that challenging one's own beliefs and behaviours – and those of others – can involve a degree of 'unlearning' (of previously held beliefs and values), which is also emotionally demanding work.

Drawing on the groundbreaking work of Hochschild (1983), writers such as James (1992), on the subject of nursing, and Hunter (2001), on the subject of midwifery, argue that providing emotional support to patients and families is very skilled work. However, **emotional labour** is not always recognized and sometimes nurses can feel ill-equipped to meet the emotional needs of patients, particularly at times of acute distress or following bereavement.

emotional labour: regulation of one's own and other people's feelings

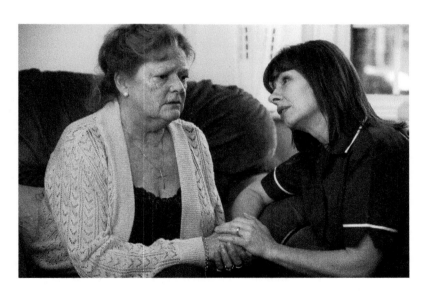

Figure 2.2 Emotional labour, such as setting patients' minds at ease or consoling patients in distress, is a definite skill that needs to be carefully developed

---

Activity 2.4 Nursing and emotional labour

Read the case study and then answer the questions below.

Laura was a student midwife on a busy labour ward. She arrived on duty one afternoon for a late shift to discover that there had been a stillbirth and that the baby's mother was critically ill following a post-partum haemorrhage. She had just been transferred to the intensive care unit. The staff members on duty were quiet and subdued by the traumatic events of the delivery. The family were still in the visitor's room on the labour ward and had requested to see the baby. Laura's first job was to wash and dress the baby and take her to the family. She had been asked to do this because she was a trained counsellor and she agreed.

As she washed and dressed the baby, Laura talked to her and then took her to meet the other members of her family. There were four people in the room, the baby's father, grandmother, grandfather and an aunt. Laura said 'hello, I have brought the baby to meet you' and lifted the baby girl out of the cot to show her to them. The baby's grandmother stepped forward and took her in her arms. Laura asked the family if they wanted to be alone with her and they nodded agreement and she left them for half an hour before returning to see if they needed anything. She noted that the family had returned the baby to her cot and were sitting in silence. With their consent, she took the baby from the room, telling the family that they could see her at any time while she was in the hospital. They asked to be taken to the intensive care unit and Laura allocated another member of support staff to go with them.

Laura returned the baby to the small treatment room where she was being kept prior to transfer to the hospital mortuary. One of the midwifery managers entered the room and spoke to Laura. On seeing her, Laura burst into tears. The manager reached out and touched Laura's arm. Laura apologized and explained that she had not realized how distressing this would be – it was her first experience in caring for a woman who was experiencing stillbirth. The midwifery manager said, 'That makes no difference, it never gets any easier.' Laura found this very comforting.

When Laura reflected on this later, she knew that she had felt confident that she would be able to respond sensitively to the needs of the family and therefore was not afraid of having to find the 'right' words. However, in the whole of her training as a nurse and so far in midwifery, she had not received any professional development in bereavement care. Without her own development in this area she would have continued to feel unqualified to help. (Komaromy et al. 2007: 32)

(a) How does Laura engage in emotional labour?
(b) Reflect on your own practice experiences and consider how, when and to whom you provide emotional labour.
(c) Do you always feel equipped to provide for the emotional needs of patients or clients?

5 The role of sociological knowledge

The aim of this section is to illustrate the value of sociological knowledge and the role it plays in examining the realities of nursing practice. Recognizing the significance of an evidence base within modern nursing, this section draws on a range of empirical studies, all of which have something to tell nurses about their relationships with patients, informal carers and other health professionals, or about their role in the workplace. A key feature underpinning sociological research is the idea that things may not be what they seem. As Berger (1963) suggests, you are 'looking behind', or 'seeing through' and generally unmasking the common facades of everyday life. As Earle (2001: 14) argues in her discussion of the role of sociology within the therapies, sociologists take the everyday and the taken-for-granted and try to look beyond obvious explanations to gain a deeper understanding of contemporary social issues.

Ellis (1992) attempts to integrate knowledge from various academic disciplines with the theory and practice bases of interpersonal professions. Following on from his discussion of a 'personal education', his model of 'semantic conjunction' can also be useful. In application to nursing, this term simply suggests that the subject matter of sociology is useful to nurses because sociologists and nurses share some common interests and concerns. Nowhere is this more clearly illustrated than in the piece of classic sociological research – described in Jeffery's *Normal Rubbish* (1979) – a study based on interviews with doctors and observation of three English casualty departments.

Perceptions of patients in casualty departments

Jeffery's study has as much to tell nurses, doctors and anyone working with vulnerable or health-compromised individuals about the truth of their work today as when it was published. It provides insight into perceptions of patients and demonstrates at best a lack of care, and at worst the wholesale neglect of and infliction of (further) damage on certain groups of patients. Via a process of **social construction**, particular patients became categorized by doctors as 'normal rubbish' (see Box 2.2). This is a good example of an interactionist approach to research (see Chapter 1), in which individual actions are subject to scrutiny.

social construction: the way in which social reality is constructed by individuals and groups

Box 2.2 'Normal rubbish'

Trivia

Patients who 'casually' pop into casualty with conditions neither traumatic nor urgent are described as 'normal trivia'. They trivialize the emergency services by presenting with conditions which should be taken to the GP.

Drunks

'Normal drunks' are abusive and usually appear in the middle of the night. If they are brought in unconscious, normal drunks are often kept in as it is unclear whether they are sleeping off the drink or whether they have received a blow to the head.

Overdoses

A 'normal overdose' is usually female and perceived as a self-harmer rather than as a 'genuine' suicide. She is usually a regular and 'does it for attention'.

Tramps

'Normal tramps' smell and wear layers of rotten clothing. They usually come in during the night in winter and are just trying to find a bed for the night. They often pretend to be sick in order to achieve this.

(Other patients defined as 'normal rubbish' include 'nutcases', and smelly, dirty and obese people.)

(Jeffery 1979: 106–7)

seminal:
research is seminal if it has a determining influence on sociological thought

reliability:
research is reliable if it can be repeated to produce the same results

validity:
research is valid if it measures what it has set out to measure

Significant for the sociological study of nursing is that although Jeffrey confined his interviewing to doctors, it is made clear that other staff working in the department – such as nurses and porters – were in a process of collusion with the medical staff about the way these particular patients were viewed. It is shown in the following comment made by a porter to a doctor after a person identified by the department staff as a 'tramp' was seen in the casualty department and discharged by the doctor. A short time later he collapsed and died outside on the pavement. In order to allay the worries of the doctor concerned, the porter says: 'It's all right, sir, I've turned him round so that it looks as though he was on his way to Casualty.' This **seminal** piece of sociological research, which so clearly demonstrates the interface between sociology and nursing, has a tremendous amount to say to nurses.

Before the results of published research can be used as evidence for practice, such research must be scrutinized in an informed way for **reliability** and **validity** – terms which will become more familiar and meaningful to you in the future.

Activity 2.5 Normal rubbish deviant patients in casualty departments

In Jeffery's study (1979), 'rubbish' was a category generated by the staff themselves. It was commonly used in discussions of the work and of the patients seen within the casualty environment:

> 'It's a thankless task, seeing all the rubbish, as we call it, coming through.'
> 'I wouldn't be making the same fuss in another job – it's only because it's mostly bloody crumble like women with insect bites.'
> 'I think the [city-centre hospital] gets more of the rubbish – the drunks and that.'

(a) It is clear from this research that nurses working in the casualty department shared the same attitude towards some patients as the doctors. If twenty-first-century nurses are educated to underpin their practice with theory, which specific aspects of the latter do you consider that the nurses of 1979 might not have been aware of?

(b) The full title of the article appears as the heading for Activity 2.5. In what sense do you think that some patients are identified by the author as 'deviant'?

(c) It is clear from Jeffrey's study that some patients are regarded as 'legitimately sick' while others are not. How do you think this impacts on the concept of 'holistic' assessment and care within contemporary nursing?

The remainder of this section continues the theme of exploring the realities of nursing work by focusing on more contemporary sociological research (but for a more recent study of 'problem patients' see the work by Shaw (2004), who explores attitudes to patients with psychiatric diagnoses). Some comparisons between the studies will be

2

self-evident as the chapter progresses and it is not the remit here to focus on them, but rather to identify and emphasize the value of socio-logical knowledge for practising nurses.

Researching the experiences of clients with learning difficulties

Richardson (2000) explores the social context of people with learning difficulties by interviewing over a period of eighteen months six people living in nurse-managed community homes. Drawing on the social model of disability, which is discussed at length in Chapter 10, he asks three questions (p. 1384):

- What do people with learning difficulties, living in the community, have to say about their lives and experiences?
- What are their views about the differences between their lives and those of non-disabled people?
- How do disablist assumptions influence the lives of people with learning difficulties and nursing practice?

The significance of this research undoubtedly lies, in part, in its inclusion of people with learning difficulties as participants, thereby reversing the stereotypical notion that 'People corralled within the frame of learning difficulties are deemed incompetent, unable to ade-quately speak for themselves, and thus requiring care, protection and treatment' (Richardson 2000: 1384).

As well as giving nurses valuable insight into participants' views, the research also reflects current policy initiatives for people with learning difficulties, which are based on the principles of rights, independ-ence, choice and inclusion. It is a useful illustration of the way that sociological research can be used by nurses to explore the experiences of specific client groups, enriching the practice base of nurses and others (for another interesting study, on end-of-life care and people with learning difficulties, see the study by Todd (2009)). The concept of research validity is implicit in Richardson's work through his focus on **autobiographical voice**.

autobiographical voice:
methodological approach which allows participants to tell their own stories

Whereas the two articles explored so far have addressed the experi-ences of patients or clients, the next takes a broader perspective and explores the role of nurses in the workplace, and their relationships with other health-care workers.

Relationships between nurses and health-care assistants

A study by Daykin and Clarke (2000) explores the relationships between nurses and health-care assistants (HCAs) in the NHS. It is based on interviews in two English hospital wards providing medical care for older adults. A sociological account of nursing is given in which various perspectives are brought to bear on aspects of the individual nursing role and the profession as a whole.

The research was carried out to evaluate a new skill-mix project which increased the number of HCAs in proportion to registered nurses and simultaneously phased out the role of primary nurses. The aim of the research was to discover what impact the project had on the staff in relation to care delivery and working conditions.

The research identified a dichotomy between professional rhetoric and professional practice (Holt and Warne (2007)) – that is, what nurses *should* do and what *really* happens in practice. Despite nurses heralding the concept of holistic care as reflecting best practice, the researchers found that in the context of the new skill mix described above, a hierarchical division of labour emerged between the two groups. This resulted in care organization by selectivity of work and task allocation. Box 2.3 outlines some of the key findings.

Box 2.3 Rhetoric vs reality

Perceptions of the skill-mix project

- a threat to the holistic delivery of care;
- detrimental to the quality of care;
- a threat to the ability to apply sophisticated skills of assessment and analysis.

Realities of the skill-mix project in practice

- staff shortages and resource constraints prevented skill-mix teams;
- qualified nurses worked below their actual skill levels;
- a hierarchical division of labour emerged.

(Daykin and Clarke 2000: 353–4).

The exposure of some of the realities of nursing practice necessarily suggests that the registered nurses did not want to deliver the essentials of hands-on care in keeping with the philosophy of primary nursing and holistic-care delivery, but rather that when faced with the realities of financial constraints, staffing shortages and so on, there is a clear theory–practice gap.

From these observations, the authors provide significant insights into the perceived value of nursing's professionalization project, described by the authors as an attempt by nurses to 'renegotiate their relationship with the state and secure greater recognition and professional status' (Daykin and Clarke 2000: 349). A key factor in this has traditionally been the claim to a distinct knowledge base from which to develop theoretical models of holistic care, professional autonomy, the selection and ownership of higher-status technical skills, and the scope to renegotiate role boundaries between nursing and doctoring.

Taking up this issue, Daykin and Clarke suggest that, given the current social context for care, where the likelihood is that nurses and HCAs will continue to do a significant proportion of the round-the-clock work, the profession might serve itself better by adopting an inclusive rather than a hierarchical 'out-group' attitude towards this group of co-workers. Not only would this help to preserve the knowledge and ownership of nursing care for nurses, but it would also acknowledge the crucial contribution to care made by health-care assistants.

A further useful insight to emerge from this research is that, although the two groups were generally united in their opposition to the skill-mix project, a range of 'multiple and apparently contradictory viewpoints' (p. 353) was expressed about respective workplace roles; health-care assistants were, on the whole, far more enthusiastic than the nurses. Daykin and Clarke attribute this again to the dichotomy between ownership of a perceived appropriate theoretical stance for nursing and the social reality of the care context, steeped as it is in day-to-day issues of staff shortages, economies of scale and financial stringency. Using a structural analysis, they suggest that a possible effect of this apparent disunity of ideas and purpose (expressed in the article as 'ambivalence') is that it represents potential for exploitation by managers if perceived as a weakness of nursing systems. Likely manifestations could be (further) imposition of routinized, ritualistic, deskilled, task-based work systems on to hospital staff, in direct contradiction to the concept of professional autonomy so prized by some sections of the contemporary nursing workforce.

Daykin and Clarke (2000) challenge some of the existing premises on which current nursing practice is based, and make an invaluable contribution to the sociology of nursing. For example, they explore issues that have the potential to raise awareness of professionalization among practising nurses; such awareness is a prerequisite for the necessary action to achieve future changes, which will ultimately improve the experiences of both patients and health-care workers (also, for an interesting study on the relationship between operating-theatre nurses and operating-department practitioners, see Timmons and Tanner (2004)).

6 Sociological knowledge and the case of diabetes

There is an increasing prevalence of diabetes in the UK and globally, and as such there is a growing body of sociological literature that focuses on the issue. Much of this literature reports on studies that seek to explore the lived experiences of people with diabetes. The work by Julia Lawton provides one such example. In a paper published in 2007, Lawton and her colleagues report on two sociological studies conducted in Edinburgh, Scotland, that explored respondents' accounts of diabetes causation. This work is interesting because respondents included women and men of white British and South Asian (Pakistani and Indian) origin; and rates of diabetes are particularly high amongst these ethnic groups. All of the respondents in both studies were interviewed in their first language (English or Punjabi). What is notable about this work is that, whilst the respondents of both studies draw on diverse accounts to explain the cause of their diabetes, there were subtle differences between the white British and South Asian respondents. In particular, the white British participants tended to attribute their diabetes to their own lifestyle choices, whereas the South Asian participants tended to contextualize their diabetes onset in relation to a wide range of external factors (see Box 2.4).

Box 2.4 Ethnicity and different accounts of diabetes onset

Christine: Probably the lack of exercise 'n eating the wrong stuff I would think that's probably what caused it. Plus, as I say, I was having chocolate, which was the wrong thing. (White British respondent)

Bushra: I got blood pressure because of worry, because my son, when he was married, he was married into my sister's home. My sister lives here, and then we had a bit of conflict. We also had a shop together and then divorce was given to the girl, and then my son and my sister and I were separated because of that . . . That's the reason why I got blood pressure . . . And that's how I got sugar. (South Asian respondent)

(Lawton et al. 2007: 895)

Lawton et al. conclude that, in describing their diabetes onset, white British participants tended to depict themselves as to blame, whereas South Asian participants generally allocated responsibility to external factors and to life circumstances in general. Lawton et al. argue that in seeking to understand these differences, both micro- and macro-factors are important (these sociological approaches are outlined in Chapter 1).

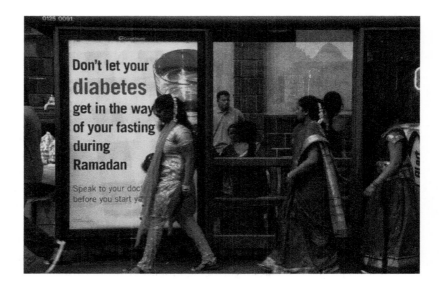

Figure 2.3 Certain groups have higher rates of illness than others – sociological consideration on the nurse's part can lead to understanding why a patient's diabetic control might be poor

What is Health?

Sarah Earle

KEY ISSUES IN THIS CHAPTER:
- ▶ Defining health.
- ▶ Modes of health.
- ▶ Social influences on health and disease.
- ▶ Experiences of illness, sickness and disease.
- ▶ Nursing, health and holism.

BY THE END OF THIS CHAPTER YOU SHOULD BE ABLE TO:
- ▶ Review official and lay definitions of health.
- ▶ Compare and contrast the biomedical and social roles of health.
- ▶ Give an account of how health and disease are influenced by social factors.
- ▶ Understand illness behaviour, sickness and stigma.
- ▶ Evaluate a holistic approach to nursing practice.

1 Introduction

Did you know that poorer people will die sooner and suffer more ill health than those who are wealthier? Did you know that women are more likely than men to be diagnosed with mental illness, and that older and disabled people are the two groups in society most likely to be refused life-saving treatment? Arguably, these facts are social rather than biological, and although the majority of sociologists would not deny the biological nature of disease, most would agree that our understanding, treatment and experience of health and ill health are socially influenced. Sociologists would also agree that the production and distribution of disease are social rather than biological matters. The purpose of this chapter is to explore how sociology can help us to understand health better, taking as its foundation the position put forward by Turner, who argues that health and ill heath are 'fundamentally a social state of affairs' (1995: 37).

2 Defining health

It may seem easy, but defining health is actually quite hard. Before you read on, think about what health means to you. Is your definition of health the same as that of your colleague? Kelman has argued that 'perhaps the most perplexing and ambiguous issue in the study of health since its inception centuries or millennia ago, is its definition' (1975: 625), but defining health is essential if we are to understand it and deliver appropriate services. It is an important issue for nurses because, to help the patient achieve health, nurses should have some understanding of the factors that contribute to 'healthiness'.

Official definitions of health

Health is often defined quite simply as an 'absence of disease'. This has been one of the most pervasive official definitions of health in the modern Western world and is one that can frequently be found within medical documentation, government reports and legislation.

Do you believe that this is a good way of defining health? How does it compare with your own definition? Health as an 'absence of disease' is also the cornerstone of the biomedical model – discussed in more detail below – which, in spite of its limits (Barbour 1995), is the most influential model of health within modern medicine. To describe health in this way is to define it in extremely negative terms; that is, you are considered healthy only if you are not suffering from any disease. However, research suggests that just as it is possible to feel unwell when one is healthy (for a discussion of the **'worried well'**, see Brodersen, Siersma and Ryle 2011), it is possible to feel healthy even when suffering from chronic or terminal illness (for example, see Falk, Wahn and Lidell 2007).

worried well:
healthy individuals who are concerned about their health and well-being

Another commonly used definition is that of the World Health Organization, which defines health as 'not merely the absence of disease, but a state of complete physical, mental, spiritual and social well-being' (WHO 1948: 1). This marks a shift away from defining health solely in relation to disease and reflects an acceptance of some of the other factors that influence health. It also reflects a more positive, although idealistic, approach to health. Here, health is perceived as a goal. Lupton has suggested that this overriding concern with health has reached the proportions of a social movement which she calls **healthism**, arguing that 'the pursuit of health has become an end in itself, rather than a means to an end' (1995: 70).

healthism:
a personal, cultural and political health movement

More recently health has been defined as a resource:

To reach a state of complete physical, mental and social wellbeing, an individual or group must be able to identify and to realize aspirations, to satisfy needs, and to change or cope with the environment. Health is, therefore, seen as a resource for everyday life, not the objective of living. Health is a positive concept emphasizing social and personal resources, as well as physical capacities. (WHO 1986: 1)

As you can see, here health is still regarded as a positive concept, but rather than being an end in itself, it is seen as a resource for living, a means to an end.

3

Lay definitions of health

Although sociologists are interested in unpacking official definitions of health, in the last twenty-five years or so sociologists have become interested in understanding **lay definitions of health** and have attempted to demonstrate how an understanding of lay definitions can be useful for health professionals. This approach has been influenced by theories of social action (see Chapter 1) that are concerned with the meaning that individuals give to their own experiences. Official, or medical, definitions are thought to be based on **universal and generalizable knowledge** in scientific terms, whereas lay definitions are thought to be unscientific and based on individual experience. Although our own health beliefs are 'unscientific', they are essential to the way in which we make sense of health and illness, and indeed the very subjective nature of health has led some researchers to argue that lay definitions are the only valid measure of health. Williams and Popay (1994) suggest that lay definitions of health and illness are organized in the following way:

lay definitions of health:
based on experience or folk knowledge, as opposed to 'official' or medical definitions

universal and generalizable knowledge:
knowledge assumed to be common

1 They do not mimic medical views.
2 They are logical and coherent.
3 They are biographical (based on lived experience).
4 They are culturally framed within particular systems of belief.

Some researchers have also argued that, whilst lay definitions of health and illness do not mimic medical views, scientific knowledge can become part of the views of lay people (Blaxter 1990; Hugher and Klein 2004). However, other sociologists disagree and argue that subjective definitions of health can be very individual, eccentric, contradictory and just plain wrong!

> ### Activity 3.1 Lay 'experts'?
>
> It seems reasonably clear (from where we stand now) that during the latter stages of the 20th century medical practitioners have been required to be more clearly and openly accountable to lay assessment and more sensitive to patient viewpoints than had previously been the case . . . These trends are undoubtedly related to the operation of other, wider, forces that have led to a

challenge on the expertise of professionals. Thus medicine – as with so many other forms of professional activity – has been confronted by something of a legitimation crisis. . . . [There has been] an increased interest in what lay people have to offer by way of knowledge of health and illness [and] there has been a tendency to argue that lay knowledge can be every bit as valuable as professional knowledge. . . . patients can have extensive knowledge of their own lives and the conditions in which they live . . . they can (and sometimes have to) turn themselves into experts in order to challenge medical hegemony. . . . [However,] for the most part, lay people are not experts . . . What is more they can often be plain wrong about the causes, course and management of common forms of disease and illness. (Prior 2003: 42–5)

(a) Do you think that nurses are accountable to lay assessment and sensitive to patient viewpoints?

(b) Does the concept of the 'lay expert' apply equally to all groups of patients (e.g., patients with learning disabilities or mental health problems, or children)? If not, try to explain why this is the case.

(c) How and why might the expertise of health professionals be challenged? Have you ever felt that your expertise has been challenged by patients? If so, how did this make you feel?

One of the most comprehensive studies of lay health in the UK is the Health & Lifestyles Survey (Blaxter 1990), involving 9,000 people. This survey asked individuals the following questions:

1 Think of someone you know who is very healthy. Who are you thinking of? How old are they? What makes you call them healthy?

2 At certain times people are healthier than at other times. What is it like when you are healthy? An analysis of responses to these questions revealed ten major lay concepts of health (see Box 3.1).

Lay definitions of health are variable and are, generally speaking, often dependent on factors including age, gender, disability and so on (see Part II). Activity 3.2 asks you to consider children's definitions of health.

Box 3.1 The health and lifestyles survey: lay concepts of health

Health as not ill

You are healthy when you do not have any symptoms of disease – a concept popular amongst people of all ages, but particularly older people, and most likely to be used to describe others.

Health as absence of disease/health despite disease

A definition focusing on disease and drawing on a medical model of health, most commonly used by those who described themselves as feeling healthy despite disease.

Health as a reserve

The idea that someone is healthy due to an inborn reserve of health.

3

Health as behaviour

A healthy person was often defined in terms of their healthy behaviour and the phrase was most likely to be used to describe the behaviour of others.

Health as physical fitness

The concept of fitness was most commonly referred to by men of all ages, although young men tended to stress strength and the ability to play sports. Young women rarely mentioned sports but often mentioned being (or feeling) slim.

Health as energy

Having energy, vitality and enthusiasm was seen by women and older men as important.

Health as a social relationship

This concept was particularly important to women who saw health in terms of having good relationships with others or the ability to help other people.

Health as function

This refers to being able to carry on with everyday tasks and was often used to describe a man. It was also used to refer to older people who could get along despite advanced age.

Health as psychosocial well-being

This category often included some of the other concepts of health, such as health as energy, or health as social relationships. However, some individuals saw health purely as a state of mind.

Negative answers

A small group of respondents were not able to define being healthy. Most of these were not interested in 'healthy behaviour'.

(Adapted from Blaxter 1990).

Activity 3.2 Understanding children's perceptions of ill/health

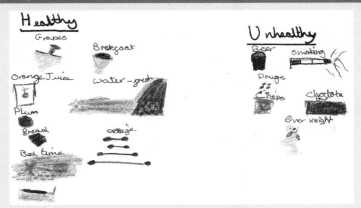

Figure 3.1 Drawing by Maria Perry, aged nine

(a) Drawing techniques are often used as a research method when exploring children's perceptions of health and illness. What does Figure 3.1 tell us about children's views of what makes us healthy and unhealthy?

(b) What are the implications of this for nursing children?

(c) In what other ways could nurses encourage children to discuss their experiences of health and illness?

3 Understanding models of health

Models of health offer nurses different ways of thinking about health and how they might offer care to patients. These models differ because they identify distinct causes of illness, sickness and disease and therefore offer different suggestions for the prevention of ill health. In this section we examine the biomedical and the social models of health.

The biomedical model

The present system of medical knowledge within modern Western societies is commonly known as the biomedical, or medical, model. This model is characterized by several features (see Box 3.2).

Box 3.2 Characteristics of the biomedical model

- Health is the absence of disease, and disease is the absence of health.
- Illness can be reduced to disordered bodily functions within the individual.
- Health services treat sick and disabled people largely within specialisms (e.g., paediatrics, obstetrics, podiatry, etc.).
- Health services are remedial and curative.
- Each disease is thought to be caused by a specific (potentially identifiable) pathogen, often leading to an over-reliance on pharmacological intervention.
- The production of medical knowledge via the use of 'scientific' research methods is valued over the use of qualitative research methodologies.
- Health professionals are the 'experts' with the power to diagnose disease and decide on treatment.

The biomedical model has been and, some would argue, still is dominant within modern Western health care. However, this perspective is not without its critics. Blaxter (1990), for example, argues that the medical model of health does not always focus narrowly on biomedical science and that more holistic concepts of health are also part of medical practice. Nonetheless, there are many who believe that a biomedical model is outmoded and unhelpful and that it acts as a 'straitjacket' for thinking about nursing care (Allott and Robb 1998; Engebretson 2003).

In response to this, alternative models of health have emerged. The next model we consider here is the social model, which identifies the role of social factors in the production and distribution of disease.

The social model

The social model of health has developed largely as a critique of the biomedical model and, whilst sociologists have offered various critiques of biomedicine, three characteristics are usually central (Annandale 1998).

First, the social model assumes that health and disease are socially produced; biomedicine is reductionist because it assumes that disease is natural and located in the individual. Second, biomedicine is characterized by the 'doctrine of specific aetiology', which refers to how the biomedical model assumes a direct relationship between pathology and disease. In contrast, the social model recognizes that other factors play a role in determining who becomes sick and why. In fact, some commentators suggest that diseases should be classified by their social causes rather than by specific aetiology.

The third critique of the biomedical model relates to the belief that medicine is neutral and scientific; this is referred to as scientific neutrality. However, the social model emphasizes the way in which health care is influenced by a range of social factors. For example, a study of the treatment of patients in accident and emergency departments (Jeffery 1979) demonstrates that certain patients – 'drunks, tramps, nutcases and self-harmers' – are not treated equally (see Chapter 2).

The social model cannot tell you how to nurse patients, but it can provide you with interesting insights into the causes of disease and the way in which social factors help to shape treatment. Whilst the biomedical model focuses on the diagnosis and treatment of disease, the social model focuses more on prevention and is a useful model for nurses involved in health promotion (see also Chapter 10 for a discussion of a public-health model) and those interested in promoting patient empowerment and partnership.

4 Social influences on health and disease

One of the most significant contributions that medical sociologists have made has been to show how health and disease are influenced by a range of social factors. In this section, we examine the relationship between changing patterns of disease and changes within society. We then explore the way in which the process of **medicalization** has had a significant impact on the way we define health and disease.

medicalization: applying a medical label to aspects of everyday life

Changing patterns of disease

Various writers have suggested that modern societies have passed through three distinct types of disease patterns:

- *Disease in pre-agricultural societies:* Before 10,000 BC, evidence suggests that most people died from environmental and safety hazards, for example, exposure. Infectious diseases and so-called 'lifestyle diseases' such as heart disease and cancer were uncommon.
- *Disease in agricultural societies:* Infectious diseases such as tuberculosis and cholera were the most common.
- *Disease in the modern industrial era:* By the mid-twentieth century infectious diseases were no longer a primary cause of death. Chronic and degenerative diseases, such as cancer, diabetes and cardiovascular disease, have become more common (Fitzpatrick 1986).

Why do you think that disease prevalence has changed? It could be argued that advances in medicine and health-care provision have had a significant impact on the prevalence of certain diseases. This may be true in some instances, but sociologists would suggest that if we examine the changing patterns of disease, we can see that they are closely related to social and economic factors. If, for example, we take the case of tuberculosis (TB), official records show that death rates began to fall quite rapidly in the first half of the nineteenth century, well before the introduction of chemotherapy treatments in the 1940s and the BCG vaccination in the 1950s, and even before the identification in 1882 of the tubercle bacillus (Department of Health 1998). It is worth noting, however, that reported cases of TB in the UK began to rise in the early 1990s, particularly amongst migrants from Africa and the Indian subcontinent and refugees (see, for example, <www.doh.gov uk>). Although the incidence of TB continues to increase in England, it has decreased again in Northern Ireland, Scotland and Wales (see Table 3.1). This reinforces the view that social and economic factors can have a significant influence on patterns of disease.

Table 3.1 Notification rates of tuberculosis											
	1996	1997	1998	1999	2000	2001	2002	2003	2004	2005	2006[1]
United Kingdom	10.7	10.9	11.3	11.4	12.1	12.2	12.2	11.7	12.1	13.4	13.2
England	11.3	11.6	12.1	12.1	13.0	13.3	13.3	12.8	13.1	14.8	14.7
Wales	5.6	6.7	5.9	7.1	6.6	4.9	4.3	4.6	6.1	5.4	5.2
Scotland	10.0	8.5	9.0	9.8	9.3	8.7	8.3	8.3	9.1	7.6	6.9
Northern Ireland	4.5	4.5	3.6	3.6	3.5	2.8	4.0	2.2	4.3	3.9	2.8

Rates per 100,000 population

[1] UK and Scotland figures are provisional.

(Adapted from: ONS 2008, Table 7.7, p. 146)

The medicalization of everyday life

Zola (1973: 261) argues that 'if anything can be shown in some way to affect the workings of the body and to a lesser extent the mind, then it can be labelled . . . "a medical problem".' Sociologists have shown that healthy physical processes, such as menstruation, pregnancy and the menopause, have become medicalized (see, for example, Patterson 2014; Katz Rothman 2014; and Rubinstein 2014). Sociologists also suggest that what comes to be defined as a disease is dependent upon a range of political and economic factors. For example, Hunt (1994) and Lee (1998) point out that the construction of the menopause as an 'oestrogen-deficiency' disease developed in the 1960s and was strongly associated with the development and availability of hormone replacement therapies. Gambling, alcoholism and sexuality have been similarly medicalized (Conrad 2014).

However, just as some healthy processes become medicalized, others become demedicalized. A good example of this is the demedicalization of homosexuality, which until 1973 was listed in the *Diagnostic and Statistical Manual of Mental Disorders* as a pathological psychiatric disorder. This demonstrates how the labelling of a process or behaviour as a disease is only tangentially related to a distinct physiological or psychological occurrence.

Medicalization has been widely criticized by sociologists. For example, Ivan Illich (1976) developed a theory of **iatrogenesis** in which he identifies three types:

iatrogenesis:
'doctor-caused illness'

- *Clinical iatrogenesis:* where individuals are directly harmed by medicine through treatment itself or through the ineffectiveness or the uncertainty of treatment. This also includes the actions taken by doctors to avoid litigation; for example, an increase in the Caesarean section rate.
- *Social iatrogenesis:* where individuals become dependent upon medicine for their understanding of natural processes and become consumers of health care.
- *Structural iatrogenesis:* where the nature of society renders people unable to care for themselves and each other without recourse to medical attention and medical concepts of health. It also refers to the way that individuals strive to achieve better health.

Activity 3.3 Medical 'problems'?		
BALDNESS	FRECKLES	UGLINESS
JET LAG	INFERTILITY	SMOKING
SHORTNESS	NAIL-BITING	BAD BREATH
SHYNESS	INSOMNIA	HAIRINESS

(a) Think about the list of 'problems' identified above. Are these medical problems?

(b) Who decides what becomes a medical problem and why?

(c) What are the implications of medicalizing such problems, for individuals, for health professionals and for society as a whole?

Most importantly, sociologists are interested in the way that obesity can be positioned as a social and structural issue rather than a personal one. Earle (2007: 360) argues:

> There is increasing awareness that obesity is not just an individual problem and a personal responsibility, but a societal issue caused by increased industrialization, urbanization and mechanization. Most people work longer hours, rely on cars to get around, have less time to prepare foods from fresh, have sedentary jobs and perform little physical activity. People live in obesogenic – or obesity-promoting – societies in which they eat more and are less physically active than is healthy to maintain an appropriate body weight.

5 Experiences of illness, sickness and disease

Whilst some sociologists have focused on the social factors influencing health and disease, others are more interested in the experiences of ill health, recognizing that responses to illness are influenced by our own experiences as much as by the biological symptoms of disease (see Chapter 2 for a discussion of the role of sociology in nursing).

Illness behaviour

Everybody feels ill at some point in their lives, but, as we all know from our own experiences, when we feel ill we don't always go to the doctor. Research suggests that most of the illness in society goes unreported as health professionals only get to see a very small proportion of all illness; this is known as the 'clinical iceberg'.

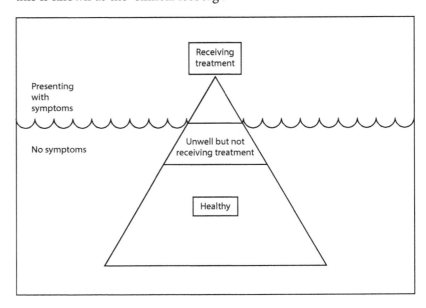

Figure 3.3 The Clinical Iceberg is a model used to explain why health professionals only see a small percentage of those who are ill in the population

Sociologists are interested in **illness behaviour** because, as Robinson argues, 'a person's readiness to consider himself, or another, ill cannot adequately be explained by reference to the severity of the symptomatic person's condition' (1971: 7). In other words, it would appear that the nature of disease has little relation to the likelihood of someone consulting their health practitioner. In a classic study carried out by Mechanic (1968), a wide range of factors could be seen to contribute to seeking help (see Box 3.3).

illness behaviour:
actions of people when they feel unwell

3

> **Box 3.3 Factors influencing help-seeking behaviour**
>
> - The extent to which symptoms are visible and recognizable.
> - Their perceived seriousness and consequent levels of anxiety.
> - The extent to which they impact on the sufferer's life.
> - Their perceived frequency and persistence.
> - The degree to which an individual can tolerate them.
> - Knowledge about what symptoms may mean.
> - Competing needs.
> - Competing explanations for the symptoms.
> - Availability of treatment and assistance.

In this context, we can see that individuals respond not just to a symptom, but to the meaning of the symptom and the effect that it has on their lives. Zola (1973) suggests that there are triggers which lead individuals to seek medical attention:

1 *The occurrence of an interpersonal crisis:* This refers to the presence of an event of some kind which calls attention to the symptoms, forcing the individual to do something about them.
2 *The perceived interference with social or personal relations:* The extent to which symptoms seem to interfere, at any given time, with daily life.
3 *Sanctioning:* This refers to when the decision to seek medical attention lies with another person, who sanctions that decision.
4 *The perceived interference with vocational or physical activity:* This usually refers to the extent to which symptoms seem to interfere with work.
5 *The temporalizing of symptomatology:* The setting of external time criteria, after which treatment will be sought.

The sick role

As we have seen above, not everyone who is ill will receive treatment for their illness, but sociologists have argued that those who do are likely to achieve the status of 'sick'. The concept of the **sick role** was developed by the sociologist Talcott Parsons, who believed that illness is 'partly biologically and partly socially defined' (1991: 431). Parsons

sick role:
the sanctioning of illness within society

deviance:
behaviour considered unacceptable within a society or culture

argued that ill health was a form of **deviance** and disruptive to the normal functioning of society (also see Chapter 1). Additionally, he suggested that the role of medicine was to ensure that only those who are truly ill are permitted to adopt the sick role. Those who claim to be sick without being truly ill are perceived as skivers and malingerers. Entering the sick role, therefore, requires that certain conditions be met; these are best understood in terms of expectations placed on the patient and on the doctor (see Box 3.4).

Box 3.4 On being sick: roles and responsibilities

The patient

- Is exempted from normal social role responsibilities, e.g., going to work.
- Is not responsible for his or her illness and cannot get well on his or her own; cannot, for example, just 'pull himself together'.
- Must want to get better.
- Must seek technically competent help and comply with treatment.

The doctor

- Must act in a professional and objective manner.
- Must do everything possible to help the patient recover.
- Must be well trained and competent.
- Must be able to examine the patient.

The concept of the sick role is perceived to be a good explanation for temporary bouts of ill health to which any of us could reasonably become susceptible; for example, influenza or a broken leg. However, there have been many criticisms of the concept of a sick role, especially in relation to its inability to explain the experiences of specific groups; for example, those with chronic illness (see Chapter 9).

Stigma and disease

stigma:
social disgrace attached to any condition

The sociology of **stigma** and disease has been particularly influenced by the work of Erving Goffman (1963), who argued that stigma is a powerful discrediting label that can change and 'spoil' the way in which the person is viewed. Goffman's work is influenced by theories of social action (see Chapter 1) and the view that individuals are active agents within the social world.

Goffman argues that there are two types of condition: discrediting conditions, which are conditions that are clearly visible to others, for example eczema, psoriasis, physical impairments or stammering, and discreditable conditions, those that are usually not visible to others, or can be easily concealed, for example epilepsy, HIV, depression or diabetes. The attention given to people with Down's syndrome provides us with a good example of the distinction between discrediting and discreditable conditions. Generally speaking, Down's syndrome

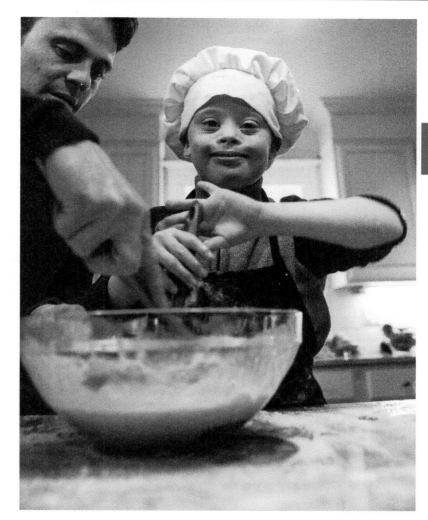

Figure 3.4 Conditions which produce visible changes to an individual can result in the individual being stigmatized by the wider society in which they live

is a discrediting condition as the facial features of the individual are distinct from those of other people, thus immediately stigmatizing that person. Media reports have highlighted cases of parents who are seeking cosmetic surgery for their children with Down's syndrome, arguing that it is the visibility of this condition which leads to stigma, rather than the condition itself.

Arguably, by changing the visible aspects of Down's syndrome, parents are turning a discrediting condition into a discreditable one. The ethics of this type of surgery on children are strongly disputed by organizations such as the Down's Syndrome Association (see <downs-syndrome.org.uk>) and others. Indeed, an article in the *Journal of Medical Ethics* likens facial reconstruction to the mutilation of female circumcision (Jones 2000).

Some conditions lead to stigma because of the moral attributes associated with a particular condition. HIV and AIDS are commonly associated with sexual promiscuity, drug use and homosexuality

(Rhodes and Cusick 2000), so individuals who are HIV-positive often experience what is known as 'enacted' stigma (Lekas, Siegel and Leider 2011); this is the type of stigma that leads to actual discrimination. People with other types of condition may experience 'felt' stigma, which refers more to feelings of shame rather than to an actual experience of discrimination. This is often relevant to people with rectal cancer (Phelan et al. 2013), epilepsy (Leaffer, Hesdorffer and Begley 2014), prostate problems (Pateman and Johnson 2000) and testicular cancer (Chapple and Ziebland 2004).

Lastly, it is worth considering the concept of 'courtesy stigma', which has been defined as a 'tendency for stigma to spread from the stigmatized individual to his close connections' (Goffman 1963: 30). There is evidence, for example, that the family and carers of those with Alzheimer's disease often experience considerable embarrassment and shame (Werner and Heinik 2008). Courtesy stigma is also relevant to others, including the family and friends of those with mental health problems and learning disabilities.

Activity 3.4 Autism and stigma

The extract below presents data from a study of stigma among parents of children with high-functioning autism, living in the Brisbane metropolitan region of Australia. The data were collected using in-depth semi-structured interviews with fifty-three parents whose children were aged between five and twenty-six years (Gray 2002: 739–41).

> As a mother, when a child sort of acts up . . . you don't want him to do it, because it's a bit embarrassing. And you feel like it reflects on you a little bit. I mean I'm intelligent enough to know that that's not the case, but it's very difficult to take yourself away from the situation. (Mother)

> I have always taken my boys shopping, always . . . Oh, it's a disaster initially. [My son] threw a jar of vegemite at an elderly lady who smiled at him, you know . . . they look at me as though I'm a mother who obviously isn't very good at being a mother. (Mother)

> Occasionally we'd ask [some] family down and we'd have a drink or whatever, but we never got invited [back] . . . we never seem to be reciprocated. They don't say, 'Well, come over'. So, yes, you do feel like they've sort of judged and thought, 'Give them a miss'. (Father)

> We went on . . . camp and we were pretty apprehensive about going . . . We were the only ones with an autistic child and . . . he performed in front of all those people there and had to take charge. And he called me an idiot in front of all those people, and swearing started to come out, and everybody just freezes. Everybody is just embarrassed. (Mother)

(a) What kinds of stigma are being experienced by these parents of autistic children?

(b) Why might mothers be more likely than fathers to experience stigma?

(c) Do you think that nurses contribute to the stigma experienced by patients and their relatives or carers? Can you think of any examples from your own practice?

(d) What role can nurses play in enabling patients and their carers to manage stigma?

entry into the emerging professions was barred to women until the end of the century, so the only occupations available to them were those of companion or governess.

To attract middle-class women into nursing with the aim of transforming it into a professional occupation, the hygiene and domestic elements of the nursing role were redefined as scientific (Rafferty 1996), and training schemes modelled on medical training were introduced. Initially this was confined to the voluntary hospitals, but the ethos spread to other forms of institution. Asylums and children's hospitals began to regard a training in general nursing as superior to a specialist training, and by the early twentieth century had made it a requirement for promotion above staff nurse level.

4

Nurse registration, with its separate registers for children's nurses, asylum nurses and male nurses amongst others, served to reinforce

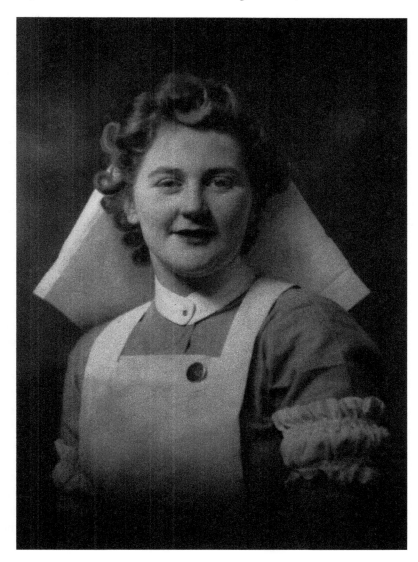

Figure 4.1 The author's mother, a trained psychiatric nurse c.1944; notice the uniform, which was adopted from the traditional general nurse uniform

these hierarchical divisions within nursing. The call for nurse registration was made by those who wanted to develop nursing as a profession (such as Ethel Bedford Fenwick), and opposed by those (including Florence Nightingale) who perceived nursing as a vocation, with 'character' as the primary requirement. Witz (1992) called the campaign for registration a female **professional project** in that pro-registrationists were attempting to create an autonomous occupation for women, on a par with medicine, aiming for **occupational closure**. Although registration was introduced in 1919, nursing failed to gain autonomy or control of entry to the occupation. The General Nursing Council (GNC) set up to certify nurses was a body with few powers.

professional project:
an attempt by an occupation to become a profession

occupational closure:
the monopoly of work to maintain power and status over other occupational groups

If nursing has traditionally been viewed as 'women's work', what does this mean for men who take up nursing as a career? In the past men mainly worked in areas such as psychiatry or the military, which were not associated with the feminine caring roles of female nurses. As men have moved into other areas of nursing (moves often resisted by female nurse leaders), this has on occasion proved problematic as certain suspicions have been raised about their motives, that they could be predatory and abuse their position of trust with vulnerable people. This is despite the fact that both male and female nurses have been convicted of abuse. Conversely, Evans (2004) states that within patriarchal society men in nursing, although in a minority, are given a special and privileged status. They gain power disproportionate to their numbers, and dominate in elite specialisms and administrative positions, which are considered more reflective of masculine values.

3 Socialization into nursing

The first time you went on placement and someone called you 'nurse', it probably felt rather strange; you may even have felt an impostor. By the end of your education you will feel quite comfortable with the term, not only because you will have more knowledge and confidence in carrying out the work, but also because you will have internalized the values and attitudes of nursing. The way that this occurs has been demonstrated by two sociological studies.

Davis in 1975 described the way in which over the course of training students are socialized into nursing. Davis states that the socialization of student nurses is 'the process by which the student passes from identification with a "lay" to a "professional" culture' (Davis 1975: 116). He argues that the socialization process comprises six stages during which the nurse passes from 'lay innocence', when his or her imagery of nursing is that shaped by previous perceptions, to 'stable internalization' where the self-image of students is that of a professional nurse.

Melia (1987) studied student nurses' experiences of education and training, and found a division existed between the way that nursing was represented in college and the way it was practised on the wards. This is

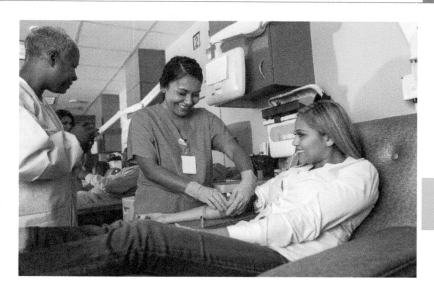

Figure 4.2 Learning from more experienced professionals is one way in which student nurses are socialized into nursing practice

4

often referred to as the 'theory–practice gap', examples of which were given in Chapter 2. Students learned to manage this tension by adopting strategies that allowed them to fit in on the wards. Melia identifies five categories by which students achieve this (see Box 4.1).

In describing the way in which student nurses internalize the values of nursing and begin to identify themselves as members of the occupation, Davis and Melia show how this is not just the result of increasing nursing knowledge, but also a social process in which the student learns the shared norms of nursing.

More recent work conducted since the status of student nurses became supernumerary has shown that similar problems still exist for student nurses. In her observational study, Wakefield (2000) found that students are now seen as external to the ward environment, and categorized as 'visitors' rather than 'belonging' to the hospital. Students themselves have problems in getting practice in skills, as health-care assistants (HCAs) now receive some training and carry out more tasks than previously, taking over what always used to be regarded as a student nurse's role. Wakefield argues that this has led to a change in power relations, with students being treated as subordinate by HCAs.

A longitudinal, qualitative study by Macintosh (2006) with student nurses in a UK university found the effect of their socialization into nursing to be largely negative. Between the first interview (six to nine months into their training) and the second (eighteen months later) the students' attitudes towards care had changed, with a reduction in its perceived importance, and 'the lessening of the caring role may be as a direct consequence of the needs of the individual to adapt and cope with this new role. It may be that nurses have to learn to care less in order to cope more effectively with the daily pressures of the nursing role' (Macintosh 2006: 960). Similarly, Curtis et al. (2012) found that socialization into compassionate practice is compromised by a dissonance between the idealism with which students entered nursing, and the realism of nursing practice. The implication of this for nursing education and practice will be discussed later in the chapter.

Box 4.1 Strategies adopted by student nurses

- 'Learning the rules' is concerned with the way in which students pass as workers to the satisfaction of permanent workers on the ward.
- 'Getting the work done' describes how nursing work is organized and achieved on hospital wards. Clarke (1978) found that student nurses feel they are judged by their success in 'learning the ropes' and 'getting through the work' – in other words, by how soon they can function effectively within the ward routine.
- Student nurses have to achieve the above within the constraints of the dual role of the third category, 'learning and working', although the situation has changed somewhat with student nurses achieving supernumerary status.
- 'Just passing through' reflects on the student's transient status, with the consequent relearning of the first and second categories on each new placement.
- Another consequence of the transient experience is the fifth category of 'nursing in the dark', where students find that they are not always given the information about patients that the permanent staff possess.

(Adapted from Melia 1987)

Activity 4.1 Socialization into nursing

Melia's study was undertaken before nurse education moved into higher education and students became supernumerary.

(a) How well do each of Melia's categories reflect your experience?
(b) Do Macintosh's and Curtis's findings about caring and compassionate practice resonate with the reality of your branch of nursing?
(c) From your placement experience can you identify with Wakefield's finding that students do not always have the opportunity to develop skills?
(d) Discuss your experience with someone from a different branch of nursing.

---

4 Nursing within the health division of labour

Profession and professionalization

Although the image of nursing as women's work discussed in Section 2 above persists, and 90 per cent of the nursing workforce is female, the position of nursing within the health division of labour today is more complex than for previous generations of nurses.

In order to examine nursing's place within the health division of labour, it is useful to review the concept of profession as it has traditionally been defined within sociology, and to consider whether we need a new way of looking at occupations in order to explain the development of nursing practice.

Sociological definitions have tended to view professions as particular types of occupation that possess specific traits or attributes that distinguish them and give them a higher status within society. Typically, these include public service, an ethical code and some form of training in higher education (see, for example, Millerson 1964). This functionalist approach is criticized as being ahistorical; that is, it does not question how or why these occupations were able to achieve these attributes and become dominant in an area of work. Nor does it take a critical approach to the motives for pursuing a professionalization agenda, but stresses the important role professions play within society, the altruistic role of medicine being a prime example.

Freidson (1970), adopting a neo-Weberian stance (see Chapter 1), defines a profession as possessing certain characteristics (see Box 4.2).

So a profession has a large amount of control over its working practices. The power that professions possess within Western societies has enabled them to lay claim to areas of work, and to dominate and constrain subordinate occupations within the same sphere. This is **social closure:** **social closure** (Parkin 1979), and it can be used to explain the actions of both dominant and subservient occupations. Exclusionary tactics include the use of entry qualifications, legislation or other means to restrict access to the occupation, and demarcation describes the placing of boundaries around the work of a subordinate occupation. For example, the medical profession fought against the introduction of nurse prescribing for several years, as it would erode the monopoly power they enjoyed.

social closure:
one social group maintaining power in society

> **Box 4.2 Characteristics of a profession**
>
> * Specialist knowledge gained through higher education and qualifications.
> * Monopoly over certain tasks and procedures.
> * Autonomy – control of working conditions and entry into the profession.
> * Possession of an ethical code, or code of conduct.
>
> *(Freidson 1970)*

---

expanded roles:
roles that include activities formerly carried out within other occupations

Subordinate occupations may attempt to adopt the same values and characteristics as the dominant one – what are known as inclusionary tactics. **Expanded roles** in nursing, where nurses take on tasks traditionally undertaken by doctors, may be defined as inclusionary strategies. Subordinate occupations may also use exclusionary tactics in order to maintain boundaries between themselves and occupations that they consider subordinate; for example, the division between the roles of qualified nurses and health-care assistants (HCAs). The latter are restricted in the tasks they may carry out, with some roles being reserved for qualified nurses. Traynor et al. (2015) demonstrated that these concepts are still useful in examining the health-care workforce. They argue in their exploration of nursing support workers that changes in health-care delivery require a reconfiguration of occupational closure to account for the rise in numbers of unqualified nurses working as paraprofessionals to the qualified nursing workforce. Law and Aranda (2010) also point to the continuing resonance of professionalization theories, and point to the existence of support workers in reigniting debates about the professionalization project and nursing.

If medicine is viewed as the archetypal profession within the health-care system, nursing has been described as a semi-profession (Etzioni 1969) because of its perceived limited knowledge base and lack of autonomy. This concept is somewhat deterministic as it implies that there is no opportunity for nursing to develop professionally. In order to counter such definitions of nursing, some feminist writers (notably Davies 1995; Witz 1992) have criticized traditional notions of profession for emphasizing power and an esoteric knowledge base that separates the practitioner from the client. Davies (1995) argues that this form of power, which relies on denying knowledge to others, is a very masculinist interpretation of profession. Within this model nursing can never be accepted as a profession, as it seeks to share expertise and to encourage empowerment and participation by patients and families through strategies such as negotiated care. Davies advocates a new model of professionalism in which partnership and reflective practice constitute the basis of professional expertise, and where nursing roles and values are acknowledged and given credibility. This is consistent with the notion of **enhanced roles** in nursing, in which the curative elements of health care are viewed as part of the specialist skills of nursing, and as an area of autonomous nursing practice.

enhanced roles:
roles that allow nurses to use expert knowledge to make autonomous decisions

Many of the enhanced and expanded roles within nursing, and within other health occupations, have been as a result of changes in the NHS, particularly the reduction in junior doctors' working hours and changing consultant and GP contracts. The increasing prominence of long-term illness has encouraged the development of specialist and consultant nurses who provide leadership in the care and management of this group (see also Chapters 13 and 15). Nurses, particularly in the community, are now trained to prescribe medicines, either independently or as supplementary prescribers. These roles have facilitated changing relationships within the health-care team as more nurses work as independent practitioners in all branches.

Elitism in nursing

elite:
small group with power and influence by virtue of its social position

The idea of an **elite** in nursing would seem to be paradoxical, as nurses are not viewed as a powerful group (Mowforth 1999). They are often marginalized when decisions are made, which in theory should preclude them from power. However, both horizontal and vertical elites exist within nursing.

Vertical elitism exists between nurses of different grades. The higher the position within the organization, the greater is the prestige. In nursing, status is gained by moving away from clinical work with patients/clients into management or education. So in order to gain promotion nurses must cease to do the work they came into nursing for. What Davies (1995) has called the polo-mint problem is created, a hole caused by a skills shortage at the bedside and in clinical teaching, as experienced nurses no longer undertake this work. As Daykin and Clarke (2000) demonstrate, this has raised questions about the relationship of nursing to basic health care, with nurses in their study demonstrating ambivalence to the changing role of the nurse. Many nurses expressed concern at the perceived threat to nurses' claim to a distinct contribution to health care if HCAs carry out much of the bedside care, albeit in a subservient position. At the same time, they recognized the reality of workplace imperatives, most crucially the shortage of qualified nurses to carry out care (see also Chapter 2 for a longer discussion of this research).

Horizontal elitism is influenced by the medical model, and the value this places on science and technology. Medicine, along with other professions, uses its possession of expert knowledge to maintain its high status. The gap between the knowledge of the doctor and that of the patient creates a mystique about medical knowledge. This is said to depersonalize, or deny the experience of, the patient, privileging the scientific over other forms of knowledge. It is those within nursing who are seen to have some insight into this scientific knowledge, such as those in intensive therapy units (ITU), special-care baby units or accident and emergency departments (A & E), who are perceived as elite by themselves and by the public. Each nursing discipline has its elite roles, but those within the high-technology areas associated with adult and children's nursing have the highest status within wider society.

New technologies which require extra monitoring and interpretation are associated with clean as opposed to dirty work. Wolf (1996) has argued that those who perform dirty work are soiled by association (see also Law and Amanda 2010). Being involved with bodily functions has little status (Latimer 2014), and Clarke (1999) states that many nurses believe that an increase in nursing status is not compatible with these tasks. So care of the elderly or chronically ill does not carry the same prestige as more high-technology specialisms (see also Chapter 8), even though it could be argued that the art of nursing (the skills that make nursing unique) is more apparent in the former. Nursing work associated with caring is seen as 'natural' and therefore not requiring intellect or education (Miers 1999). Nurses within highly technologized areas do carry out 'dirty work', such as continence care; however, they are characterized not by this, but by their work with the technology.

Within mental health nursing, status is aligned to the clean work of psychotherapy with short-term patients, or forensic psychiatry, rather than to what is often regarded as the menial work of care of long-term patients (Godin 2003).

The concept of expanded roles within nursing, such as nurse prescribing or acting as a surgeon's assistant, adds status by taking nurses further away from the caring role of nursing, and towards cure, which is a feature of clinical medicine. These roles remove the nurse from the 'dirty work' of nursing and into the 'clean' world of medicine. A consideration of the roles that nurses have taken on shows most to be fairly routine, repetitive tasks, which doctors themselves do not find as rewarding as other parts of their job. However, they do give some nurses the opportunity to work more autonomously as part of multidisciplinary teams. Paradoxically these new roles also bring nursing further under the control of medicine, as the medical profession defines the terms of nursing involvement, and circumscribes and supervises the work that the nurse takes over (Denny 2003). This can be demonstrated by the changes that have taken place within mental health nursing, where Brimblecombe (2005) argues that a shift to community care from the 1970s provided a catalyst for a new interest in greater professional autonomy and status amongst mental health nurses. This resulted in greater independence for nursing, being outside of the direct influence of psychiatry, and taking direct referrals from GPs. This move, however, also led mental health nurses away from a focus on severe mental illness, and it was the return to working more with this client group that reinforced the link between mental health nurses and psychiatry, with the latter continuing to exert influence over the former, both at a policymaking and a clinical level (Brimblecombe 2005).

Case Study: Nursing people with dementia

Dementia is an important and growing area of health care in the UK and in most other countries. Figures from the Alzheimer's Society (<www.alzheimers.org.uk>) suggest that there are currently 850,000 people in the UK living with dementia, and by 2025 this will rise to 1 million. Around two thirds of these are women and 25,000 are from minority ethnic groups. Around 670,000 people in the UK are caring for someone with dementia.

In a review of the literature on discrimination against older people with dementia and its impact on student nurses' professional socialization, Chan and Chan (2009) argue that age discrimination is embedded in society and is reflected in the care system. Much of the care of people with dementia is carried out by poorly paid care assistants with little training, which challenges the idea of dementia care as a specialism. It is therefore ascribed low professional status. Berry (2012) concurs, stating that working with older people is seen as a job, not a specialism, and Happell (2002) adds that working with older people is the least preferred area of practice for student nurses, and the least desirable career option (see also Robinson and Cubit 2007).

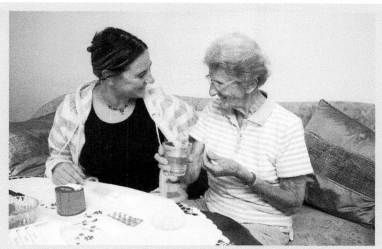

Figure 4.3 An important part of the health-care worker's role is to seek to share expertise and encourage patient empowerment

The student nurses' tale

A number of studies have considered student nurses' experience of working with people with dementia, in acute and nursing home settings. Baillie et al. (2012), in their qualitative study with adult nursing students in hospitals in England, identified three sets of challenges to providing care for people with dementia in the hospital setting.

1   *An inappropriate hospital environment*

   Neither the physical environment (which was not conducive to people moving around freely and safely) nor the organizational culture of a busy ward was seen as appropriate to nursing people with dementia. Watts and Davies (2014), in their study with final-year nursing students in Wales, also reported that other demands on the ward meant that there was not enough time to care for dementia patients adequately.

2   *Deficits of knowledge, skills and attitudes of staff and students*

   This is a consistent theme in the literature with students typically feeling out of their depth, unprepared for issues such as dealing with aggression, and being left, often unsupervised, to care for dementia patients (Watts and Davies 2014; Robinson and Cubit 2007; Baillie et al. 2012). However, staff in acute wards were reported by students as not providing expert guidance, as they saw a dementia patient as not fitting in, and a nuisance (Baillie et al. 2012), or as a hazard prone to wandering or interfering with equipment (Watts and Davies 2014).

3   *The struggle to provide care*

   Problems of communication, aggression, difficulties in assessing levels of pain and assuring good nutrition were all problems that students grappled with and reported in all of the studies. Students found residents' behaviour disturbing in a nursing home study and felt scared and intimidated at times (Robinson and Cubit 2007). They felt out of their depth in trying to manage people with dementia, although most recognized their need for good-quality, individualized care (Baillie et al. 2012).

The daughter's tale

The author Nicci Gerrard started John's Campaign (<www.johnscampaign org.uk>), following the experience of her father, John, who had dementia and was admitted to hospital for treatment to persistent leg ulcers.

> *Five weeks. He went in strong, mobile, healthy, continent, reasonably articulate, cheerful and able to lead a fulfilled daily life with my mother. He came out skeletal, incontinent, immobile, incoherent, bewildered, quite lost. There was nothing he could do for himself, and this man, so dependable and so competent, was now utterly vulnerable. He could not sit up. He could not turn over. He could not put one foot in front of the other. He could not lift a fork or a glass to his mouth. He could not string words into a sentence – indeed, he could barely make a word (except to say hello, to say thank you, to say that he was lucky). He did not know where he was, who most of his friends were, sometimes perhaps he no longer knew who he himself was. . . .*
>
> *It wasn't really the fault of the doctors and the nurses. They healed his infection, they put food and drink beside him, almost all of them treated him with respect and genuine kindness. But they left him to himself and couldn't spend hours making sure he ate and drank. They couldn't brush his teeth and shave him and comb his hair and read poetry to him, do crosswords, play chess, talk to him, hold his hand, tell him he was safe, keep him anchored to the world he loved. (Gerrard 2014)*

John's Campaign aims to secure the right for a carer to stay in hospital with a person with dementia and care for them, in the same way that parents enjoy the right to stay with their child.

Activity 4.2 Identifying challenges and solutions

Student nurses in the studies above recognize the challenges in caring for people with dementia, and Nicci Gerrard also identifies that, on hospital wards focused on acute care, the time needed to spend with patients with complex needs is limited.

(a) What is your experience of caring for patients with dementia on hospital wards? Did you feel adequately prepared and supported? What was done well or badly in the university and hospital setting to promote care of people with dementia?

(b) Is care of the elderly person with complex needs 'just a job' or, as some students in Watts and Davies' study reported, 'a privilege'?

(c) What can be done to tackle age discrimination in nursing, when it remains prevalent within society?

(d) If you are a children's branch nurse can you identify a group of patients that evokes similar negative reactions to those discussed in the studies above?

Working within the organization

Earlier in the chapter we considered the nineteenth-century image of doctors as powerful and nurses as obedient and subservient. This emanated from the relative position of men and women in Victorian society, which no longer applies. Relationships are now less rigid; for example, mental health nurses tend to see their role as complementary to that of psychiatrists, and learning-disability nurses view themselves as the expert workers in an area where the closure of institutions has seen the decline of the medical specialist (Denny 2003).

In the past, sociological research into relationships within health-care settings tended to focus on the doctor/nurse relationship, and Porter (1999) summarizes these studies. One of the first to consider this issue was Stein (1967), who viewed matters as more complex than the traditional power relationship, and described them as a game. Doctors are trained in a manner that creates certainty (in diagnosis, and in treatment), and for nurses to question or comment on their decisions would undermine this. Stein showed how nurses often had more knowledge of patients and their treatments than doctors who rotated through the specialisms, but they would never openly contradict them. Instead, the nurse would put forward suggestions, which the doctor could present as his or her own idea. The subservient nurse would not risk disagreement with the more powerful doctor. The notion of the doctor/nurse game as a process of negotiation is taken up in Chapter 14.

More recently, other writers have reviewed the doctor/nurse game and found that it has evolved as roles have developed. Carmel (2006) and Stein et al. (1990) noted that in many hospital settings nurses were challenging medical decisions. These studies support Wicks' (1998) findings that structural factors, such as power relationships, may be overcome by individual agency in certain circumstances, most usually

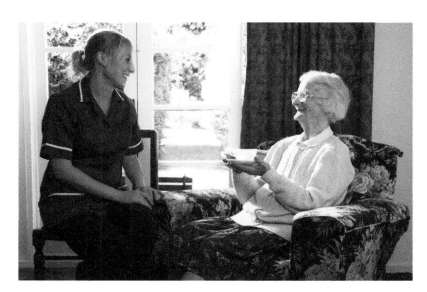

Figure 4.4 A home visit; nurses work in a variety of environments

when nurses have expertise derived from experience and specialist education.

Despite examples such as these, which demonstrate that nurses act more autonomously, NHS reforms and changing management structures have restricted the ability of nurses to deliver care to patients. Some of the problems highlighted above around the status of nursing and the responsibility for caring are explored in a guest editorial by Joanna Latimer. She argues that nurses have to balance competing agendas (political, managerial, professional) in order to provide care, none of which they can influence or control. For example, what she calls the 'demise of the figure of the ward sister' (Latimer 2014: 540) demonstrates the demotion of status and authority, with the ward manager preoccupied with administrative and financial responsibilities rather than overseeing patient care. However, nurses are rarely in a position of influence or power to engage in, let alone set, the agenda. Second, she argues that the delivery of health care by targets and performance measures removes the permission to care in an individualized way from nurses, who are accountable to a management hierarchy that is centralized and top down. Allen (2015) adds that it is through its relationship with patients that nursing is defined, yet there is a mismatch between professional values, in terms of nursing expertise in its caregiving role, and the everyday reality of nursing work. However, the rationalization of nursing work and the reduction in qualified nursing numbers have led to more caring tasks being undertaken by unqualified support staff, and nurses carrying out tasks delegated by junior doctors. Nurses are increasingly distant from undertaking direct patient care, and are undertaking more tasks that contribute to information flows and external scrutiny.

Activity 4.3 Nurse staffing and patient outcomes

Having read the section above, read the extract below, which demonstrates that the issues raised by Davina Allen have been identified for some years.

> In a study of 30 hospital trusts in England, which looked at the relationship between nurse staffing levels and patient outcomes, Rafferty et al. found a large and consistent effect of nurse staffing on mortality outcomes in surgical patients as well as on nurse job outcomes and nurse ratings of quality of care. Hospitals in which nurses cared for the fewest patients each had significantly lower surgical mortality and FTR [failure to rescue] rates compared to those in which nurses cared for the greatest number of patients each. . . .
>
> In addition to better outcomes for patients, hospitals with higher nurse staffing levels had significantly lower rates of nurse burn-out and dissatisfaction. The nurses in the hospitals with the heaviest patient loads were 71% more likely to experience high burn-out and job dissatisfaction than hospitals with the most favourable nurse staffing. . . .
>
> The findings suggest that quality of care and nurse retention would improve if staffing levels across the NHS were brought more into line with those in the best-staffed hospitals in this study.

(Rafferty, Clarke and Coles et al. 2007: 175–82)

The following questions can be completed with reference to placements that you have already done, but you can also think about them on future placements. Discuss your findings with colleagues who have had placements in different clinical areas.

(a) How many nurses are on duty at different times of the day and night? Do different types of clinical areas, and different NHS Trusts, have different staffing levels?

(b) How many of the nurses are qualified and how many are health-care assistants?

(c) Which nurses appear to experience burn-out, and which have a high level of job satisfaction?

(d) Apart from the effect on patient mortality and nurse burn-out, what other benefits do you think would come from the improved staffing levels called for in this research?

4

5 Nurse education

One of the factors that has facilitated changing roles within nursing has been the shift from an apprentice style of training to an education system based on a university model. However, these moves have not been uncritically accepted. Meerabeau (2001: 431), in her review of the literature on the debate over pre-registration nursing, points to critics within the press who denounced the need for a degree programme, frequently citing the 'pollution' involved in nursing work (referred to above as 'dirty' work), 'bedpans and bottoms' and what are classified as 'basic tasks', as justification for their argument that a degree is unnecessary for such menial work.

Miers (2002) points to cultural factors inhibiting the entry of nursing into higher education. Attitudes within higher education concerning the status of practice-based professions, particularly care professions, have seen many nursing departments viewed as less than academic (see also Latimer 2014). Within nursing, there exists an anti-intellectualism, where nursing research is viewed as 'ivory tower', removed from the real work of nursing. So nurses themselves are often hostile to degrees in nursing, and have used sanctions against those who expressed individuality, questioned or challenged existing practices. Miers argues that this has been a consequence of an education system where practical caring courses, more often undertaken by students from lower social classes, have the lowest status in the educational hierarchy. The anti-intellectualism within nursing may be viewed as a defensive reaction against a culture that values abstract thinking more highly than practical activity.

Nurses with degrees have been particularly affected by this anti-intellectualism, as was discussed by Sarah Earle in Chapter 2. Meerabeau (2001) and Latimer (2014) further argue that nursing has remained a marginal subject in higher education. Unlike other university courses, it is not funded by the Department of Education and Skills, but is commissioned by the devolved health services, to whose expressed needs universities respond when developing curricula.

Activity 4.4 Nurses and caring

The criticisms of graduate nurses continue in the press, in headlines such as that from the *Daily Mail* in February 2013: 'Why have nurses stopped CARING?', citing the move of nurse education into higher education as one reason, with a focus on the technical rather than caring aspects of nursing. Similarly, the *Daily Telegraph* in August 2011 stated: 'Nursing is no longer a caring profession', claiming that the move into higher education had professionalized what had been a vocation.

(a) Do you view caring and professionalism as mutually exclusive attributes?

(b) Why do you think that nursing is the caring profession that incurs most criticism?

(c) How do you think that leaders in nursing (the RCN, NMC) can counter such claims?

(d) How long do you think it may take for nursing to be accepted as a graduate profession?

In order to address the alleged association between changes to nurse education and declining standards of nursing care, which has been persistently restated, in 2012 the Royal College of Nursing commissioned a study to address the question:

• What essential features of pre-registration nursing education in the UK, and what types of support for newly registered practitioners, are needed to create and maintain a workforce of competent, compassionate nurses fit to delivery future health and social care services? (<www.williscommission.org.uk>)

The Willis Commission reported that patient-centred care should be at the centre of nurse education and continuing professional development. It went on to state that there were no major shortcomings in the provision of nurse education that could be held responsible for poor practice or decline in standards of patient care. On the contrary, the move to higher education helped to drive up standards, but has also become a lightning conductor for disquiet, often fuelled by the media. It called the suggestion that kindness and intelligence are not compatible an irrational argument, and not one that is levelled at other graduate caring professions. The Commission supported a graduate nursing workforce, acting as clinical team leaders to a nursing assistant workforce educated to NVQ level. It identified the positive impact of qualified nurses on patient outcomes and argued that the enhanced skills of the emerging graduate workforce need to be seen as an opportunity to raise standards of care (Willis 2012). This reflects the findings of the empirical research by Rafferty et al. (2007), discussed above. The education of health-care assistants was also a key recommendation of the Cavendish Report (2013), which was set up in the wake of the Francis Inquiry. The Francis Reports identified, among other things, poor standards of care and supervision among unqualified nursing staff, but also a preoccupation of hospital management with finance and targets, and a neglect of patient care (see Chapters 13 and 14; and Latimer 2014, above). Camilla Cavendish, a journalist and now head of the Number 10 policy unit for the UK government, was asked by the Secretary of State for Health to investigate the recruitment, training, supervision and support for the 1.3 million unregistered support staff who provide most of the hands-on care in the NHS. She found that, although this group of workers are in the frontline of care, they have no compulsory training, different job titles in different work environments, and undertake a range of duties. Like Willis, Cavendish recommended a structured training programme for health-care assistants, but she went further and argued that this group of workers should not be seen as separate from the qualified nursing workforce, and that elements from the nursing degree programme should be incorporated into their education (Cavendish 2013). The government at the time, however, rejected a formal training programme for care assistants.

In the wake of reports such as those cited above, a new division of labour may be emerging within nursing. We may also in the future witness a recognition that what has been derogated as 'women's work' is in fact highly skilled.

Summary and Resources

Summary

▶ The present occupation of nursing developed from the domestic role of women in caring for the sick in institutions and the community.

▶ The idea of nursing as 'women's work' has led to advantages for men in nursing as they are deemed to possess qualities required for leadership, but they may also be treated with suspicion, particularly when working with vulnerable groups.

▶ Nurses have attempted social closure strategies in order to raise the status of nursing, and to lay claim to a distinct contribution to health care.

▶ Although nursing has traditionally been constrained in its development by a powerful medical profession, recent nursing developments have made occupational relationships more complex.

▶ Nurse education has shifted from an apprenticeship model of nursing training in health-care institutions, to an academic, professional education producing an all-graduate workforce.

Questions for Discussion

1 Historically, nursing was considered as 'women's work' because of the association between women and caring work. Does this have any relevance for nursing today? Do men and women have different expectations from a career in nursing?

2 'In all branches of nursing status is gained by moving away from direct care, creating the "polo mint problem"' (Davies 1995). What can nurses do to raise the value of caring roles within society?

3 Debates continue over whether the move of nurse education into higher education better prepares nurses for present and future roles than the old apprenticeship training. What are the benefits to nursing of a combination of an academic education and learning in practice?

Glossary

elite:	a minority group that has power and influence and is generally recognized within society as being superior; traditionally, elites have been viewed as those who rule over others, but more recently elites within structures of society have been identified
enhanced roles:	enhanced roles give nurses more discretion in using their expertise in order to provide care for patients; they allow for autonomy in decision-making within areas where nurses have traditionally had a role
expanded roles:	nurses have expanded the number of roles they are engaged in, by taking on tasks delegated by junior doctors, or by becoming involved in management; this has involved nurses shedding some roles in order to accommodate the new ones, which has usually led to direct care being provided by health-care assistants
occupational closure:	if an occupational group can lay claim to an area of work and prevent others from carrying out that work it offers them monopoly power; doctors have been very successful in laying claim to diagnosing sickness and prescribing treatment, while preventing other occupational groups from carrying out this work
professional project:	occupations may wish to professionalize by using strategies aimed at enhancing power and status; this is achieved by closure (see 'social closure' below) which will maximize the

	advantages, both social and monetary) to the group engaged in the project
social closure:	the means by which one social group maintains power and status in society by closing entry to other groups; in occupational closure, control of entry into the occupation and monopoly over an area of work are the means usually adopted

4

Further Reading

M. Traynor: *Nursing in Context: Policy, Politics, Profession.* Basingstoke: Palgrave, 2013.
This book is written to prepare student nurses for the complexities of their chosen profession, by attempting to answer the question 'What is nursing?' It includes topics such as history, care, education, policy and politics.

S. Proctor: *Caring for Health.* Basingstoke: Palgrave, 2000.
Caring is a fundamental part of nursing and yet has become increasingly marginalized. This volume uses nursing and sociological knowledge to examine the role of caring, and the link between caring and health.

R. Simpson: *Men in Caring Occupations.* Basingstoke: Palgrave, 2009.
This book considers how men in caring occupations manage gender and identity in feminized occupations. Part 1 draws on theoretical concepts, while Part 2 uses specific occupational settings (including two chapters on nursing) to explore the experience of men in these occupational roles.

Also useful are the following online resources:

Royal College of Nursing (<www.rcn.org.uk>). The nursing professional association that campaigns on nursing and wider health matters, and represents nurses and nursing. Other nations have their own associations, such as the American Nurses Association (<www.nursing world.org>) and the Australian Nursing and Midwifery Federation (<www. anmf.org.au>).

The Nursing and Midwifery Council for the UK (<www.nmc.org.uk>). The professional regulator for nurses and midwives throughout the UK.

Nursing history (<www.rcn.org.uk/library>). The history and archives of British nursing held by the Royal College of Nursing. A similar website for American nursing history is at: <www.upenn.edu>.

References

Allen, D. 2015 Nursing and the future of 'care' in health care systems. *Journal of Health Services Research and Policy* 20: 129–30.

Baillie, L., Cox, J. and Merritt, J. 2012 Caring for older people with dementia in hospital: Part one: challenges. *Nursing Older People* 24/8: 24–7.

Berry, L. 2012 Working with older people seen as job not specialism. *Nursing Older People* 24/5: 5.

Brimblecombe, N. R. 2005 The changing relationship between mental health nurses and psychiatrists in the United Kingdom. *Journal of Advanced Nursing* 49/4: 344–53.

Carmel, S. 2006 Boundaries obscured and boundaries reinforced: incorporation as a strategy of occupational enhancement for intensive care. *Sociology of Health and Illness* 28/2: 154–77.

Cavendish, C. 2013 *An Independent Review into Healthcare Assistants and Support Workers in the NHS and Social Care Settings.* London: Department of Health. Available from: <www.gov.uk/publications>.

Chan, P. A. and Chan, P. 2009 The impact of discrimination against older people with dementia and its impact on student nurses' professional socialization. *Nurse Education in Practice* 9: 221–7.

Clarke, J. 1999 The diminishing role of nurses in hands-on care. *Nursing Times* 95/27: 48–9.

Clarke, M. 1978 Getting through the work. In R. Dingwall and J. Macintosh (eds), *Readings in the Sociology of Nursing.* Edinburgh: Churchill Livingstone, pp. 67–86.

Curtis, K., Horton, K. and Smith, P. 2012 Student nurse socialization into compassionate practice: a grounded theory study. *Nurse Education Today* 32/7: 790–5.

Davies, C. 1995 *Gender and the Professional Predicament in Nursing.* Buckingham: Open University Press.

Davies, C., Stillwell, J., Wilson, R., Carlisle, C. and Luker, K. 2000 Did Project 2000 training change recruitment patterns or career expectations? *Nurse Education Today* 20: 408–17.

Davis, F. 1975 Professional socialization as subjective experience: the process of doctrinal conversion among student nurses. In C. Cox and A. Meade (eds), *The Sociology of Medical Practice.* London: Collier-Macmillan, pp. 116–31.

Daykin, N. and Clarke B. 2000 'They'll still get the bodily care.' Discourse of care and relationships between nurses and health care assistants in the NHS. *Sociology of Health and Illness* 22/3: 349–63.

Denny, E. 2003 The class context of nursing. In M. Miers (ed.), *Class, Inequalities and Nursing Practice.* Basingstoke: Palgrave, pp. 77–97.

Dingwall, R., Rafferty, A. M. and Webster, C. 1988 *An Introduction to the Social History of Medicine.* London: Routledge.

Etzioni, A. 1969 *The Semi-professions and their Organization.* New York: Free Press.

Evans, J. A. 1997 Men in nursing: issues of gender segregation and hidden advantage. *Journal of Advanced Nursing* 26: 226–31.

Evans, J. 2004 Men nurses: a historical and feminist perspective. *Journal of Advanced Nursing* 47: 321–8.

Freidson, E. 1970 *The Profession of Medicine: A Study in the Sociology of Applied Knowledge.* New York: Dodd Mead.

Gerrard, N. 2014 My father entered hospital articulate and able. He came out a broken man. *Observer*, 29 November. Available from: <http://www.theguardian.com/society/2014/nov/29/nicci-gerrard-father-dementia-hospital-care-elderly>.

Godin, P. 2003 Class inequalities in mental health nursing. In M. Miers (ed.), *Class, Inequalities and Nursing Practice.* Basingstoke: Palgrave, pp. 125–43.

Happell, B. 2002 Nursing home employment for nursing students: valuable experience or a harsh deterrent? *Journal of Advanced Nursing* 39/6: 529–36.

Healthcare Commission 2005 *Ward Staffing.* London: Commission for Healthcare Audit and Inspection.

Latimer, J. 2014 Nursing, the politics of organization and meanings of care. *Journal of Research in Nursing* 19: 537–45.

Law, K. and Aranda, K. 2010 The shifting foundations of nursing. *Nurse Education Today* 30: 544–7.

Macintosh, C. 2006 The socialization of pre-registration student nurses: a longitudinal, qualitative, descriptive study. *International Journal of Nursing Studies* 43/8: 953–62.

Meerabeau, E. 2001 Back to the bedpans: the debates over preregistration nursing education in England. *Journal of Advanced Nursing* 34/4: 427–35.

Melia, K. 1987 *Learning and Working: The Occupational Socialization of Nurses.* London: Tavistock.

Miers, M. 1999 Nursing teams and hierarchies: nurses working with nurses. In G. Wilkinson and M. Miers (eds), *Power and Nursing Practice.* Basingstoke: Palgrave, pp. 64–79.

Miers, M. 2002 Nurse education in higher education: understanding cultural barriers to progress. *Nurse Education Today* 22/21: 2–9.

Millerson, G. L. 1964 *The Qualifying Association.* London: Routledge and Kegan Paul.

Mowforth, G. 1999 Elitism in nursing. In G. Wilkinson and M. Miers, *Power and Nursing Practice.* Basingstoke: Palgrave, pp. 51–63.

Parkin, F. 1979 *Marxism and Class Theory: A Bourgeois Critique.* London: Tavistock.

Porter, S. 1999 Working with doctors. In G. Wilkinson and M. Miers, *Power and Nursing Practice.* Basingstoke: Palgrave, pp. 97–110.

Rafferty, A. M. 1995 The anomaly of autonomy: space and status in early nursing reform. *International History of Nursing Journal* 1: 43–56.

Rafferty, A. M. 1996 *The Politics of Nursing Knowledge.* London: Routledge.

Rafferty, A. M., Clarke, S. P., Coles, J. et al. 2007 Outcomes of variation in hospital nurse staffing in English hospitals: cross-sectional analysis of survey data and discharge records. *International Journal of Nursing Studies* 44/2: 175–82.

Robinson, A. and Cubit, K. 2007 Caring for older people with dementia in residential care: nursing students' experiences. *Journal of Advanced Nursing* 59/3: 255–63.

Snelgrove, S. and Hughes, D. 2002 Perceptions of teamwork in acute medical wards. In D. Allen and D. Hughes (eds), *Nursing and the Division of Labour in Healthcare.* Basingstoke: Palgrave, pp. 53–74.

Stein, L. 1967 The doctor/nurse game. *Archives of General Psychiatry* 16: 699–703.

Stein, L., Watts, D. T. and Howell, T. 1990 The doctor–nurse game revisited. *New England Journal of Medicine* 322/8: 546–9.

Traynor, M., Nissen, N., Lincoln, C. and Buus, N. 2015 Occupational closure in nursing work reconsidered: UK health care support workers and assistant practitioners: a focus group study. *Social Science & Medicine* 136: 81–8.

Wakefield, A. 2000 Tensions experienced by student nurses in a changed NHS culture. *Nurse Education Today* 20: 571–8.

Watts, T. E. and Davies, R. 2014 Tensions and ambiguities: a qualitative study of final year adult field nursing students' experiences of caring for people affected by advanced dementia in Wales, UK. *Nurse Education Today* 34: 1149–54.

Wicks, D. 1998 *Nurses and Doctors at Work.* Buckingham: Open University Press.

Willis, Lord P. 2012 *Quality with Compassion, the Future of Nurse Education. Report of the Willis Commission on Nursing Education.* London: Royal College of Nursing. Available at: <www.williscommission.org.uk>.

Witz, A. 1992 *Professions and Patriarchy.* London: Routledge.

Witz, A. 1994 The challenge of nursing. In J. Gabe, D. Kelleher and G. Williams (eds), *Challenging Medicine.* London: Sage, pp. 23–45.

Wolf, Z. R. 1996 Bowel management and nursing's hidden work. *Nursing Times* 92/21: 26–8.

Researching Health

Carol Komaromy

KEY ISSUES IN THIS CHAPTER:

▶ Sociological research methods.
▶ The research process.
▶ Quantitative research methods.
▶ Qualitative research methods.

BY THE END OF THIS CHAPTER YOU SHOULD BE ABLE TO:

▶ Distinguish between quantitative and qualitative research.
▶ Recognize which research method is suited to which method of data collection.
▶ Be familiar with key limitations and strengths on specific methods.
▶ Apply the principles of research to the case of coronary heart disease.

---

1 Introduction

Sociological research seeks to explain aspects of social life. It goes beyond description to offer explanations. It is located in the discipline of sociology, which is concerned with the way that societies are organized. This means that the key features of sociology – concern with the way society is organized, the role of groups of people within society, and the relationship between the two – are focused on big ideas such as social class, power and social divisions, and the way that people experience these features (O'Brien 1993). All sociological research will be about those big ideas or within the context of them.

However, sociology goes beyond offering common-sense explanations of the way that societies are organized and experienced, to challenge assumptions about taken-for-granted notions and to highlight patterns in society. For example, sociologists would challenge the notion that societies are organized around a so-called 'natural' order of things, and would look for other explanations. Indeed, sociologists argue that the way certain groups in society are less powerful than others is not because it is 'natural', but because of the way society is organized to privilege one group over another.

O'Brien (1993: 5) argues that the role of sociology is to '(D)isrupt myths and the apparently fixed and immutable characteristics of the world we live in'. Further, looking for patterns involves making connections, and the way in which phenomena are connected can be explained by different theories, or ways of seeing the world, that are based on evidence, and are critical and coherent. Feminism is an example of a sociological theory that has changed the way society can be viewed. It is based on gender differences in society, and challenges the idea that biology can fully explain the position of men and women in society by highlighting the way that power operates. Many sociologists would argue that power is a key aspect of all sociological research and that power impacts not only on the way societies are organized, but also on what aspects of social life get funded for research. This is the focus of the next section.

2 The politics of social research

The evidence base for health and social care is mainly derived from research. Sociological research in health and social care uses research that is based on a variety of types of evidence but which broadly reveals social patterns, challenges definitions such as the meaning of health, explains the way health and illness are distributed in society, and keeps the social explanation central. Statistical information on health and illness is routinely collected on such things as the number of deaths from what cause, who is suffering from what condition, hospital admissions, waiting lists and so on. This collection of information in itself is not research, but a way of monitoring and evaluating health care and treatment.

However, the information also raises questions that are often seen as problems worthy of solving. For example, the rising number of people with dementia, not just in the UK but worldwide, presents a problem to health and social-care providers that requires a solution. Likewise, the long-term conditions associated with ageing are set to increase demands on limited resources. The focus of research initiatives is on finding a cure, with some funding offered to improve the quality of life for people with dementia to enable them to avoid hospital admission. Thus, from these data sets, where successes and challenges are highlighted, sociological research endeavours to offer some sort of explanation as well as recommendations for practice.

The strength and validity of any explanation depends upon the quality of the information gathered and the extent to which it is reasonable to generalize from the findings in similar situations. In this process, not only does the method need to be sound but also any other

variables:
factors that vary, such as gender, age, social class

variables need to be taken into account. For example, research into the relationship between lifestyle and certain conditions (such as diabetes or heart disease) needs to capture the impact of all other possible factors in this relationship, even though one aspect of lifestyle such as smoking might appear to be the most significant contributory factor. Further, research might not find answers to questions but will raise further questions or highlight areas in need of investigation. This in itself is a significant research finding.

Activity 5.1 Variables

Consider the issues raised in Section 2 above, then answer the questions below.

(a) What variables might impact upon lifestyle, other than smoking?

(b) How would you factor them into an inquiry?

5

The above points are true for all types of research, whether it is about groups in society and how the social dimensions of life affect health and illness, or whether it is at the level of cells in the body and how they might respond to biomedical processes. In Western societies, the scientific method has tended to dominate what counts as truth. Social scientists would argue that seeing individuals as being reducible to sets of cells and biological systems fails to take into account the reality that they exist within society and that social factors play a significant role in health and illness. Nevertheless, research in health care has been, and largely continues to be, dominated by clinical and biomedical research.

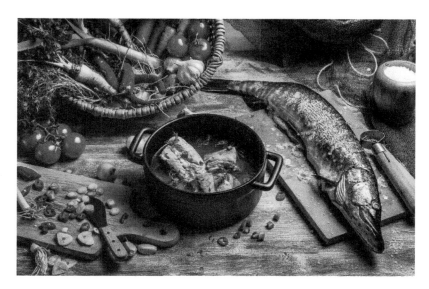

Figure 5.1 Diet is a key lifestyle variable, and it is often the focus of encouraging behavioural change

While it is self-evident that prevention is better than cure, the reality is that most of the government funding for research is awarded to a process of health-care evaluation of the impact of health interventions and focuses mainly on clinical trials, including randomized-control trials (RCTs), the evaluation of the effectiveness of new technologies, setting standards for clinical care and economic evaluation. Examples of this type of measurement can include managing symptoms through the use of medications, evaluating the effectiveness of more invasive interventions such as surgery and evaluating more widely the factors that aid recovery from illness and those that might prevent people becoming ill in the first place. Most of the examples fall into the category of clinical research. However, overall, evaluations fall largely into two categories:

(i) clinical products such as drugs; and
(ii) surgical procedures and clinical processes and the ways in which health care is organized.

Both of these types of evaluation are inextricably linked but pose different challenges for researchers.

The focus on evaluating effectiveness as a priority is not surprising since most NHS spending is on ill health rather than maintaining health and well-being. Further, given that resources are finite, the tension within national commissioning funding bodies, including the NHS, is in choosing between priorities. This involves negotiating between competing interests. Overall, the National Institute of Health Research has a focus on outcomes that are nationally relevant and the political rhetoric at least emphasizes a commitment to equity of access to high-quality care.

In sum, given that sociology is concerned with societies, it follows that social research in health care will be concerned with taking into account the wider social context. For example, as you will see, there is much evidence to show that inequalities in health impact on health outcomes. However, it does not follow that social research attracts adequate funding. For the purpose of this chapter, you should note that the way in which types of research are valued and funded carries a heavy clinical, scientific bias.

3 Researching social life

In his seminal text on researching social life, N. Gilbert (1993) argues that there are three major aspects of social research: first, theory and its construction; second, data collection; and, third, the methods with which to collect that data (p. 18). Medical sociologist Gayle Letherby (2015) highlighted how these aspects are part of the research process, so that not only do funding bodies influence or even dominate what

theory:
a set of explanatory concepts

methods:
the data-collection tools

methodology:
the research approach and the knowledge base, including what counts as knowledge

research is done, but **theory**, **methods** and **methodology** affect the outcome, which includes the findings and how they are interpreted. Further, she claims that the process and the product are intimately connected – which means that the notion of scientific objectivity is not only impossible but might be undesirable. This is because researching people's lives within specific social contexts involves making their subjective experience part of the data you want to collect.

Social theory in health and illness research would draw on answers to such questions as why divisions in illness exist. For example, one explanation about why women suffer less coronary heart disease (CHD) than men could be because they have biological protective factors, or lead different lifestyles, which could relate to their behaviour in a wider social context, taking into account their position in society. This could form a basis from which to test out a social theory, and data collection would need to provide sufficient data and be appropriate for that theory. For example, if the theory is about lifestyle, then finding out from a large enough and representative sample of women how their lifestyle differs, by asking questions or making observations, would be appropriate. Alternatively, research into mental illness might highlight the disproportionate numbers of black and minority ethnic (BME) people diagnosed with mental illness compared to their non-BME counterparts (see Box 5.1), where surveying those practitioners responsible for diagnosing mental illness might be appropriate.

Box 5.1 Experiences of mental health

This is an extract from the mental health foundation about BME people living in the UK, which claims that, in general, they are:

- more likely to be diagnosed with mental health problems
- more likely to be diagnosed and admitted to hospital
- more likely to experience a poor outcome from treatment
- more likely to disengage from mainstream mental health services, leading to social exclusion and a deterioration in their mental health.

(Available at: <http://www.mentalhealth.org.uk/help-information/mental-health-a-z/b/bme-communities/>)

These differences may be explained by a number of factors, including poverty and racism. They may also be because mainstream mental health services often fail to understand or provide services that are acceptable and accessible to non-white British communities and meet their particular cultural and other needs.

It is likely that mental health problems go unreported and untreated because people in some ethnic minority groups are reluctant to engage with mainstream health services. It is also likely that mental health problems are over-diagnosed in people whose first language is not English.

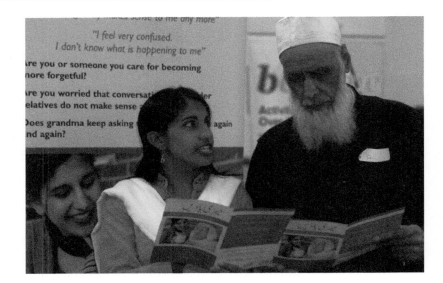

Figure 5.2 Different ethnicities have different rates of illness, which may be explained through sociological research

Divisions in society and how they might impact upon life experiences, including health and illness, are key to large sociological studies. Exploring the impact of divisions in society through such things as class, ethnicity, gender and age are core sociological approaches that have held key traditional positions in social research. They are particularly suited to large collections of data. Broadly, in social research there are two main ways of gathering information, which are quantitative and qualitative approaches. The first focus is on quantitative methods.

Social research in health and illness: quantitative methods

Quantitative methods set out to collect data in answer to questions about things that can be measured, such as how many people are diagnosed with mental illness each year at what age, and their ethnicity and gender, with results often presented in numbers and percentages. Such measurements can relate to the incidence (e.g., the number of new diagnoses of CHD in a period of time), and the prevalence (the total number of people at a particular moment with the diagnosis). In identifying a problem that requires further research, such as CHD, diabetes, dementia and mental illness, and given that data sets are routinely collected which reflect social divisions, it is relatively straightforward to compare groups, such as men and women or younger and older people, and look at any statistical differences. The next step might be to highlight why there are such differences – and here the attempt is to offer explanations. Box 5.2 illustrates the importance of sociological dimensions to such research.

In the sociological method, it is the researcher who designs the questions and the options for any answers, providing limited possibilities for participants to respond freely. Within quantitative research the

Box 5.2 The importance of sociological research in health

The following abstract from a journal article highlights why health research needs to include the sociological dimensions of gender in health research.

Abstract

Health research has failed to adequately explore the combination of social and biological sources of differences in men's and women's health. Consequently, scientific explanations often proceed from reductionist assumptions that differences are either purely biological or purely social. Such assumptions and the models that are built on them have consequences for research, health care and policy. Although biological factors such as genetics, prenatal hormone exposure and natural hormonal exposure as adults may contribute to differences in men's and women's health, a wide range of social processes can create, maintain or exacerbate underlying biological health differences. Researchers, clinicians and policy makers would understand and address both sex-specific and non-sex-specific health problems differently if the social as well as biological sources of differences in men's and women's health were better understood. *(Bird and Rieker 1999: 745)*

5

main methods employed are surveys, attitude measurements using a scale that asks for the degree of agreement with key statements in a multiple-choice survey (called a Likert scale), and direct observations. Direct observations involve some sort of counting; for example, making quantitative observations of the number of interactions between patients and staff on a ward. The results will reflect the reality that findings are based on people with opinions, preferences and different interests and the diverse behaviours of the people being studied. In other words, both the views of the researchers and those of research participants are subject to interpretations based on the different values that people hold. Further, since the 1960s, within the social sciences, the assumption that the social world could be studied in the same way as the natural world has been disputed alongside the idea that **objective** scientific knowledge (that can be demonstrated to be true, and is value-free) is the most important type of knowledge. Indeed, core to calling for recognition of the failings in objective knowledge was the notion that social life is not value-free – rather, how life is arranged and how people behave is **subjective** and open to interpretation. Given the subjectivity of behaviours and the need for research to capture this within broad social structures, it poses dilemmas about the value of any claims that are made. Therefore, sociologists try to ensure that the process of any measurement and interpretation is transparent.

Most research builds on the work of others – so researchers might extend work already carried out or take a fresh approach. For example, if researchers wanted to explore gender differences in CHD, they might begin by exploring biological, lifestyle or other factors that determine this difference. This would involve a review of existing knowledge on the subject and writing a review of that literature, which would form part of any research proposal and also part of a final report. You will be aware that much research has been conducted on CHD and its

objective: knowledge that can be demonstrated to be true, that is value-free

subjective: people's personal opinions, preferences, interests and behaviours, which may differ from those of others

potential causes. There is no simple explanation of what causes CHD, but data on individual behaviours suggest that there are key biological and lifestyle factors that play a part. You might begin to explore these direct causes, taking into account other variables, such as age, gender, ethnicity, social class and so on. Likewise, if you wanted to explore the relationship between ethnicity and mental illness, you would not assume that ethnicity was the key variable.

Activity 5.2 Exploring gender difference

Consider the points raised in Section 3 above, then answer the questions below.

(a) If you wanted to explore gender differences using a quantitative research approach, what might be your key concerns about focusing solely on gender?

(b) How would you deal with the concerns raised in order to ensure that the research was useful? Would you modify your approach and, if so, in what ways would you do this?

For the more complex variable of lifestyle, with many values within each significant aspect, researchers would need to select a sample of people who represent the larger group about whom they want to make any claims and to explore key behaviours related to the risk factors associated with the specific illness. This might involve exploring such things as diet, work, exercise, alcohol consumption and smoking habits. The values within the variable of diet could be any number of different types of food intake, but might be classified here according to fat levels, sugar levels, the number of calories and so on. If a survey has been selected as the most effective method, then, having chosen the representative sample and designed a survey questionnaire, the next step would be to conduct the survey. Surveys can be conducted face-to-face, on the telephone, by post or online. There are logistical and practical advantages and disadvantages to each. Finally, the data from the survey would be analysed. Part of this analysis would involve looking at the missing returns and deciding if the sample of returned questionnaires is representative.

Activity 5.3 Choosing the right survey method

(a) What are the advantages and disadvantages of collecting data using the following methods: face-to-face, by post, on the telephone or online?

(b) What might be some of the concerns associated with missing data in terms of how representative the sample is?

(c) What might be the association between the means of servicing the survey and its response rate?

Data from the survey is then coded, with codes collapsed into categories and then related to an overarching theory. For quantitative data analysis, a software data-analysis package is often used so that the data can be manipulated in various ways – and presented in various forms.

For example, it is possible to produce charts and tables using various commands in the software package, as well as making comparisons between variables – you might want to see the relationship between age and exercise, for example. It is important to recognize that direct associations (correlations) do not necessarily have a causal link. Finally, the results might answer the research questions, be inconclusive and/ or raise further questions. This very simplified version of the research process would involve a much more rigorous approach as well as an explanation of its limitations in any published results, so that people who might want to apply its recommendations or build on it could evaluate its usefulness and recognize its limitations. One of the ways in which sociological research can overcome accusations of bias is to make each stage of the process as **transparent** as possible.

transparent:
open and candid, easily recognized

5

> **Activity 5.4 Choosing the right quantitative method**
>
> The NHS Frameworks document on cancer includes a statement of the strategy for risk reduction, stressing that about a third of cancers are caused by smoking, diet, alcohol or obesity. To help people reduce their risk of getting cancer, the NHS has plans for:
>
> • reducing smoking
> • reducing obesity and improving diet
> • reducing harmful drinking
>
> *(Source: NHS 2011)*
>
> (a) What quantitative research method would you use if you wanted to collect data on smoking behaviour?
> (b) What might be one of your concerns about the validity of the data?

There are requirements laid down by most research councils for findings to be disseminated and to demonstrate impact on key stakeholders. For example, a study into the benefits of weight loss in reducing blood pressure carried out in one NHS Trust could provide useful information on the pros and cons of such an initiative, which would be useful to other NHS Trusts. The government has a duty in 'universalizing the best'. One of the ways in which it does so is discussed next, in Section 4.

4 Putting research into practice

National Service Frameworks (NSFs) are NHS initiatives developed in response to problems that are deemed to be a national priority. With a foreword by the Secretary of State, the Framework provides the government's plan for tackling particular health problems. The National Service Framework for Mental Health (1999) was selected as a priority. Box 5.3 shows an extract from the framework on the standards, with one area expanded to show the detail of one standard.

Box 5.3 The National Service Framework for Mental Health 1999

This National Service Framework sets out standards in five areas; each standard is supported by the evidence and knowledge base, by service models, and by examples of good practice. Local milestones are proposed; timescales need to be agreed with NHS Executive regional offices and social care regions, and progress will be monitored.

Standard one addresses mental health promotion and combats the discrimination and social exclusion associated with mental health problems.

Standards two and three cover primary care and access to services for anyone who may have a mental health problem.

Standards four and five encompass the care of people with severe mental illness.

Standard six relates to individuals who care for people with mental health problems.

Standard seven draws together the action necessary to achieve the target to reduce suicides as set out in *Saving Lives: Our Healthier Nation*.

Aim

To ensure health and social services promote mental health and reduce the discrimination and social exclusion associated with mental health problems.

Standard one

Health and social services should:

- promote mental health for all, working with individuals and communities
- combat discrimination against individuals and groups with mental health problems, and promote their social inclusion.

Rationale

Mental health problems can result from the range of adverse factors associated with social exclusion and can also be a cause of social exclusion. For example:

- unemployed people are twice as likely to have depression as people in work
- children in the poorest households are three times more likely to have mental health problems than children in well-off households
- half of all women and a quarter of all men will be affected by depression at some period during their lives
- people who have been abused or have been victims of domestic violence have higher rates of mental health problems
- between a quarter and a half of people using night shelters or sleeping rough may have a serious mental disorder, and up to half may be alcohol dependent
- some black and minority ethnic groups are diagnosed as having higher rates of mental disorder than the general population; refugees are especially vulnerable
- there is a high rate of mental disorder in the prison population
- people with drug and alcohol problems have higher rates of other mental health problems
- people with physical illnesses have higher rates of mental health problems.

Available at: <https://www.gov.uk/government/uploads/system/uploads/attachment_data/file/198051/National_Service_Framework_for_Mental_Health.pdf>.

Activity 5.5

When you have read the Framework details shown in Box 5.3, consider the list of nine bullet points at the end.

(a) Which of the examples of social exclusion listed in these bullet points do you think would be suited to a sociological approach to research? Give reasons for your choice.

(b) Select one of the issues raised in the list of bullet points and consider various approaches to research this. Which method do you think might be particularly effective?

Such an enquiry cannot be based solely on quantitative measurements. Many of these adverse factors require a different approach to establish an explanation. Indeed, all could benefit from enquiring further about the behaviours and motivations of the key actors. The NSF mentions the role of service users throughout, and this is best suited to qualitative research methods which are considered next, in Section 5.

5

5 Qualitative research methods

Qualitative methods are not concerned with measurements, but rather with the meanings of behaviour. Qualitative research can provide more in-depth explanations of what is happening, taking experience into account. In particular, recognizing that people are social actors whose behaviour is determined by the wider context, it is clear that the best way to understand reasons for actions is to ask the people involved. This approach involves exploring 'what is really going on here' – and finding out from the social actors involved what meaning they attribute to their actions.

The research findings need to be related to social theory in some way. For example, if a researcher thought that the way in which women are positioned in society in terms of money and power affects their health outcomes, then that would affect the research design (see Annandale and Clark 2000). It would not mean that the research findings would necessarily support that theory, but it would show the extent to which they might.

While qualitative interviews are best suited to an exploration of why social actors behave in the way that they do, it does not necessarily mean that the explanations that people offer are a true representation of their actions. For instance, family members living with someone who has a mental illness might not want to disclose details of their experience.

As with quantitative surveys, qualitative interviews can be conducted remotely, by post or online, face to face or by telephone, and comprise different types. For example, interview questions can be tightly structured, with each interview following a specific pattern;

semi-structured interviews allow for the same areas to be covered in each interview but include more scope for participants to offer explanations or expand points in their own words. Unstructured interviews might involve the interviewer in offering one basic question such as 'tell me about your health' and the occasional prompt or probing question. The researcher using an unstructured interview schedule will usually have a guide to what areas he or she wants to cover.

In sociological research into health and illness, a particular type of interviewing taken from biographical methods has been used to explore the part that people's illness plays in their life. The term 'illness narrative' has been applied to this qualitative approach. Fundamentally, interviewees are asked to give an account of something – here their illness – allowing them to structure the interview, with the interviewer asking questions of clarification or for further detail once they have told their stories. A narrative method is used to highlight overtly the relationship between illness and social context.

Other types of qualitative research include what is broadly termed an **ethnographic approach**. The word 'ethnography' is founded in groups (*ethno*) and writing (*graphy*). This method involves recording every detail of what is happening, including the words that people use, in sets of field notes. The level of detail in recording field notes is called 'thick description', and the method is derived from anthropological studies.

ethnographic approach: observation of what is taking place, experiencing the world from the participants' point of view

Observational methods can use participant or non-participant observation. The researcher uses informal conversations, written documents and direct observations, in an attempt to think him or herself into the situation and to see the world from the actors' point of view. In other words, the ethnographic approach can be used to see people in action rather than hear about their actions. Historically, more 'exotic' groups were studied by social anthropologists, usually in inaccessible settings (see Malinowski 1884–1942). Fundamentally, the analysis of such groups in 'natural settings' reveals regular patterns.

This approach adopted by social scientists is used effectively in research into health and illness, a good example of which is a seminal ethnographic study conducted in the 1960s by the sociologist J. A. Roth, who observed patients in a TB sanatorium in the US and explored the ways in which they interpreted what was happening to them (Roth 1963). Specifically, he was interested in how they managed the uncertain trajectory of their long-term illness and long hospital stay. His ideas drew on his own experiences of being a TB patient when he noted that fellow patients did not base their understanding on the logical, rational, scientific approach of the medical profession, but used lay interpretations of what was taking place and within which they located themselves. Roth drew on Parsons' theory of the 'sick role' (Parsons 1951), to show how patients used their own criteria to interpret what was happening to them in their illness trajectory.

A similar ethnographic study by Bluebond-Langner (1978) explored how children with leukaemia (in the US) who were protected from the seriousness of their diagnosis, at a time when outcomes were much poorer, interpreted events around them. She found that even very young children recognized they might be dying but followed the social rules about not discussing death. She described this as part of 'mutual pretence', which had been developed as a theory about communication in caring for dying adults by Glaser and Strauss (1965) in their ethnographic work on dying trajectories. In this way, she used a theory developed by a sociologist studying the experiences of dying adults and applied it to children.

These examples highlight the role of theory in social qualitative research. Unlike the scientific method, the process does not prove or disprove a theory; rather, it builds on a theory that is useful – either by extending it or by evaluating the extent of its usefulness. Also, sociological research tends to highlight areas that are not explained by particular theories.

5

Activity 5.6 Applying ethnography to practice

Consider the types of ethnographic study described in Section 5, above.

(a) Can you find more examples of this type of study, either from the recommended reading lists or by researching online?

(b) What similarities or differences can you find between different types of ethnographic study?

(c) How might the types of ethnographic study described in Section 5 above apply to practice?

---

6 A focus on coronary heart disease

Statistics about health and illness play a significant role in setting research agendas and health-care priorities. As in most countries, there is a legal requirement to register all deaths and attribute a cause of death. In the UK, all deaths are registered in civil registration records, which are collected and collated by the Office of National Statistics. These UK statistics show that coronary heart disease (CHD) is the biggest cause of death (ONS 2014). Indeed, in the UK each year, just under 500,000 people die and CHD is responsible for around 73,000 of these deaths. Further, CHD is also the leading cause of death worldwide (NHS Choices 2014).

Therefore, it is unsurprising that a key government priority in health care is to reduce the number of deaths from CHD. However, the inequalities in the incidence and outcomes of CHD reflect the political tension between whose business health is, and thus whose responsibility it is to consider the wider social context – such as social determinants of health (see, e.g.: <http://www.local.gov.uk/health/-/journal_content/56/10180/3510830/ARTICLE>).

Coronary heart disease most typically affects the coronary arteries that supply the heart muscle with blood, and can cause angina and heart attacks. If the blood supply to part of the heart is diminished, as in angina, pain symptoms can be relieved by using a vasodilating drug. Further treatment for angina involves the insertion of a stent (or stents) to widen the affected artery or arteries, or the replacement of damaged coronary arteries, which is a more intensive surgical intervention that is sometimes undertaken. If the coronary artery is blocked by a clot, as in a heart attack (myocardial infarction, MI), pain and symptoms cannot be relieved and the person requires emergency hospital admission. Effectively a segment of the heart muscle, the myocardium, has died because its blood supply has been cut off. It might be possible to

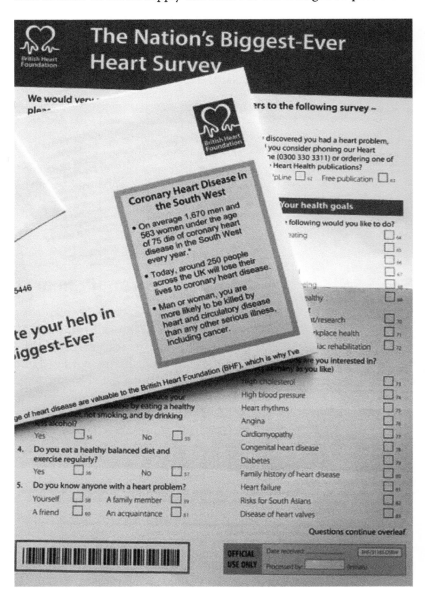

Figure 5.3 Surveys can be a useful way of measuring social factors which impact disease

remove or dissolve the clot, to halt damage to the heart muscle, or at least to provide coronary care while the damaged heart muscle repairs itself. As with strokes, a further MI or an extension of the current MI damage is a potential likelihood. However, despite advances in acute coronary heart care, according to Department of Health statistics, about a third of people who have a myocardial infarction (MI) die as a result (NHS Choices 2014).

At any one time, it is estimated that 2.3 million people are living with CHD.

The prevention, detection and management of CHD is not just concerned with exploring and building evidence on what works by drawing on clinical research, but also with understanding the way that social factors impact on the disease. For example, it is one of the diseases most strongly associated with inequalities in health (see Marmot 2013). There is a clear north–south divide, with death rates being highest in Scotland and the north of England and lowest in the south, and also a division along gender (one in six men and one in ten women die from CHD) and ethnic lines, with lower socioeconomic groups, men and minority ethnic groups being over-represented (BHF 2015). Therefore, given the degree of inequality associated with this disease, CHD has been the focus of much health research – both in terms of obtaining clinical evidence about what treatments might be most effective and efficient, and examining the social determinates of CHD. Such inequalities sit uncomfortably with the NHS principles of care, which state that it should be universal, free at the point of delivery and provide a good quality of service for everyone in need of health care.

Box 5.4 Sociological research on gender and CHD

The following abstract from an article on gender differences and CHD illustrates how qualitative sociological research suits an exploration of the more detailed aspects of quantitative findings.

Although there has been considerable research on psychosocial working conditions and their effect on physical and mental health, there has been little research into the effects of psychosocial domestic conditions on health. The association between psychosocial working conditions (and control at work in particular) and coronary heart disease (CHD) is not as strong for women compared to men. Other research suggests that household and domestic factors may have an important effect on women's health. Some studies have shown that low control at home affects psychological well-being. However, there has been little research into its effects on physical health. Furthermore, similar to results analysing low control at work, low control at home may form part of the pathways underlying social inequalities in health. The study investigates the meaning of control at home, the effect of control at home on incident CHD events and whether this explains some of the social inequalities in CHD events in men and women. Data from phases 3–5 of the Whitehall II study, London, UK, were analysed (N=7470). The results indicate that low control at home predicts CHD among women but not among men. Furthermore, low control at home may explain part of the association between household social position and CHD among women. There is some evidence suggesting that low control at home among women results from a lack of material and psychological resources to cope with excessive household and family demands. Psychosocial domestic conditions may have a greater effect on the health of women compared with men (Chandola et al. 2004: 1501).

As stated earlier, quantitative and qualitative approaches are not mutually exclusive. Using a multi-method approach can provide a much fuller explanation about such things as divisions in coronary heart disease. The various methods produce different types of data in answer to different questions.

Activity 5.7 Understanding risk factors for coronary heart disease (CHD)

The NHS Choices website summarizes the direct causes of CHD as:

Coronary heart disease (CHD) is usually caused by a build-up of fatty deposits on the walls of the arteries around the heart (coronary arteries).

The fatty deposits, called atheroma, are made up of cholesterol and other waste substances.

The build-up of atheroma on the walls of the coronary arteries makes the arteries narrower and restricts the flow of blood to the heart muscle. This process is called atherosclerosis. Your risk of developing atherosclerosis is significantly increased if you:

* smoke
* have high blood pressure (hypertension)
* have a high blood cholesterol level
* do not take regular exercise
* have diabetes

Other risk factors for developing atherosclerosis include:

* being obese or overweight
* having a family history of CHD – the risk is increased if you have a male relative with CHD under the age of 55 or a female relative under 65

(NHS Choices 2014)

(a) How might the risk factors listed above, from the NHS Choices website, be researched using a sociological approach?
(b) In what ways do you think a sociological approach might influence the results of any research?
(c) Consider and list ways of using a multi-method approach to researching the risk factors listed above from the NHS Choices website, noting the different types of information you want to obtain and the method best suited to each type of information required.

In a multi-method approach the first step of the research endeavour, as in all research, is to identify a problem to which to offer a solution, or at least an explanation, and this is done using a combination of data sources. The next step is to design research questions that need to be answered, from the broad overarching ones to more detailed questions within them, then to consider what method or methods will best answer the questions. A large quantitative survey can provide the basis from which to explore in more detail a purposive sample for semi-structured interviews which will yield both demographic quantitative and qualitative data. Following analysis of these first stages, it would be possible to choose aspects that would benefit from an ethnographic approach, giving a much more in-depth insight into the experience of the social actors.

In conclusion, social research adds to knowledge in two key ways. First, it provides empirical data, and, second, it adds to, extends, refutes or develops social theory. In this way, research both builds on and extends the base on which further research can be conducted. It is usual for social research into health and illness, like other forms of research, to offer recommendations for practice based on the findings. As stated earlier in this chapter, making research relevant to practice is an increasing demand of research funding bodies. Given the statistical evidence on the divisions in society of the incidence of CHD and the poorer outcomes associated with these divisions, coronary heart disease provides an example of an area of illness which would benefit from a sociological and multi-method approach to understanding and explaining such differences, hopefully changing outcomes to redress the inequalities.

5

Summary and Resources

Summary

▷ Social research includes the social context as part of its exploration.

▷ Social research is informed by and informs social theory as a body of coherent knowledge.

▷ Despite the strong evidence of social divisions and inequalities in health, most funding research is awarded to clinical/biomedical research.

▷ Social research uses two fundamental approaches, quantitative and qualitative, within which is a range of approaches.

▷ Coronary heart disease (CHD) is a condition that reflects social divisions and inequalities in incidence and outcomes.

▷ Multi-method approaches within social research provide an effective means of producing rich explanatory data from which to offer recommendations for practice.

Questions for Discussion

1 From your practice experience, what are the key issues that matter most to health service users?

2 How does the way that research is conducted influence research findings?

3 How does qualitative research inform nursing practice?

4 What specific aspects of CHD does clinical research fail to explain?

Glossary

ethnographic approach: observation of what is taking place, experiencing the world from the participants' point of view which involves making very detailed observations of what people do and say, while not assuming an understanding; to do this, researchers have to spend time in the field and experience the world of the participants

methodology: the research approach and the knowledge base, including what counts as knowledge and which needs to fit with the theory and methods; a set of practices within a system of knowledge or discipline.

methods: the data-collection tools that are used in any study and include such things as postal surveys, structured interviews, participant observation and so on

objective: knowledge that can be demonstrated to be true, that is value-free and that does not show an interpretation that is weighted by particular interests; it might be difficult for practitioners heavily involved in certain areas to be objective

subjective: people's personal opinions, preferences, interests and behaviours, which may differ from those of others and affect the interpretation of research findings, making them biased; the potential to be subjective lies in research participants who might present a view of events that reflect their own beliefs and values, and also in the researcher

theory: a set of explanatory concepts which are often tested or added to by research studies; an example is the anthropological theory that boundaries such as death can be symbolic, explaining rituals and practices at the time of death as ways to keep the life/death boundary safe; a theory offers an explanation of the social world

transparent: open and candid, easily recognized; this involves the researcher being aware of and recording his or her own biases

variables:
factors that vary, such as gender, age and social class, and which can account for differences in data and which therefore need to be taken into account during analysis and interpretation; social class is a variable that often features in health inequalities

Further Reading

M. Saks and J. Allsop: *Researching Health: Quantitative, Qualitative and Mixed Methods*, 2nd edn. London: Sage, 2012.
This book provides a comprehensive guide to both quantitative and qualitative research methods in health and illness for students new to research.

J. Seymour: *Death and Dying: Critical Moments in Intensive Care*: Oxford: Oxford University Press, 2001.
This book is based on an ethnographic study of end-of-life care in an intensive care unit. It explores how care staff decide when someone in intensive care who is close to death is dying and how that is managed. It provides an example of qualitative research, how this relates to social theory and also how this knowledge might impact upon practice.

UK Research Analysis Report, 2012: Available at: <http://www.ukcrc.org/research-coordination/health-research-analysis/uk-health-research-analysis/>.
This report provides a detailed breakdown of the key public and charity funders of health research to show how much is allocated to what type of funding. It provides an understanding of what type of research is funded, which itself is part of the social context of health and illness.

References

Annandale, E. and Clark, J. 2000 Gender, postmodernism and health. In S. J. Williams, J. Gabe and M. Calnan (eds), *Health, Medicine and Society: Key Theories, Future Agendas*. London: Routledge, pp. 51–66.

Bird, C. E. and Rieker, P. P. 1999 Gender matters: an integrated model for understanding men's and women's health. *Social Science and Medicine* 48/6 (March): 745–55.

Bluebond-Langner, M. 1978 *The Private Worlds of Dying Children*. Princeton, NJ: Princeton University Press.

British Heart Foundation 2010 Available at: <https://www.bhf.org.uk/publications/statistics/ethnic-differences-in-cardiovascular-disease-2010>.

British Heart Foundation 2015 Available at: <https://www.bhf.org.uk/~/media/files/research/heart-statistics/cardiovascular-disease-statistics---headline-statistics.pdf>.

Chandola, T., Kuper, H., Singh-Manoux, A., Bartley, M. and Marmot, M. 2004 The effect of control at home on CHD events in the Whitehall II study: Gender differences in psychosocial domestic pathways to social inequalities in CHD. *Social Science and Medicine* 58/8 (April): 1501–9. Available at: <http://www.sciencedirect.com/science/article/pii/S1359178913000037>.

Gilbert, N. (ed.) 1993 *Researching Social Life*. London: Sage.

Glaser, B. G. and Strauss, A. L. 1965 *Awareness of Dying*. Chicago: Aldine Publishing Company.

Letherby, G. 2015 Methods, methodology and epistemology. In R. Deery, E. Denny and G. Letherby (eds), *Sociology for Midwives*. Cambridge: Polity, pp. 38–55.

Malinowski, B. 1884–1942 Available at: <http://www.oxfordbibliographies. com/view/document/obo-9780199766567/obo-9780199766567-0096. xml>.

Marmot, M. 2013 *Heart UK Report*. Available at: <http://heartuk.org.uk/files/ uploads/Bridging_the_Gaps_Tackling_inequalities_in_cardiovascular_ disease.pdf>.

Mental Health Foundation 1999 *The National Service Framework for Mental Health, 1999*. Available at: <http://www.mentalhealth.org.uk/ help-information/mental-health-a-z/b/bme-communities/>.

NHS 1999 *National Service Framework for Mental Health*. Available at: <http://www.nhs.uk/Conditions/Coronary-heart-> and <https://www.gov. uk/government/uploads/system/uploads/attachment_data/file/198051/ National_Service_Framework_for_Mental_Health.pdf>.

NHS 2000 *National Service Framework for CHD*. Available at: <https:// www.gov.uk/government/uploads/system/uploads/attachment_data/ file/198931/National_Service_Framework_for_Coronary_Heart_Disease. pdf>.

NHS 2011 *Improving Outcomes: A Strategy for Cancer*. Available at: <http:// www.cancerscreening.nhs.uk/breastscreen/improving-outcomes-strategy- for-cancer.pdf NHS, 2011>.

NHS Choices 2014 *Risk Factors for Coronary Heart Disease*. Available at: <http://www.nhs.uk/Conditions/cardiovascular-disease/Pages/Risk- factors.aspx>.

O'Brien, M. 1993 Social research and sociology, in N. Gilbert (ed.), *Researching Social Life*. London: Sage, pp. 1–17.

Office for National Statistics (ONS) 2014 Available at: <https://www.gov.uk/ government/organisations/office-for-national-statistics>.

Parsons, T. 1951. *The Social System*. Glencoe, Ill: Free Press

Rassin, M. 2009 The cardiac patient: a gender comparison via illness narratives. *Journal of Nursing and Healthcare of Chronic Illness* 1/1 (March 2009): 20–8.

Roth, J. A. 1963 *Timetables: Structuring the Passage of Time in Hospital Treatments and Other Careers*. Indianapolis, IN: Bobbs-Merrill.

Part II
Inequalities and Diversity in Health and Health Care

It is important to be aware of diversity amongst patient/client groups and the impact of this on health and health care. Part II examines health inequality and diversity, focusing specifically on gender, age, family, long-term conditions, disability, class, and race and ethnicity.

In Chapter 6, 'Gender', the emphasis is on the significance of sex and gender for health and illness. The chapter provides a definition of sex and gender and a historical overview of some key gendered concerns, emphasizing how 'gender issues' do not relate just to women and girls, but also to men and boys. While it is often the case that 'women get sick and men die', the picture is much more complex than that, and this chapter unpacks some of the key issues. The concepts of masculinity and femininity are explored and the question 'What makes women and men sick?' is addressed. The chapter concludes by arguing that, just as sexism affects perceptions of what makes women and men sick, it also affects service provision. You are encouraged to think about how gender and sexism influence the treatment and care you offer to patients.

Chapter 7, 'The Family, Health and Caring', focuses on the contribution made by the family both to health and well-being *and* to ill health. It begins by unpacking 'common-sense' views of the nuclear family, demonstrating the diversity that exists within family life. It then introduces some key sociological perspectives on the family. This chapter considers the role of the family in maintaining health, focusing on the care and caring work carried out both within and by family members. The chapter concludes by exploring the ways in which families can cause ill health, for example, via domestic violence, or the burden of caring for the chronically ill.

'Age and Ageing', Chapter 8, suggests that while we may think about 'ageing' solely in relation to older people, the study of age and ageing is relevant to all nurses. Nurses work with patients of all ages, and may be influenced by the assumptions made in wider society about health care in relation to age. Drawing on a life-course perspective, this chapter challenges some of these assumptions and explores the social construction of ageing. The chapter explores definitions of 'age' and examines the changing structure of the population. You will be introduced to both traditional and more contemporary theories of ageing and will examine the impact of ageism on health. The chapter encourages you to explore your own stereotypes about 'age', to reflect on anti-ageist policies and to consider how these might affect your nursing practice.

Chapter 9 considers long-term conditions within the population and begins by looking at the health challenge of the increase in chronic (or long-term) illness. It introduces students to the sociological research on long-term conditions, in particular interpretive narrative accounts. The enduring and influential concept of biographical disruption is explored, with some of the more recent developments that have built on the original work. Pain is a common feature of long-term conditions and the chapter examines this from a sociological perspective, including the importance for people in pain of having that pain believed, in particular by receiving a medical diagnosis. People who live with a condition over a long period become experts in their own situation and may decide to adapt the way that they use medical advice and treatments to reflect their social context. The way this is interpreted and judged is the final section in this chapter.

Disability is the topic under discussion in Chapter 10. The classification and definition of disability and impairment are considered, and you are introduced to some of the sociological theorizing on disability. The chapter discusses the social model, which has been very influential within sociological thinking on disability; the social model makes a distinction between 'impairment' and 'disability' and suggests that disability is socially constructed. It also looks at the barriers that disabled people face in receiving good health care, and the role of the disability movement in campaigning for change. Throughout the chapter the experience of people with disability is utilized to illustrate concepts.

In Chapter 11, 'Social Class and Health', we explain the traditional sociological concept of class and discuss the more contemporary measurement of socioeconomic differences. The chapter maps the history of the relationship between class and health and considers the widening gap in inequalities between the richest and poorest. The chapter then turns to a discussion of the evidence relating to class inequalities in health. Some of the policies used to tackle health inequalities in the twenty-first century are discussed and the explanations for such inequalities are evaluated. Chapter 11 encourages you to investigate and understand the significance of class and health for nursing practice.

Chapter 12, 'Race and Ethnicity', draws the distinction between the concepts of 'race' and 'ethnicity'. Although ethnicity relates to both individual identity and structural or cultural differences, this chapter highlights that it is important for nurses to recognize the considerable individual and social diversity within and between ethnic groups. This chapter provides a brief history of immigration in Britain, which now boasts over 4.5 million people who describe themselves as belonging to a minority ethnic group. The relationship between ethnicity and health and health care is examined, and there is some discussion of the methodological issues involved in measuring the relationship between health and ethnicity. This chapter encourages you to reflect on the implications of ethnic diversity for nursing practice.

All of the chapters within this section share certain features. First, they each explore the significance of definition and classification, demonstrating not just how this has changed over time, but also how the definition of difference and diversity can affect treatment and care. Second, they also share methodological concerns and highlight the fact that we cannot separate what we know to be true from the way in which that 'truth' has emerged. Although there is consensus on the existence of inequalities in health, there is considerable debate on the extent and nature of these inequalities and how they should be measured. Finally, all of the chapters within this section encourage you to reflect on the way in which diversity affects your practice and how inequalities in health may influence treatment and care.

CHAPTER 6

Gender

Gayle Letherby

> ### KEY ISSUES IN THIS CHAPTER:
> ▶ Definitional and historical issues.
> ▶ The significance of sex and gender in relation to health and illness.
> ▶ The gendered experience of health care.
> ▶ The relationship between gender and other 'measures' of stratification.
>
> ### BY THE END OF THIS CHAPTER YOU SHOULD BE ABLE TO:
> ▶ Explain how historical definitions and expectations of men and women affect contemporary definitions and experiences.
> ▶ Explain how historical views on the relationship between gender and health affect contemporary views and experiences.
> ▶ Understand the significance of sex and gender for patterns of health and illness.
> ▶ Explain the relationship between gender roles, masculinity and femininity, and health and illness.
> ▶ Recognize the need to take a gendered perspective, whilst acknowledging that other differences are also relevant.

1 Introduction

This chapter begins with some definitions. When considering issues of gender in relation to health and illness (or to family life, work and leisure, education, crime – in fact, in relation to anything), it is important to understand what gender means. **Gender** does not (as some people mistakenly think) refer only to the experiences and perspectives of women, but to the significance of similarities and differences

gender:
cultural differences between males and females

sex:
the biological differences between males and females

between female and male experiences. It is also important to remember that gender is a concept distinct from the concept of sex: '**sex**' is a term referring to biological differences between men and women, and 'gender' a term referring to cultural differences (Oakley 1972). Gender, then, refers to culturally prescribed expectations of women and men and differs over time and place. Thus, gender is not a fixed aspect of our identity, but is fluid, negotiated on a daily basis and something that we 'do' as well as 'have' (also see Marchbank and Letherby 2014).

In this chapter the relationship between sex and gender, and health, illness and caring, is considered, for an understanding of gender is relevant to all four branches of nursing. The chapter is divided into four main sections, which focus on historical definitions and contemporary concerns, challenging myths, the relationship between gender and caring, and diversity and difference. This is followed by a brief summary of the main issues.

2 Historical definitions and contemporary concerns

The sixteenth and seventeenth centuries were particularly significant in their effect on understandings of gender and health in the Western world. The scientific knowledge that emerged at this time was argued to be objective knowledge. As Gunew (1990) and Wajcman (1991) note, historically and to date (see Ahmed 2004), men are believed to be capable of objectivity and women are not.

The dominant message then was that women were not just different from men but physically, psychologically, emotionally and socially inferior to men (Doyal 1995; Letherby 2003), and characterized as 'sensitive, intuitive, incapable of objectivity and emotional detachment and . . . immersed in the business of making and maintaining personal relationships' (Oakley 1981: 38). Thus, women were considered naturally weak and easy to exploit, and their psychological characteristics implied subordination; for example, submission, passivity and dependency. From this perspective women are more like children than adults, in that they are immature, weak and helpless (Oakley 1981; Evans 1997). If women adopt these characteristics they are considered well adjusted (Oakley 1981), but being considered well adjusted clearly comes with a price; in the eighteenth and nineteenth centuries, defining women as weak justified their exclusion from the world of work and education.

hysteria:
a term first coined by Hippocrates derived from the Greek word *hystera* or 'uterus'

emotion work:
coping with one's own and others' feelings

However, although women have historically been constructed as weak and prone to **hysteria**, they have always performed large amounts of physical labour both in the home and outside of it, and on top of this they have been, and still are, held responsible for the dominant share of domestic and **emotion work** (Frith and Kitzinger 1998; Marchbank

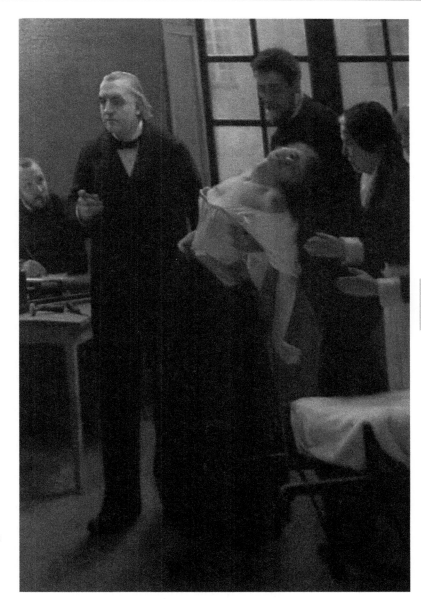

Figure 6.1
Nineteenth-century neurologist Jean-Martin Charcot was one of the key proponents of the theory of hysteria

6

and Letherby 2014; Deery et al. 2015). Despite this, the image of women as inferior is still significant in defining women's lives (for example, Coppock, Haydon and Richter 1995; Doyal 1995).

Activity 6.1 Gendered definitions: the case of hysteria

The word 'hysteria' is usually used to describe a woman as though she were simply behaving according to expectations . . . Hysteria now refers to a specific psychoneurosis that may affect anyone, male or female. In popular usage it is a state of excessive fear or other emotion in individuals or masses of people, but in this sense men – whether individually or in groups – are seldom said to be hysterical. After a series of rapes at a large college in 1974, news stories repeatedly described a 'mood of hysteria' among women students on the campus. The description, according to the dean of women, was totally false. 'The mood of the women is one of concern and anger,' she told reporters. 'When men feel concern and anger, it is called concern and anger, never hysteria.' (Mills 1991: 127)

(a) Can you think of some more examples of women being described as hysterical?

(b) Do you think that the association of hysteria with womanhood affects the ways we popularly define women's and men's, and girls' and boys', mental health and well-being? If so, what are the implications for the treatment and care of women and men with mental health problems?

(c) The Hysterectomy Association recently introduced an annual women's fiction competition in an attempt to raise money and awareness. The publication that results is called *Hysteria*, available at: <http://www.hysterectomy-association.org.uk/hysteria-writing-competition/>. Do you think this kind of irony is helpful? If so, why?

All of this has implications for women in terms of their health and of general perceptions of women as healthy or not. In the nineteenth century, middle-class women were thought to be particularly weak and susceptible to illness: menstruation was thought to be an 'indisposition' or illness that sapped women's energy, making it necessary for them to rest; childbirth was termed 'confinement', and a long period of bed rest was thought necessary after the birth of a baby; and the menopause was considered a disease which marked the beginning of senility (Webb 1986).

Oddly, working-class women were not seen as being susceptible to the same problems. They were considered to be physically stronger, emotionally less sensitive, and well able to work fourteen hours a day outside of the home and still be able to 'cook, clean and service their husbands, and bear children without such suffering' (Webb 1986: 6). Furthermore, working-class women were seen as potentially polluting through their work in the kitchen, the nursery and the brothel (Abbott et al. 2005). The harshest reading of this is that working-class women were not viewed as women at all, and the most generous that, whereas middle-class women were 'sickly', working-class women were 'sickening'.

Current lay and medical definitions of the gendered significance of health seem to continue the sexist view of women as 'sickly'. When asked to think of someone they consider healthy, both men and women are more likely to choose a man (Blaxter 1990; Marchbank and Letherby 2014). Psychologists and clinicians are more likely to define women's than men's health problems as psychological, and definitions of mental health are often related to traditional notions of **masculinity and femininity**: healthy men are thought to be independent, logical and adventurous, and healthy women less aggressive, more emotional and easily hurt (Webb 1986; Miers 2000; Ahmed 2004; Marchbank and Letherby 2014).

masculinity and femininity:
ways in which men and women are expected to behave, think and feel

Evidence from research also suggests that women make more use of health services and appear to feel less healthy than men (Annandale and Clark 1996). However, in some interpretations of data where comparisons are made between males and females, the health status of men is glossed over or informed by simplistic, stereotypical approaches (Miers 2000; Watson 2000). This construction of women's health as poor has consequences for men too, in that there is an implicit assumption that men's health is 'good'. The result of this is that men's poor health remains invisible and differences between men are not considered (Annandale and Clark 1996; Watson 2000; Featherstone, Rivett and Scourfield 2007). One reaction to this has been the presentation of men as a disadvantaged group whose health needs have been previously disadvantaged (Courtenay 2000; Bradby 2012). But as Hannah Bradby (2012: 66) notes, this type of discourse 'tends to re-inscribe gender in deterministic terms', leading to unhelpful arguments about who is sicker.

The seeking of professional help for both physical and mental health needs is gendered, and it is well known that men are generally less likely to seek professional help than women (Featherstone, Rivett and Scourfield 2007). In fact, men's denial of illness can be so strong that even the pain associated with a heart attack can be ignored so that the victim will not be seen as weak or effeminate (Courtenay 2000; Emslie and Hunt 2008). However, stressing men's reluctance to access medical care can support the problematic view that the health and well-being of men and children is the responsibility of women:

> They [women] are seen as responsible for bringing up healthy children and maintaining the health of their men for the nation. Health visitors, social workers and other professional state employees 'police' the family to ensure that women are carrying out their task adequately. (Abbott et al. 2005: 196)

Furthermore, there is evidence that self-help designed specifically with men in mind – for example, in the areas of mental health and young fatherhood – can be beneficial (Galdas, Cheater and Marshall 2005; Featherstone, Rivett and Scourfield 2007).

So, historically and to date, lay and medical perceptions of the relationship between sex, gender, health and illness are based on sexist assumptions of what women and men are and should be like.

3 Challenging myths: masculinity, femininity, and health and illness

The phrase 'women get sick and men die', which historically has been central to research findings in the area of gender inequalities in health, still holds some truth, but it oversimplifies the complex relationship between gender and health. Abbott and her colleagues (2005) note that a gendered pattern is found in all societies, with women, on average, living longer than men. Yet Bradby (2012) points out that in a few countries, where there is a high prevalence of infectious disease, women have no mortality advantage over men (e.g., in Bangladesh and Zimbabwe). Further, there are social class differences between women within societies, and the male–female gap in life expectancy varies significantly between countries – for example, Russia has the largest male–female gap in life expectancy, whereas in some countries in Southeast Asia and parts of sub-Saharan and West Africa the gap is much smaller or even virtually eliminated. As health service use increases with age in societies where women do live longer, not surprisingly they have higher consultation rates over a lifetime, especially when we take into account the visits related to menstruation, pregnancy, childbirth, post-natal care and menopause. Furthermore, women appear to find it easier and more socially acceptable to discuss their own health, and there may also be important psychosocial factors, such as how men and women evaluate symptoms (Watson 2000; Featherstone, Rivett and Scourfield 2007; Bradby 2008).

The main causes of lower life expectancy for men lie in higher death rates from coronary heart disease, lung cancer and chronic obstructive airways disease, accidents, homicides, suicides and AIDS (Miers 2000). Men are more likely to die of occupationally related illnesses, men engage in more physical risk-taking than women, and accidents and homicides have always been a feature of masculine rather than feminine experience (Featherstone, Rivett and Scourfield 2007). Cigarette smoking has, hitherto, been a major cause of death among men (although in the 1990s male and female smoking rates in the UK began to even out), and men drink more than women (although this is changing too, and gender is not the only signifier of differential substance use). For example, King and McKeown (2003) report high levels of alcohol and substance misuse among (especially young) lesbian, gay and bisexual (LGB) people, and link this to the importance of pubs and clubs in LGB social life.

The poorer aspects of men's health are often associated with stereotypical male gender roles: trying to live up to a macho image and lifestyle, which is itself dangerous to health. From this perspective, much ill health among men is a consequence of lifestyle, which nurses and other health professionals can address in their role as health educators. However, the challenge to change male behaviour and resist stereotypical masculinity is problematic because men's experience (just like women's) is affected by other aspects of their identity, such as age, dis/ability, ethnicity and so on (Featherstone, Rivett and Scourfield 2007; Dolan 2007).

Cancer: experience and awareness

In 2012 there were 281,118 cancer diagnoses in England. Of these, there was a total of 143,406 male diagnoses, with the top three types being prostrate, lung, and colon and rectum cancer, and a total of 137,712 female diagnoses, with the top three types being breast, lung, and colon and rectum cancer (ONS 2014).

In 2013, the following appeared in the Telegraph Online:

> Prostate cancer is simply not on the radar in the UK. Even though it kills one man every hour, that's 10,000 men each year . . . We need to follow the lead of the successful female movement against breast cancer and create a real change for men. (At: <http://www.telegraph.co.uk/news/health/news/9772648/Prostate-cancer-research-underfunded.html>)

Since this piece was written, attention has been given to this issue, in the Men United (keep friendship alive) Prostate Cancer UK campaign.

In 2002, Clare Moynihan published an article in the *European Journal of Cancer Care*, arguing for a 'gender relational approach' to cancer care. This type of approach acknowledges that the experience of cancer, just like any experience, does not occur within a vacuum, and therefore dominant conceptions and expectations of masculinity and femininity (including those within and perpetuated by medical institutions) affect the ways in which individuals – as male and female – respond and cope with their illness.

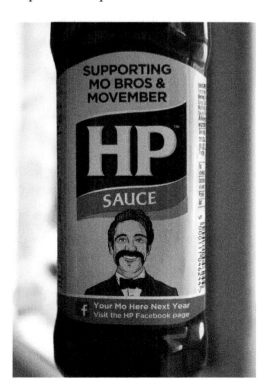

Figure 6.2 Campaigns such as Movember are focused on men's health

Activity 6.2 Cancer: a gendered experience and a gendered approach

Visit the breast cancer page on the Cancer UK web pages, then go to the one for prostate cancer. See what other pages you can find that focus on these two forms of cancer.

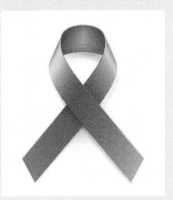

Figure 6.3 Coloured ribbons are used as fundraising and awareness symbols for several charities, including organizations focused on breast and prostate cancer

(a) Make a note of the similar and different language and images that are used to encourage issues such as cancer awareness, experience and fundraising. Do these conform to or challenge gender stereotypes? If so, in what ways? Do you think this helps or hinders the campaign?

(b) Design your own website for cancer awareness. Ensure that you pay attention to issues of gender as well as adult/child and mental health and learning disability issues as they appertain to cancer experience and cancer care.

In common with stereotypical views, just as men's 'dangerous lives' are thought to be detrimental to their health, women's mental and physical weaknesses are thought to be of major significance to women's ill health. Statistics suggest that about twice as many women as men suffer from a mental disorder. However, yet again, in reality things are more complex, as there are distinctive gender patterns associated with different mental phenomena. For example, anorexia nervosa is a predominantly female condition, and women report anxiety, phobias and depression more often than men, while substance-use disorders, personality disorders and suicide are more common among men (Featherstone, Rivett and Scourfield 2007). An evaluation of the Swedish Level-of-Living Survey by Katarina Boye in 2010 suggests that time spent on housework in part explains gender differences in psychological distress, leading Boye to argue for the need to tackle men's unequal contribution to housework. As with physical ill health, not all men and not all women are the same, and the labelling of an illness or a condition as 'women's' or 'men's' business is often inaccurate and has serious medical, social and emotional consequences.

Activity 6.3 Reproductive health

In contemporary Western society there are higher levels of infertility than ever before. At the same time there are more women (and couples) choosing to remain childless. Those who do have children are having fewer, later, and increasing numbers of babies are born following some form of 'assistance' from self-administered donated sperm to medically sophisticated procedures (Marchbank and Letherby 2014). Increasing numbers of individuals and couples are participating in 'reproductive tourism', travelling from one institution, jurisdiction or country where the treatment they require is not available to another where it is (Inhorn and Patrizio 2009). At the same time, 20 million women submit to unsafe abortion every year, and in some countries it is the most common cause of maternal death, while there is evidence of (worldwide) forced sterilization of women and girls because of HIV status, poverty or mental disability (Zampas and Lamackova 2011; Essack and Strode 2012).

- Very little information is available on the risks and benefits of various forms of contraception for women with disabilities.
- Only certain types of disabilities interfere with fertility in women.
- Some believe that eugenics and general perceptions of women with disabilities as asexual are responsible for the high rate of hysterectomy in younger women with disabilities.
- Women with disabilities may not receive the same amount of sexuality and reproductive health information from the same sources, as non-disabled women.
- Minority status and sexual orientation both have disproportionately negative impacts on women with disabilities. (Improving the Health and Wellness of Women with Disabilities: A Symposium to Establish a Research Agenda, Houston, Texas, June 2003)

Look online to see what sites you can find that focus on the health, especially reproductive health, needs of women (and men) with disabilities, including learning disabilities?

Overall, then, the expectations of both men and women and their roles and responsibilities have consequences for health. As noted earlier, despite enduring stereotypical views of women as weak and helpless, work, both paid and unpaid, is a significant aspect of women's lives. However, most research into the relationship between paid work and ill health has focused on male-dominated occupations. It is widely believed that female jobs are neither physically hazardous nor stressful, but research demonstrates otherwise (for example, Hochschild [1983] 2003; Doyal 1995; Morgan, Brandth and Kvande 2005; Bradby 2012). On your next placement, it is worth considering the extent to which you find nursing work hazardous or stressful. The sexist bias in occupational health research is further extended by traditional assumptions of women's weaknesses. For example: 'Researchers have been concerned for some time to determine whether or not menstruation interferes with women's capacity to work. They have been much less interested in how women's work affects their experiences of menstruation' (Doyal 1995: 169). The hazards of domestic work are even more hidden, although we know that being a 'good' wife and mother can make women sick. Evidence suggests that women prioritize the needs of other family members, allocating them more resources and caring for them to the detriment of their own health – not least because, as argued earlier, this is expected of them (for example, Doyal 1995; Abbott et al. 2005; Boye 2010).

Furthermore, many women and children live in danger of ill health, even death, as the result of men's emotional, psychological, sexual and physical violence (Stanko 1990; Letherby et al. 2008). Both Kelly's (1988) and Daly and Wilson's (1988) careful examination of homicide reveal men's use of violence to control their female partners across industrial and non-industrial societies. While they argue that the killing of women is relatively rare, the use of violence is not. While men's violence to women is usually characterized as 'losing control' or flying into a 'blind rage', all the evidence suggests that both battered women and the men who batter tell the same story, that men's behaviour is used as a means of control. Intimate partner violence is recognized to include acts of physical violence, such as slapping, hitting, kicking and beating; sexual violence, including forced sexual intercourse and other forms of sexual coercion; emotional (psychological) abuse, such as insults, belittling, constant humiliation, intimidation (e.g., destroying things), threats of harm, threats to take away children and controlling behaviours, including isolating a person from family and friends, monitoring their movements, and restricting access to financial resources, employment, education or medical care (WHO 2012). Although men do experience violent attacks by women, this constitutes the smallest proportion of assaults on men, and men are much more likely to be victims of physical and sexual violence from other men (Newburn and Stanko 1994; Marchbank 2008). Recent research also identifies women-to-women sexual violence (see Twinley and Addidle 2012) as a more significant issue than was previously recognized.

Overall, although differences between male and female patterns of health and illness do have some basis in biology (for example, the protective effects of oestrogen in pre-menopausal women), these patterns are more complicated than biology alone. As noted in Chapter 1, whilst sociologists accept the significance of biology, they look for social explanations of health and illness that do not rely on sexist stereotypes of 'male' and 'female' illnesses and problems. It is important that health-care practitioners understand and respond to gendered differences in health, as noted by Kelly and Hillard (2005) whose review of female genital mutilation is written with the specific aim of aiding the health-care practitioner to ensure care of affected women.

Gender and caring

Just as sexism affects the dominant views on what makes men and women sick, so it affects the treatment and care individuals receive. With reference to waiting lists, there is evidence that women are disproportionately affected in particular areas – for example, family-planning services have been significantly reduced in many parts of the UK – and their longer life expectancy means that older women are more likely than older men to be affected by the withdrawal of continuing-care beds. Domestic responsibilities, lack of transport and cultural or linguistic barriers may also affect women more (Doyal 1998; Boye 2010).

It has long been argued that diseases and illnesses that proportionately affect men in greater numbers receive more resources than those that more often affect women. More recently it has been suggested that it is not only that 'men's diseases' are taken more seriously but male patients are too. For example, in the US, men on dialysis are significantly more likely than women with the same symptoms to obtain a kidney transplant, and men with cardiac symptoms are more likely than women to be given diagnostic catheterization. The continuing failure to include women in sufficient numbers either in epidemiological research or in clinical trials has also made it difficult to investigate gender differences or to assess the overall significance of gender in the delivery of effective care (Doyal 1998; Lockyer 2009).

paternalism/paternalistic: the sexist treatment of subordinates by those in authority

In 1986 Webb suggested that **paternalism**, sexism and stereotyping formed the hallmark of much health care. For example, the cultural emphasis on breasts as objects of male sexual interest and male sexual pleasure is significant within treatment for breast cancer (Wilkinson and Kitzinger 1994) and in relation to breast augmentation (Conrad and Jacobson 2003), and women often report feeling infantilized during consultations relating to various aspects of reproduction (for example, see Earle and Letherby 2003).

When dissatisfaction with treatment is an issue, complaining can be difficult. Patients who resist may be labelled a nuisance and become unpopular with medical staff (for example, see Denny's (2009) discussion of 'heartsink patients'), which could in turn affect their experience of treatment. The 'gratitude factor' (Coyle 1999) has also been identified as a barrier to patients complaining or expressing dissatisfaction. Given assumptions of and socialization into 'appropriate' feminine behaviour, it would be easy to think that women are more likely to find it difficult to resist and complain than men. However, it is important not to view patients – male or female – as passive victims. Research suggests that both patients and doctors attempt to control and direct the consultation along their own desired line in order to persuade the other of their preferred solution (Annandale and Hunt 2000), and research on lay people's use of the Internet suggests that the information discovered is used to understand and sometimes question medical decisions (Broom 2005; Foroushani 2008).

Activity 6.4 Improving on biology/challenging nature?

Read the extract from the news story below (you may like to access the full version on the Internet) and answer the following questions.

> There's been a surprising explosion in vanity surgery for men . . . from Botox to liposuction, nose jobs to breast implants. The domain of cosmetic surgery is often associated with vain women . . . [but] a growing number of men are willing to pay thousands of pounds to improve what God, genetics or exercise couldn't! [. . .]
>
> Steve King, editor of *Men's Health* magazine, explains that this barrage of images of 'perfection' has resulted in a rush of men desperate to go under the knife . . . 'I hate to say it,' says Steve, 'but women are putting pressure on men. They want us to look like the guy from the Calvin Klein advert.' [. . .]
>
> **Facial MOT**
>
> Mike Wood is a car dealer from Stockport. He's been around the block a few times and feels his face needs an MOT. Mike decided to have Botox and Restylane to iron out his wrinkles. Mike says, 'I'm a bit of a sucker for the ladies. I'm not getting any younger so maybe I'll be able to go for a younger girl.' (BBC 2003)

(a) What gender stereotypes are supported and challenged by this extract?

(b) When is cosmetic surgery a physical/mental health care issue and when is it 'vanity'? Is this different for men and for women?

(c) Should gender reassignment (sex-change) surgery, bariatric (weight-loss) surgery, surgery for Down's syndrome children to make eyes look more 'normal' and tongues less protruding, and skin whitening for black and Asian people be funded by the NHS? Would the sex of the person concerned affect your decision?

(d) Find some more surgery news stories and reflect on the significance of gendered stereotypes, roles and responsibilities to the decisions and experiences of all those involved.

The response to sexism in health care has a history of at least thirty-five years. A number of books with the aim of informing women about their own bodies and their own health hit the bookshops in the 1970s (perhaps the best known being *Our Bodies Ourselves*, first published by the Boston Women's Health Book Collective in 1973). These were written by women and were grounded in women's experiences. However, as Hockey (1997) notes, these early texts were relevant mostly for white middle-class audiences, and it was not until the 1980s that books aimed at black, lesbian, working-class and older women began to appear. There are fewer books even today specifically concerned with men's health, although during the 1990s men's health was an increasing concern within the media, with reports on increasing stress and incidences of cancer, declining fertility and reluctance to visit the doctor (Watson 2000). In turn, all of this has led to further

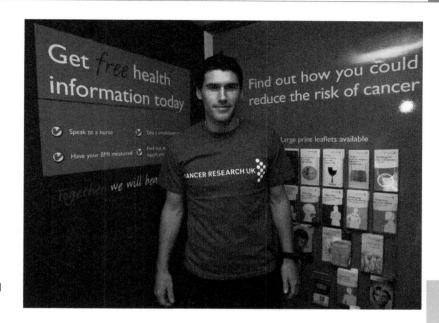

Figure 6.4 Men are sometimes reluctant to seek health advice; health promotion campaigns featuring footballers are designed to appeal to men

debate on the state of men's health and what to do about it. Attempts in the UK to encourage men to pay more attention to their health have included the production of a men's health manual modelled on the car manuals produced by Haynes (and the reference to a 'facial MOT' in Activity 6.4 perhaps demonstrates a different use of the analogy of the man's body as a car).

With their emphasis on empowerment, many of the personal health texts stress the fact that individuals should take control of their own bodies and minds and be active rather than passive. Empowerment from this perspective, then, often suggests resistance to the dominant medical model and supports 'alternative' health care. Yet there is a problem here, as the dominant message from many alternative health-care self-help books and tapes is that we become ill because of unhealthy attitudes and that we can cure ourselves.

Activity 6.5 Gender, health and media

Compare these two adverts for magazines promoting health and fitness:

- *Men's Health* is the best-selling men's lifestyle magazine in the world! Every month we're on hand with all the tips and expert advice you'll ever need to get you in peak condition. In *Men's Health* every month you'll find: Fitness, Health, Style, Gear, Sex & Relationships, Weight-loss, Grooming & Food & Nutrition. So if you're looking for success in the style stakes, to be the fittest in the field, the best in the boardroom and the bedroom or simply the happiest and healthiest you can be, make *Men's Health* your choice.
- *Women's Health* is the first UK lifestyle magazine to provide her with the best in health, beauty, fashion, weight loss, fitness, nutrition, celebrity, love and sex, all wrapped up in one super glossy lifestyle title.

(a) Look at a paper or online copy of *Men's Health* and *Women's Health*. What issues, in addition to health, are being advertised here? These and other magazines report regularly on health issues. What are the implications of this for individuals' understanding and your experience as providers of health care?

(b) Find some other examples of women's and men's magazines that have articles on health. Can you identify any differences in the articles aimed at men from those aimed at women?

One of the most important attractions of complementary and alternative medicines (CAM) is that they offer the possibility of 'stepping out of the victim role'. However, Wilkinson and Kitzinger (1994) argue that this deflects attention from the state's failure to provide health services for all society's members. Furthermore, the medical profession's authority as the arbiter of 'truth' in health care creates barriers for the professionalization of CAM groups (Kelner et al. 2004) and for general public perceptions of CAMs. Wilkinson and Kitzinger (1994), by contrast, recognizing the problems inherent in both traditional and alternative health-care provisions, note that a **feminist** analysis of health and illness begins by acknowledging that women (and some men) are victims of a patriarchal world which perpetuates gendered inequalities in health. Different foods and food groups are categorized as 'good' or 'bad', and increasingly food is being considered as CAM. In her research on everyday foodways (which she defines as the multiplicity of ways of 'doing' food, including all aspects of everyday food practices, from acquiring food, growing it, shopping for it, preparing, cooking, sharing and eating in/outside the domestic sphere), Parsons (2015) found that, perhaps not surprisingly, it is usually mothers, rather than fathers, who take responsibility for feeding the family appropriate food, including CAM foods. Feminists advocate campaigns and community action to change current medical, social and political attitudes (e.g., Wilkinson and Kitzinger 1994; Lorber and Moore 2002). Theories of social structure are relevant here, in that the structure of society is seen to perpetuate gendered inequalities in health (see also Chapter 3).

Obviously, it is not only women who are disempowered by the health service. Male members of economically and ethnically marginalized or disadvantaged groups are likely to find it hard too. Such groups are increasingly being brought within the policy gaze (Watson 2000; Featherstone, Rivett and Scourfield 2007). In addition there remains the problem in unequal help-seeking practices (between men and women), with heterosexual middle-aged men (Watson 2000) and both younger and older men (Featherstone, Rivett and Scourfield 2007) being identified as less visible groups in practice.

feminist:
relating to the political theory and practice that challenges the oppression of women

4 Diversity and difference

As Di Stephano (1990: 78) argues, gender is significant and functions as 'a difference that makes a difference' to our lives. However, when we do consider differences between men and women we need to remember that 'Much of what it is to be human and live in societies is the same for men and women' (Carpenter 2000: 48). Also, as you will become aware from the other chapters in this part of the book, gender is not the only 'difference' that we need to take seriously. Differences of age, class, sexuality, ethnicity, and physical and learning disability are also relevant to our experience of health, illness and health care.

Taking ethnicity as an example, we know that 'race' adversely affects black women's and men's experiences in relation to health (and, indeed, all other areas of social life). Yet 'race' is not a coherent category (see also Chapter 12), and the lives of those usually classified together under the label 'black' can be very different. Thus, culture, class, religion, nationality, sexuality, age and so on, in addition to gender, can all have an impact on women's and men's lives, and it is necessary to challenge the homogeneity of experience previously ascribed to women by virtue of being 'black'. For example, as Douglas (1998) notes, the health status of black and ethnic-minority women in the UK reflects the interaction between their experiences of race, gender, class and culture (see also Chapter 12). So health and well-being are determined in these groups of women by a complex mixture of social and psychological influences and biological and genetic factors.

Ethnic-minority women are not a homogeneous group with uniform needs: 'They may be South Asian, Asian, Chinese, Vietnamese, African or African-Caribbean. They may have been born in the UK, may have migrated recently and may be refugees. They may have disabilities, be older, be lesbian' (Douglas 1998: 70). Further, as Maynard (1994) points out, individuals do not have to be black to experience racism, as attention to the historical and contemporary experience of Jewish and Irish people demonstrates.

The issue of HIV/AIDS not only demonstrates further the need to consider gender in connection with other differences, but also indicates the political complexity of health inequalities and responses to these:

> professionals and volunteers in the HIV field worked hard in the late 1980s and early 1990s to get across the message that anyone could contract HIV through unsafe practices and that it was unprotected sex or shared needles that posed risks rather than so-called 'high risk groups'. This was a conscious attempt at an anti-discriminatory strategy and was understandable in the context of homophobic discourse of gay men being to blame for HIV/AIDS. However, activists such as Gay Men Fighting AIDS set out to challenge this consensus among those working in care and prevention on the basis that by far the greatest number of people getting ill and dying were in fact gay men. (Featherstone, Rivett and Scourfield 2007: 122)

6

Thus, as the examples in this section indicate, in addition to taking gender seriously, other aspects of difference should be taken equally seriously, remembering to consider when and how gender intersects and overlaps with other aspects of difference.

Summary and Resources

Summary

▶ The historical definition of women as weaker – both physically and emotionally – affects contemporary definitions, and, when asked to think of a healthy person, most people choose a man.

▶ The view that men die but women are more likely to get sick simplifies the complex relationship between gender and health.

▶ Women's and men's roles and responsibilities do have consequences for health, so patterns of health and illness relate to more than biological differences. Having said this, it is important not to rely on sexist stereotypes of 'male' and 'female' illnesses and problems, and to remember that gender is a fluid and not a fixed category.

▶ Dominant views on what makes men and women sick also affect the treatment and care individuals receive, and there is some evidence to suggest that 'men's diseases' and male patients are taken more seriously. However, both men and women are able to challenge and resist medical dominance.

▶ It is clear that gender is significant to the health and well-being of men and women, and boys and girls, but it is also important to consider how gender intersects with other aspects of difference, such as age, class, sexuality, ethnicity, and physical and learning dis/ability.

Questions for Discussion

1 Why and how is gender significant when we consider issues of health and illness?

2 Why and how is gender significant when we consider the care of the sick? To what extent have you been aware of this significance during your placements?

3 Why is it important to consider the relationship between gender and other aspects of difference and diversity when considering health and illness and the care of the sick?

Glossary

emotion work:	the regulation, management and care of one's own and others' feelings and emotions; a related term is 'emotion labour'; some authors use the term 'labour' with reference to paid work and 'work' for such endeavours within personal relationships, while others use the terms interchangeably
feminist:	relating to the political theory and practice that challenges the oppression of women; the belief that all people are entitled to the same civil rights and liberties regardless of gender
gender:	cultural differences between males and females which relate to societal norms, values and expectations; often mistakenly confused with 'sex' (the biological differences between males and females)
hysteria:	a term first coined by Hippocrates, derived from the Greek word *hystera*, or 'uterus'; the theory of female hysteria gained popularity in the works of Sigmund Freud in the early twentieth century and then by Jean-Martin Charcot, a French neurologist; hysteria is often defined as exaggerated or uncontrollable emotion or excitement
masculinity and femininity:	the ways in which men and women are expected to behave, think and feel; as such, masculinity and femininity relate to gender, rather than to biological differences (sex)
paternalism/paternalistic:	the sexist treatment of subordinates by those in authority; often presented in the supposed interest of subordinates (in this case women and girls)
sex:	the biological differences between males and females; thus, a physiological descriptor

6

Further Reading

H. Bradby: *Medicine, Health and Society*. London: Sage, 2012.
A useful book all round. See Chapter 4 for a discussion of the relationship between gender, health and feminism.

E. Annandale and K. Hunt (eds): *Gender Inequalities in Health*.
Buckingham: Open University Press, 2000.
A useful book that focuses on both male and female experience. The book not only provides detailed insight into gender differences but considers the relationship between sex and gender and other differences. Thus, attention is given to (amongst other things) social class, age and cross-cultural issues.

J. Lorber and L. J. Moore: *Gender and the Social Construction of Illness*,
2nd edn. New York: AltaMira Press, 2002.
Difference and diversity are also a key theme within this text, as are agency and resistance in relation to health care.

J. Marchbank and G. Letherby: *Introduction to Gender: Social Science Perspectives*, 2nd edn. London: Routledge, 2014.
Useful as a general introduction to the study of gender.

World Health Organisation (WHO) Gender page: <http://www.who.int/topics/gender/en/>
This page is useful for international concerns and issues, and for access to useful publications.

Also useful are the following website resources:

CHANGE: Centre for Health and Gender Equity <http://www.genderhealth.org/>.

eldis: <http://www.eldis.org/go/topics/resource-guides/gender/websites/gender-and-health#.Va_NnvlViko> Look here for access to a whole raft of web-based resources.

References

Abbott, P., Wallace. C. and Tyler, M. 2005 *An Introduction to Sociology: Feminist Perspectives*. London: Routledge.

Ahmed, S. 2004 *The Cultural Politics of Emotion*. London: Routledge.

Annandale, E. and Clark, J. 1996 What is gender? Feminist theory and the sociology of human reproduction. *Sociology of Health & Illness* 18/1: 17–44.

Annandale, E. and Hunt, K. (eds) 2000: *Gender Inequalities in Health*. Buckingham: Open University Press.

BBC 2003 Cosmetic surgery for men. *Inside Out*, 6 January; available at: <www.bbc.co.uk/insideout/northwest/series2/cosmetic_surgery_men_vanity_botox_restylane.shtml>.

Blaxter, M. 1990 *Health and Lifestyles*. London: Tavistock/Routledge.

Boston Women's Health Book Collective [1973] 1998: *Our Bodies Ourselves*, 25th anniversary edn. New York: Touchstone.

Boye, K. 2010 Time spent working: paid work, house work and gender differences in psychological distress. *European Societies* 50/10: 419–42.

Bradby, H. 2008 *Medical Sociology: An Introduction*. London: Sage.

Bradby, H. 2012 *Medicine, Health and Society*. London: Sage.

Broom, A. 2005 Virtually he@lthy: the impact of internet use on disease experience and the doctor–patient relationship. *Qualitative Health Research* 15/3: 325–45.

Carpenter, M. 2000 Reinforcing the pillars: rethinking gender, social divisions and health. In E. Annandale and K. Hunt (eds), *Gender Inequalities and Health*. Buckingham: Open University Press, pp. 36–63.

Conrad, P. and Jacobson, T. J. 2003 'Enhancing' biology: cosmetic surgery and breast augmentation. In S. J. Williams, L. Birke and G. Bendelow (eds), *Debating Biology: Sociological Reflections on Health, Medicine and Society*. London: Routledge, pp. 223–34.

Coppock, V., Haydon, D. and Richter, I. 1995 *The Illusions of 'Post-Feminism': New Women, Old Myths*. London: Taylor & Francis.

Courtenay, W. H. 2000 Constructions of masculinity and their influence on men's well-being: a theory of gender and health. *Social Science and Medicine* 50/10: 1386–401.

Coyle, J. 1999 Exploring the meaning of 'dissatisfaction' with health care: the importance of 'personal identity threat'. *Sociology of Health & Illness* 21/1: 95–123.

Daly, M. and Wilson, M. 1988 *Homicide: Foundations of Human Behaviour*. New York: Aldine de Gruyter.

Deery, R., Denny, E. and Letherby, G. 2015 *Sociology for Midwives*. Cambridge: Polity.

Denny, E. 2009 Heartsink patients and intractable conditions. In E. Denny and S. Earle (eds), *The Sociology of Long Term Conditions and Nursing Practice*. Basingstoke: Palgrave Macmillan, pp. 246–65.

Di Stephano, C. 1990 Dilemmas of difference: feminism, modernity and post-modernism. In L. Nicholson (ed.), *Feminism/Postmodernism*. London: Routledge, pp. 63–82.

Dolan, A. 2007 'Good luck to them if they can get it': exploring working-class men's understandings and experiences of income inequality and material standards. *Sociology of Health & Illness* 29/5: 711–29.

Douglas, J. 1998 Meeting the health needs of women from black and minority ethnic communities. In L. Doyal (ed.), *Women and Health Care Services*. Buckingham: Open University Press, pp. 69–82.

Doyal, L. 1995 *What Makes Women Sick: Gender and the Political Economy of Health*. Basingstoke: Macmillan.

Doyal, L. (ed.) 1998 *Women and Health Services: An Agenda for Change*. Buckingham: Open University Press.

Earle, S. and Letherby, G. (eds) 2003 *Gender, Identity and Reproduction: Social Perspectives*. Basingstoke: Palgrave.

Emslie, C. and Hunt, K. 2008 'Gender and health': their influence on menences in psychological distress. *Social Science and Medicine* 67: 808–16.

Essack, Z. and Strode, A. 2012. 'I feel like half a woman all the time': the impacts of coerced and forced sterilizations on HIV-positive women in South Africa. *Agenda: Empowering Women for Gender Equity* 26/2: 24–34.

Evans, M. 1997 *Introducing Contemporary Feminist Thought*. Cambridge: Polity.

6

Featherstone, B., Rivett, M. and Scourfield, J. 2007 *Working with Men in Health and Social Care*. London: Sage.

Foroushani, P. S. 2008 The internet: a place for different voices in health and medicine? A case study of attention deficit hyperactivity disorder. *Mental Health Review Journal* 13/1: 33–40.

Frith, H. and Kitzinger, C. 1998 'Emotion work' as a participant resource: a feminist analysis of young women's talk-in- interaction. *Sociology* 32/2: 299–320.

Galdas, P. M., Cheater, F. and Marshall, P. 2005 Men and help-seeking behaviour: literature review. *Journal of Advanced Nursing* 49/6: 616–23.

Gunew, S. (ed.) 1990 *Feminist Knowledge: Critique and Construct*. London: Routledge.

Hochschild, A. R. [1983] 2003 *The Managed Heart: Commercialization of Human Feeling*, 20th anniversary edn. Berkeley, CA: University of California Press.

Hockey, J. 1997 Women and health. In D. Richardson and V. Robinson (eds), *Introducing Women's Studies*, 2nd edn. London: Macmillan, pp. 250–71.

Inhorn, M. C. and Patrizio, P. 2009 Rethinking Reproductive 'Tourism' as Reproductive 'Exile'. *Fertility and Sterility* 92/3: 904–6.

Kelly, E. and Hillard, P. J. A. 2005 Female genital mutilation. *Current Opinion in Obstetrics and Gynecology* 17/5: 490–4.

Kelly, L. 1988 *Surviving Sexual Violence*. Cambridge: Polity.

Kelner, M., Wellman, B., Boon, H. and Welsh, S. 2004 Responses of established healthcare to the professionalization of complementary and alternative medicine in Ontario. *Social Science and Medicine* 59/5: 915–30.

King, M. and McKeown, E. 2003 *Mental Health and Social Wellbeing of Gay Men, Lesbians and Bisexuals in England and Wales*. London: Mind.

Letherby, G. 2003 *Feminist Research in Theory and Practice*. Buckingham: Open University Press.

Letherby, G., Williams, K., Birch, P. and Cain, M. (eds) 2008 *Sex as Crime*. Cullompton, Devon: Willan.

Lockyer, L. 2009 Coronary heart disease: moving from acute to long term accounts. In E. Denny and S. Earle (eds), *The Sociology of Long Term Conditions and Nursing Practice*. Basingstoke: Palgrave Macmillan, pp. 108–26.

Lorber, J. and Moore, L. J. 2002 *Gender and the Social Construction of Illness*, 2nd edn. New York: AltaMira Press.

Marchbank, J. 2008 War and sex crime. In G. Letherby, K. Williams, P. Birch and M. Cain (eds), *Sex as Crime*. Cullompton, Devon: Willan, pp. 238–52.

Marchbank, J. and Letherby, G. 2014 *Introduction to Gender: Social Science Perspectives*, 2nd edn. Abingdon: Routledge.

Maynard, M. 1994 'Race, gender and the concept of 'difference' in feminist thought. In H. Afshar and M. Maynard (eds), *The Dynamics of 'Race' and Gender: Some Feminist Interventions*. London: Taylor & Francis, pp. 9–25.

Miers, M. 2000 *Gender Issues and Nursing Practices*. Basingstoke: Macmillan.

Mills, J. 1991 *Womanwords*. London: Virago.

Morgan, D., Brandth, B. and Kvande, E. 2005 *Gender, Bodies and Work*. Aldershot: Ashgate.

Moynihan, C. 2002 Men, women, gender and cancer. *European Journal of Cancer Care* 11/3: 166–17.

Newburn, T. and Stanko, E. A. 1994 When men are victims: the failure of victimology. In T. Newburn and E. A. Stanko (eds), *Just Boys Doing Business? Men, Masculinities and Crime*. London: Routledge, pp. 153–65.

Oakley, A. 1972 *Sex, Gender and Society*. London: Temple Smith.

Oakley, A. 1981 *Subject Women*. Oxford: Martin Robinson.

Office for National Statistics (ONS) 2014 *10 Most Common Cancers among Males and Females*. Part of the Cancer Statistics Registrations, England, No 43, 2012. Available at: <http://www.ons.gov.uk/ons/rel/vsob1/cancer-statistics-registrations--england--series-mb1-/no--43--2012/info-most-common-cancers.html>.

Parsons, J. M. 2015 'Good' food as family medicine: problems of dualist and absolutist approaches to 'healthy' family foodways. *Journal of Food Studies* 4/2: 1–13.

Stanko, E. A. 1990 *Everyday Violence: How Women and Men Experience Sexual and Physical Danger*. London: Pandora.

Twinley, R. and Addidle, G. 2012 Considering violence: the dark side of occupation. *British Journal of Occupational Therapy* 75/4: 202–4.

Wajcman, J. 1991 *Feminism Confronts Technology*. Cambridge: Polity.

Watson, J. 2000 *Male Bodies: Health, Culture and Identity*. Buckingham: Open University Press.

Webb, C. 1986 *Feminist Practice in Women's Health Care*. Chichester: John Wiley.

Wilkinson, S. and Kitzinger, C. 1994 Towards a feminist approach to breast cancer. In S. Wilkinson and C. Kitzinger (eds), *Women and Health: Feminist Perspectives*. London: Taylor & Francis, pp. 124–40.

World Health Organization (WHO) 2012 *Understanding and Addressing Violence against Women: Intimate Partner Violence*. Available at: <http://apps.who.int/iris/bitstream/10665/77432/1/WHO_RHR_12.36_eng.pdf?ua=1>.

Zampas, C. and Lamackova, A. 2011 Forced and coerced sterilization of women in Europe. *International Journal of Gynecology & Obstetrics* 114/2: 163–6.

6

The Family, Health and Caring

Elaine Denny

KEY ISSUES IN THIS CHAPTER:

▶ The concept of the family.
▶ Sociological perspectives on the family.
▶ Health and the family.
▶ The family and caring.

BY THE END OF THIS CHAPTER YOU SHOULD BE ABLE TO:

▶ Understand the nuclear family and family diversity.
▶ Discuss sociological perspectives on the family.
▶ Explore the link between family life, health, illness and caring.
▶ Recognize the need to challenge common-sense ideas around the family.

1 Introduction

This chapter considers the relationships between the family, health, illness and caring. It begins by exploring some of the debates around families and then moves on to highlight some of the relevant issues when considering the impact of the family on health, illness and caring. The aim of the chapter is to draw your attention to the fact that sick people are often part of a family, and families can play an important role in patient care. However, families also hold the potential to make people sick!

In recent times, there has been an ideological shift in thinking about the family and health. In particular, there has been a conscious move away from all-encompassing, state-provided health care, to an emphasis on self-care and care by families. It appears that the family has a greater role in health care than ever before, but what are the consequences of this shift? How are families coping with this increased pressure to care for sick, frail or disabled family members and maintain the health of the nation? Arguably, with increases in unemployment, poverty and one-parent families and the greater involvement of women in paid work, the ability of the family to take on an even bigger role in health care is in question. The family has an increasingly major role in health care; however, before considering this, it is important to ask: what is 'the family'?

Activity 7.1 Defining 'the family'

It is useful, before you even begin to read further in this chapter, to start thinking about how you would define the family.

(a) Write down what immediately comes to mind when you think about the family.
(b) Who are the members of your family?
(c) How important are the people you have identified as members of your family in your everyday life?

---

2 The concept of 'the family'

Most of us are born into families and, whether we choose or not, we spend most of our childhood and teenage years within 'our family' (Bernardes 1997: 1).

Look at what you have written down for Activity 7.1. What is important to recognize is that definitions of the family change and 'the family' can mean different things to different people, according to their personal circumstances and life experiences. Writing about the challenges of diversity when working with families, Doane and Varcoe note:

> At times we find ourselves in situations where we are working with families who come from backgrounds, religious faiths, or life situations different from our own. As nurses we provide care to people and/or families whose values we do not share and who we may see making choices different than those we would make. We may find ourselves in relation with families where members harm one another or where it is difficult to connect because some family members are absent. (Doane and Varcoe 2006: 7–8)

Common sense and 'the family'

There is a common-sense understanding of what we mean when we talk of 'the family'. Common-sense understandings of the family mask the complexities of family life (see Chapter 1 for further discussion of 'common-sense' understandings). This masking perpetuates and maintains images of supposedly normal families and the naturalness of roles ascribed to individual family members. It prevents us from understanding the impact of differences such as gender, class, ethnicity, racism, sexuality, and so on, on family life. Thinking about the family sociologically enables us to unpick these overarching common-sense understandings. Sociological explanations of the family challenge common-sense assumptions and understandings and allow us to recognize that society, today, throughout history and across cultures, encompasses a diversity of family forms. It also enables us to question the 'natural' roles assumed by individual family members; for example, women's innate ability to care. With specific reference to the purpose of this chapter, understanding the diversity of family life is important; as Bond and Bond (1994) argue, the family is the context within which health is maintained and where illness occurs and is resolved.

For health professionals who are moving beyond common-sense understandings, recognizing the complexities of family life is important when providing a more holistic approach to health care.

3 Sociological perspectives on the family

The 'universal' nuclear family

An important starting point is to recognize that families are social, not natural, phenomena; therefore, they change over time and are influenced by social, economic and political developments. However, in Western societies there has existed a powerful assumption of a universal family form. The concept of 'the family' has rested on the image of a **nuclear family** consisting of a husband, wife and their dependent children, living together and connected by mutual affection, care and support (Scott, Treas and Richards 2004). This family type has been powerful and influential and exists as a standard of how sexual, emotional and parental responsibility should be structured. There now exists an enormous body of work that contains many different explanations pertinent to the existence, the functions and the role of 'the family' in society, some of which are considered below.

nuclear family:
this comprises merely parents (or parent) and their dependent child(ren)

Functionalist perspectives on the family

One of the most prominent and influential sociological attempts to explain the existence of the family was put forward by Talcott Parsons (1955) (see also Chapter 1). Parsons' theory about the family was prominent in the 1950s and 1960s and was based on research carried out with American middle-class families. From Parsons' perspective, it is argued that families exist because of the functions they perform, and, consequently, families have evolved over time because of the role they play in helping us meet the social and economic demands of society. However, what is crucial in the functionalist analysis is the notion of the evolution of the nuclear family. These small **kin groups**

kin groups:
social relationships based on blood ties and marriage

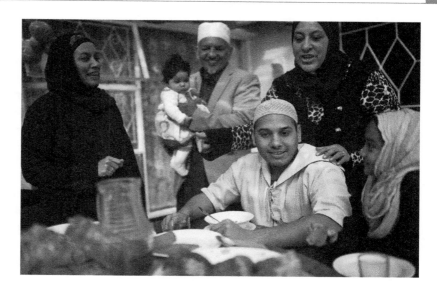

Figure 7.1 An extended kin group

7

have evolved to fit the needs of an industrial economy. Prior to the rise of industrialization, Parsons suggests, there existed large kin groups that performed a variety of functions vital to the group's survival. The smaller kin group – the nuclear family – emerged from the fact that the family was no longer required to perform many of the functions required before industrialization; for example, economic, education, health and welfare functions. The functions were increasingly shifting away from the family to become the responsibility of the newly developing state institutions, such as education and health care. It is these smaller kin groups that Parsons argues were better able than large kin groups to perform the specialized functions essential to the maintenance of society.

The nuclear family consists of a breadwinner/husband and a homemaker/wife and dependent children. There is a clear distinction between the roles of the wife/mother and the husband/father. The husband/father role is to provide economically for his family. The wife/mother role is primarily concerned with looking after the well-being of the husband and children. In the functionalist account, these roles arose out of the biological differences between women and men and primarily out of women's reproductive capability. For example, Parsons (1955) argues that the two most important functions performed by the nuclear family are the socialization of children and the provision of psychological support for adults. As Cheal (2002) argues, functionalism is a theoretical approach that emphasizes the positive benefits of families; that is, the socialization of children enables them to grow into valuable, productive, law-abiding members of society.

Critiques of functionalist perspectives

Functionalist accounts, like those of Parsons, have not been without their critics. The assertion made by Parsons that industrialization brought about a decrease in family size has been challenged. Research done by Laslett (1972), for example, demonstrates that household size remained fairly constant and that even before industrialization the nuclear family was predominant. He suggests that from the Middle Ages the most common family form was that of the nuclear family, and this appears to have been the norm even in the most rural of families. There is also the suggestion that geographical mobility was a common occurrence in pre-industrial society; for example, children were often sent away to go into domestic service or take up apprenticeships. This challenges Parsons' notion that the nuclear family evolved to fit the needs of an industrial society. With regard to the **extended family** or wider kin networks, Laslett points out that, owing to high mortality rates, very few children were likely to have parents alive when they got married, again challenging the idea that the nuclear family evolved from larger kin groupings. Laslett argues that the pre-industrial nuclear family was able to adapt relatively easily to industrialization.

extended family: three or more generations of relatives living together or in close proximity

In contemporary Western societies, the maintenance of health and well-being is sometimes not believed to be a vital function of the modern nuclear family. In Britain, the National Health Service (NHS) dominates the provision of health care, yet, despite this, we know that the health services do not act alone. For example, when we are ill, our contact with the NHS is often limited to making a brief visit to the doctor's surgery. Indeed, there are few of us requiring long-term specialist hospital care. The tending of those who are ill and recovering from illness and the care of the long-term sick and disabled is, on the whole, done by families and, in particular, women. There is an implicit recognition that without this informal care, medical institutions would not be able to cope. Furthermore, with policy developments within the health arena, for example community care and its underlying principles, it is possible to argue that this function has never been lost and the assumption remains that care will be provided by the family (see Chapter 15 for further discussion of non-institutional care). It is also important to note that the duty on the family to care is not imposed just upon the nuclear family, but on all families, and particularly on all wives, mothers and daughters.

Feminist perspectives on the family

Not all sociologists have described the family in a positive light. Feminist accounts have recognized the implications of the nuclear family for all women's lives (see also Chapter 6). The separation of the home from the workplace that emerged in the nineteenth century has implications for all women and their role within families. The legacy of nineteenth-century domestic ideology and the image of the 'angel in the home' (Hall 1982: 18) impact upon women's roles today. Victorian middle-class ideology (see Chapter 1 for a definition of ideology) identified mothers and wives who went out to work as endangering the whole of society. Engels (1845), for example, wrote that the wife's employment would not dissolve the family entirely but turn it upside down. If the wife supports the family and the husband sits at home and looks after the children and performs domestic tasks, the result would be the unsexing of the sexes. Engels goes on to argue that men would be left without their masculinity and women without their 'true' femininity (see Chapter 6 for a definition of these terms). What is evident here is the linking of masculinity to paid work and femininity to domestic labour and childcare. It is important to note the similarities with functionalist allocation of gender-specific roles, with the emphasis on the 'naturalness' of women's role as rooted in her biology.

When talking about families, Engels was not referring to all family forms but to a specific family form, the nuclear family. Engels' thoughts reflect those held by many middle-class commentators of the time. These sentiments were reinforced through legislation; for example, the Factory Acts of the 1840s limited children's and women's employment. This further reinforced the notion of women's role and encouraged their economic dependence upon the husband/father (Barrett and McIntosh 1991).

At the end of the nineteenth century, with the recognition in political circles that the working-class male child was a national asset, the health and welfare of children became entrenched in state practices. Connections were made, not to structural inequalities, but to immoral mothers who neglected their children by going out to work. The responsibility for the health of children and, implicitly, the future health of the nation, was placed firmly in women's hands. It became increasingly clear that a woman's role within the family was to care not just for dependent children but also for her husband.

By the twentieth century, normal family life had come to be defined by the breadwinning husband and the domesticated wife. Women's role was firmly located within the private sphere and women were responsible for caring for the family in health and, usually, in sickness. The role of men was located within the public sphere, as the economic provider responsible for financial stability and the **material** well-being of the family. These gender-specific roles have implications when we consider issues relating to family life, health, illness and caring.

Feminist critics of the family have highlighted how male breadwinning and the accompanying family-wage ideology have prohibited, and continue to prohibit, women from gaining equal access to paid work. The dependence of women and children on a male breadwinner creates a damaging power imbalance within the family. These inequalities are maintained by the state through social and economic policies that assume families contain a male breadwinner and a woman who is

material:
relating to economic factors

7

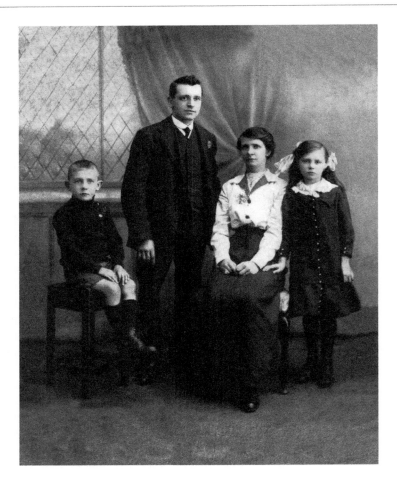

Figure 7.2 The traditional nuclear family

responsible for childcare and domestic work (Budig 2004). As Jackson (1997: 328) argues, 'family ties are ties of economic co-operation of support and dependency, but also inequality and exploitation'.

The representation of the family as heterosexual (whereby the only sexual relations to be sanctioned were those between husband and wife for the purpose of reproduction), class-specific (the family form of the new middle classes), and gender-specific (with its particular division of labour), has had far-reaching consequences. While this ideal may not have been the reality for many poor working-class families in the twentieth century, it was pervasive at that time, and while it is not the reality for a great many people today, its legacy lives on (Weeks, Heaphy and Donovam 2004).

Activity 7.2 The legacy of the nuclear family

(a) How important do you think the legacy of the nuclear family is today?

(b) Can you think of any examples of how the ideology of the nuclear family impacts on everyday life?

(c) How might the legacy of the nuclear family affect patient care?

4 Diversity and family form

This ideal becomes problematic when one takes into consideration the diversity of family life that exists in the UK today. The statistical bulletin for 2014 (ONS 2014) gives us an indication of this diversity. It shows there are 26.7 million households in England and Wales, and 28 per cent of these are one-person households. Of these, 4.1 million were aged sixteen to sixty-four, and 58 per cent were male. This may be due to a higher number of men never marrying or marrying later, or because following a relationship breakdown women are more likely to live with the children from that relationship (ONS 2014). The number of dependent children living in a one-parent household remained fairly static between 2004 and 2014, with 91 per cent of those headed by a woman. In 2004, 11 per cent of children lived in heterosexual cohabiting-couple families, and, by 2014, this was 14 per cent. This is the biggest change in household type for dependent children. Increasingly, families are 'blended'; that is, children living with one natural parent, but also with a step-parent, and possibly step-siblings, as new relationships form following the break-up of the parental one. The Marriages (same-sex couples) Act 2013 allowed for same-sex couples in England and Wales to marry from March 2014, and so this may lead to other changes in family form, with homosexual couples adopting children or using a third party to assist them in having their own children.

7

So it is evident that a large number of people do not live in a traditional nuclear family. The issue here is that if welfare, and in particular health policy, rests on the implicit assumption that maintaining health and caring are important functions of the family, and 'the family' is viewed in the context of the nuclear family, then we need to consider the implications for all those people who do not live in this type of family and do not have access to the resources the nuclear family provides.

It is acknowledged that health care comes from a variety of sources; for example, the state, private markets, volunteers, family and friends. However, the care provided by family and friends is recognized to be the most fundamental (Graham 1999). In what is now a landmark document, the Griffiths Report (1988: 5) states, 'Families, friends and other local people provide the majority of care in response to needs that they are uniquely well placed to identify and respond to. . . . The proposals take as their starting point that this is how it should be.' So it is clear that, while in the UK we do have state-provided health care in the form of the National Health Service, state-provided health care cannot exist without the large amount of caring work carried out in and by the family. We could suggest that it is important to draw on informal sources of caring, and indeed families can be a vital source of support to some people. But, as will be demonstrated, these normative assumptions can have serious consequences for individuals caring and being cared for within the family. Relying on the family to provide an

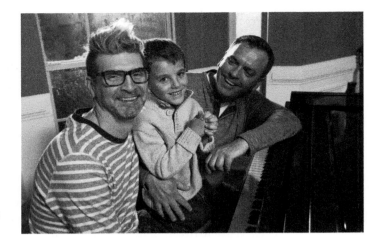

Figure 7.3 Families are becoming increasingly diverse, which has implications for nursing practice

informal network of care can be problematic. It is important not to assume that all families have the propensity to provide informal care.

Activity 7.3 Diversity, the family and health

The following extract is taken from an article published in the *Guardian Online* as part of a series on 'the world in 2020'. Read the extract and then answer the questions below.

> [A]ll are agreed that by 2020 it will be very hard to talk of a 'typical family', such will be the variety of shapes and types of families.
>
> The most marked characteristic of families since the 1960s has been that the traditional conception of the British family has disintegrated. The married couple with 2.4 children is disappearing. The sequence of life events – marriage, sex and children – has been radically reordered. Marriage rarely comes first and increasingly does not happen at all. Over the past 30 years, levels of cohabitation have trebled, the number of babies born outside marriage has quintupled, and the number of single-parent families has trebled.
>
> The most dramatic change, however, has been to the 'happy ever after' bit in the picture of family life. In the past 30 years, the rate of divorce has doubled; and half of all children now experience their parents' divorce before they are 16.
>
> All four trends – cohabitation, divorce, births outside marriage and single parents – are likely to be even more pronounced by 2020 . . . There will be dozens of different types of co-parenting arrangements, with combinations of stepfamilies, or adults with children from previous relationships entering long-term relationships with others in the same position but choosing not to live together . . .
>
> One of the most dramatic social changes of the past 30 years has been in women's patterns of employment. In the UK the proportion of women in full-time employment has trebled in the past 30 years and maternal employment has leapt from 57% to 65% during the 1990s . . . The norm in families now is for one male full-time worker and one female part-time. By 2020, more women will be the primary breadwinner . . . (Bunting, 2007, online)

(a) Consider the implications for future health-care provision by the family.

(b) What significance might this have for nurses (in their professional *and* personal lives)?

5 The family, health and caring

Families play an important role in caring for sick, frail and disabled people. As mentioned previously, most of us have minimal contact with formal health institutions, and when we are ill the majority of our care takes place within the family. It is estimated that there are 6.5 million **carers** in the UK and that one in eight adults is a carer (Carers UK 2014), saving the public purse an estimated £119 billion per year (Carers UK 2011). Caring for others can often be very demanding and time-consuming. While it may involve the normal daily tasks we associate with caring for the well, these often need to be performed more frequently. In addition, although family carers do not constitute a homogeneous group and there are clear generational and cultural differences, amongst others, there are some general characteristics that can be identified amongst carers. For example, a survey of people caring by Carers UK in 2014 found:

carers:
people who help a partner, friend or relative without payment

- high levels of stress, depressed mood and sleep disturbance;
- reduced earnings, and a struggle to pay household bills;
- employment difficulties, including juggling work and caring
- poor health and difficulty in accessing health care for themselves;
- inability to provide for their own future;
- social isolation;
- feeling undervalued by society.

(Carers UK, 2014)

7

The role of caring for others often becomes the responsibility of female family members, as this role can be perceived as an extension of the normal caring that women perform within the family; and this holds true across all ethnic groups (Department of Health 2008). Some of the factors identified above may adversely affect women to a greater extent than other family members. While most illnesses may be considered minor and requiring a relatively short period of care, caring for people who are frail, chronically ill or disabled can be a long-term commitment that can have a significant impact on family life. Families often take on this role because there is a lack of appropriate services for those with complex health-care needs.

To illustrate the point we are making here, it will be useful to consider the effect of childhood asthma on families. Statistics suggest that one in eleven children (1.1 million) in the UK has asthma and, in 2011, eighteen children aged under fourteen died from it (Asthma UK online). The prevalence of asthma is increasing in most countries, especially amongst children (GINA 2007). Research carried out with families with children with asthma and other respiratory conditions (Fiese 2008; Marchant et al. 2008) identifies the multiple impact such conditions have on family life, demonstrating how the health status of one family member can adversely affect both the material and emotional well-being of all family members. For example:

- Parents often take less well-paid jobs closer to home to be nearer their children.
- Emergency care can mean a loss of earnings due to time off work.
- One-off costs (e.g., new bedding) and regular costs (e.g., hospital visits) can be a financial drain.
- Asthma attacks can cause disrupted sleep for all family members, leading to tiredness, irritability and lack of concentration.

Caring is often perceived to be a natural means of demonstrating love and support, and something that is carried out unstintingly. However, while families can offer a significant amount of support in times of ill health, the burden of caring for a family member or being cared for by the family can exacerbate existing illness or make other family members sick.

Writing about terminal illness, Jocham et al. (2006) suggest that the whole family should be the focus of care and recommend that nurses should be aware of, and adjust their practice to take account of, the disruptive effects of illness on family functioning. Arguably, such a focus is not only applicable to families caring for someone with a terminal illness, but to all families with caring responsibilities. The role that carers play in providing health care, and the implications for health policy, are discussed more fully in Chapter 15.

Over the past forty years there has been an increasing amount of literature highlighting what has been called the 'hidden side' of family life. This literature has put the family under scrutiny and uncovers the risks many women, and children, face every day from family life; there is also now an increasing body of work that focuses on violence perpetrated against men. What is increasingly evident is that sociology, together with other disciplines, has been instrumental in challenging the dominant ideology that portrays family life as nurturing and harmonious. Giddens (1989) claims that home is, in fact, the most dangerous place in modern society.

domestic violence: abuse that takes place within the household setting

If we look first at **domestic violence**, it estimated that one in four women will experience domestic violence at some point in their lives. Domestic violence features in at least one in every four divorces, and two women die each week at the hands of their current or former partner in England and Wales (Refuge 2008). The crime survey for England and Wales 2013/14 reports that 1.1 million (8.5 per cent) women and 700,000 men (3.3 per cent) had been the victim of some type of domestic abuse in the previous year. For the majority (1.1 million women and 500,000 men) this was intimate partner abuse. In women, incidence of any domestic abuse was higher for younger (under twenty-five) than older (over forty-five) women, and the highest prevalence was in women who were separated from their partner. Women with a long-term illness or disability were particularly at risk: 11.3 per cent compared with 4.9 per cent (ONS 2015) without such illness. In 2001, in a speech given to the Women's Aid Federation in England, the Minister for Women, Sally Morgan, said that 'a man who is capable of violence towards his wife or partner is also capable of violence towards his children'.

There is a wealth of research on the effects of domestic violence on women's health and some research on the impact of domestic violence upon the health of children in the family. For example, a study exploring the effect of domestic violence on children under five shows that such children can suffer from emotional, physical and behavioural problems, including speech and language difficulties, regression and post-traumatic stress (Refuge 2005).

A report on the role of health professionals in tackling domestic violence (Taket 2004) highlighted the importance of routine enquiry into domestic violence, pointing out the advantages of this as:

- Giving all women basic information about the unacceptability of domestic violence in all its forms.
- Giving all women information that will be relevant, not just to them, but to their friends, family members and neighbours.
- Helping to reduce the stigma of abuse and the taboo nature of domestic violence.
- Giving a clear message to women that they are not alone, that abuse is unacceptable, and that there are services available to help them.

7

However, it is important when thinking about abuse within the family that we recognize that this abuse is not always perpetrated by men against women or by parents against their children, but can also take the form of women abusing men or a child abusing a parent, and can occur within same-sex relationships, or between siblings (Bernardes 1997).

Activity 7.4 Domestic violence: the role of nurses

Read the case study and then consider the questions below.

Lakshmi is twenty-seven and lives in the West Midlands with her husband of seven years; she works in a call centre. They have two children: a daughter aged four and a son aged six. When her eldest son reached his second birthday, Lakshmi became very worried about his behaviour but her husband told her 'it was nothing'. Lakshmi wanted to take him to the doctor but her husband wouldn't allow this. When her son started school, teachers began to express concern and he was soon referred to an educational psychologist. After some time, and after consultation with other specialists, her son was diagnosed with autism. Lakshmi told her husband but he did not believe that there was anything 'wrong' with his son. He told Lakshmi not to tell anyone about their son's condition, especially members of their family.

> Lakshmi felt that she needed to tell members of her own family and told her mother and sister. When she told her husband that she had done this he became really angry. He beat her unconscious, breaking her arm in two places, fracturing her cheekbone and burning her with a cigarette.
>
> While Lakshmi was hospitalized with these injuries, he told both their families that she was a liar and that she was frequently aggressive and had tried to kill him. Both families disowned her. Later that week, when Lakshmi was beginning to recover from some of her injuries, her brother-in-law was overheard by a nurse on the hospital ward threatening to kill her after she was discharged.
>
> (a) Define domestic violence and explain how and why Lakshmi was subjected to domestic violence.
>
> (b) Imagine that you are the nurse who overheard Lakshmi's brother-in-law threatening to kill her. What would you do? Explain your reasons.
>
> (c) More generally, think about the role that you can play in the prevention of domestic violence and its consequences (in a personal and professional capacity). Make a list of these.

As most physical abuse occurs in the privacy of the family home it often remains invisible. It is suggested that most physical assaults on children are not reported as crimes, and parents who perpetrate these assaults are not defined as abusive. However, what is important to note is that when children are killed it is usually by their parents. Cheal (2002) suggests abusive parents kill children of all ages, but those at greatest risk are very young children, who are more likely to die when they are exposed to severe physical abuse. Accurate figures on abuse as a cause of death in children are very difficult to come by, but the implication for children's physical health and emotional well-being cannot be overstated.

The state has always had a responsibility for the safety of children, and in England this is currently exercised through Local Safeguarding children boards. Parton (2010), however, has noted how this responsibility has shifted over time and ideologically, often as an immediate response to the death of a child at the hands of its parents. The discourse moved from ideas of dangerousness in the 1970s and 1980s to notions of risk in the 1990s; that is, away from identifying individuals (parents or carer) who are prone to violence, instead focusing on the identification of certain risk factors in an individual in the absence of any evidence from their behaviour or circumstances, such as drug- or alcohol-dependent parent(s) living in insecure housing. Ideas about when the state should intervene have also changed over this period, from intervening on the basis of suspicions/evidence of physical, sexual or emotional harm to optimizing the life chances of children by intervening earlier in their lives. This involves screening for 'high risk' in individuals, which is prone to producing **false positive** results, and leads to services that focus on prevention and surveillance, which undermines privacy and confidentiality for parents and children

false positive:
a result that indicates the presence of a condition that is not actually there

(Parton 2010). More recently, Parton (2014) has argued that, since 2010, child protection, as opposed to enhancing life chances, has again taken centre stage in safeguarding. Reductions in public expenditure, particularly in local government, have led to a downgrading in priority of family and children's services. Families with children have seen reduced income levels, and children's charities have suffered the biggest reductions in government grants (Parton 2014). The priority now is to rescue children, which often involves removing more children from their parents, and to make efforts to increase adoption rates of such children. This, states Parton (2014), has replaced state control of families by means of surveillance with coercion and authoritarian control.

Activity 7.5 Families can harm your health

In 2007, the National Centre for Social Research, together with researchers at King's College London, produced a report on behalf of the charity Comic Relief and the Department of Health, which focused on the prevalence of abuse and neglect of older people. Figure 7.4 shows some of the findings of this research. The commentary that follows shows the reaction to this report by the charity Carers UK, an organization which campaigns for the rights of carers.

Examine the bar chart in Figure 7.4 and read the commentary, then answer the questions below.

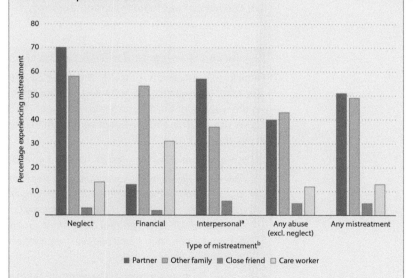

Figure 7.4 Bar chart: the mistreatment of older people (*O'Keefe et al. 2007*)

[a] Interpersonal abuse included psychological, physical and sexual abuse.
[b] Respondents were able to give more than one answer.

Carers UK reaction to elder abuse report, 14 June 2007

Commenting on the UK Study of Abuse and Neglect, Imelda Redmond, Chief Executive of Carers UK, said: 'This is the first in-depth study of elder abuse that has been undertaken and it challenges some of the prejudices that people have that domestic abuse stops when someone gets older.'

This survey shows, quite clearly, that it continues into older age. This is wholly unacceptable and needs to be urgently tackled. We welcome the measures being announced today by Ministers, such as the registers of abuse.

The research highlights some shocking facts such as the level of sexual abuse. It also raises critical questions about the nature of relationships between the older person and their abuser. For example, if the person carrying out the abuse is supposed to be caring for them, what agreement do they have about caring?

Is the abuser withholding support to make the older person suffer on purpose or are they simply not able to provide the level of care and support that the older person wants them to? For example, they may not be able to visit as often as the older person would like. Whilst systematic abuse needs to be firmly and swiftly dealt with, we must also recognize that in some cases there is a mismatch between expectations and the support that can actually be provided.

This research is helpful because it challenges prejudices. We also need more research to unpick some of these more complicated questions to look at the real risks of abuse and we need urgent action to tackle persistent abuse for people of all ages, including older people. (Carers UK 2007, online)

(a) To what extent do you think that the family can make you sick?
(b) What do you think might be some of the methodological problems encountered when researching abuse of older people, or other vulnerable groups? (It might be useful to reread parts of Chapter 1.)
(c) To what extent is the home the most dangerous place in modern society?
(d) Can nurses contribute to making the family a safer place?

Case Study: Families and mental health

Families play an enormous role in providing care for others, but families can also harm your health. The following case study from experiences posted on the website of the mental health charity MIND (<www.mind.org.uk>) shows the positive and the negative part that families can play in a person's ill health.

Louise (whose story featured in Activity 1.4) wrote:

I'd been struggling with anxiety since the death of a very close loved one and depression was clouding my mind, making me tearful and not as robust as I usually am . . . I always believed my immediate family loved me unconditionally, regardless of my 'flaws' or my mental health. But it turns out for one non-blood relative, they were simply masking how they truly perceived me.

'She's an attention seeker; she wants all the focus on her. She's a weak person. She needs to grow a spine. Everyone thinks she's a hypochondriac.' . . . I had no idea that someone who'd been there, who'd been supporting me through most of my life really saw me as weak for having mental health problems . . .

But this isn't the first time I've felt unaccepted by my own family; I was previously told to hide my mental health from prospective employers as according to a certain relative, they themselves wouldn't hire someone with depression.

Violet posted about her experience of the stigma of mental illness and how it made her feel worthless and despised.

> *When you are unwell you hope that people will be there to support you. However, during my struggle with mental health problems I have found that some people are not supportive and can make things considerably worse. . . . Luckily my parents were completely supportive of me. They often said it was 'us three against the world', which reassured me that no matter what anyone else said, they would be there for me. My parents were also the target of horrible comments . . . I found that the stigma surrounding mental health problems doesn't just affect the person with the illness but all those who support them too.*

Summary and Resources

Summary

▶ The ideology underpinning the nuclear family is still pervasive, but the reality today is that many of us live in families that bear little resemblance to this form.

▶ The ideology of the nuclear family has played an important role in informing the organization and delivery of health care in Britain. Nurses should be sensitive to this and avoid stereotyping families according to this ideology.

▶ Families are pivotal to the maintenance of health, but at the same time are facing an increasing responsibility to care for sick, frail and disabled people; this can place an increasing pressure on family members, of which nurses should be aware.

▶ Some family members, particularly women, are perceived to be 'naturally' more inclined to caring and nurturing roles, with the majority of the health task role being deemed their responsibility.

▶ While families can be of vital support for many individuals, there are also occasions when families can affect health negatively, and it is important to recognize that experience of family life is not always positive.

Questions for Discussion

1 Is it important for health professionals to challenge common-sense (or traditional) ideas about 'the family'? How may they do this?
2 Why and how do families play an important role in maintaining health?
3 Why is it important to consider the diversity of family life in nursing work?

Glossary

carers:
: people who carry out caring roles without pay for friends, a partner, neighbours or relatives, are often called 'informal carers', but this phrase underplays the importance of this group of people in maintaining the frail and sick within the community; spouses and adult children form the largest group of carers, but a significant number of children are primary carers for a parent

domestic violence:
: domestic violence includes physical violence as well as psychological, emotional, sexual and economic abuse; it can be perpetrated within intimate relationships as well as by other family members; it can include forced marriage, genital mutilation and honour killings

extended family:
: extended families are united not only by proximity, but by a series of networks and obligations such as childcare and social occasions; in modern societies contact may be by social media, and therefore physical proximity is less important than in the past

false positive:
: a medical test for the presence or absence of a disease normally gives a positive result when the disease is present or a negative result when it is not; if a disease is detected by the test that the person undergoing it does not actually have, then it is a false positive

kin groups:
: the social relationships and lineage groups bound together through a system of well-defined customs, rights and obligations; kin relationships may either derive from descent or be established through affinity

material:
: materialism is part of Marxist ideology and in sociological terms refers to the notion that social phenomena are linked to the production of material things

nuclear family:
: nuclear families of parents and dependent children are often thought to have evolved as the dominant household structure to service the Industrial Revolution; it is now recognized that high death rates in the past, and high divorce and separation rates in the present, mean that family forms have always been fluid

Further Reading

D. Chambers: *A Sociology of Family Life*. Chichester: Wiley, 2012.
The growing diversity of family life is explored in this book. It covers a wide range of topics, including gender, ethnic identity and new sexual lifestyles in analysing modern family life. It also highlights both the continuity and changes that have taken place within the family, and points to future developments.

E. Dermot: *Intimate Fatherhood: A Sociological Analysis*. London: Routledge, 2008.
A really interesting book which focuses on contemporary fatherhood and men's parenting behaviour, allowing you to explore this aspect of family life in more depth.

C. Gatrell: *Hard Labour: The Sociology of Parenthood, Family Life and Career*. Buckingham: Open University Press, 2002.
An innovative book exploring fatherhood, motherhood and family life.

H. Graham: *Women, Health and Family*. Brighton: Wheatsheaf, 1984.
A classic text that considers the relationship between women's role in the family and health.

References

Asthma UK online. Available at: <www.asthma.org.uk>.
Barrett, M. and McIntosh, M. 1991 *The Anti-Social Family*. London: Verso.
Bernardes, J. 1997 *Family Studies: An Introduction*. London: Routledge.
Bond, J. and Bond, S. 1994 *Sociology and Health Care: An Introduction for Nurses and Other Healthcare Professionals*, 2nd edn. Amsterdam: Elsevier.
Brannen, J., Dodd, K., Oakley, A. and Storey, P. 1994 *Young People, Health and Family Life*. Buckingham: Open University Press.
Budig, M. 2004 Feminism and the Family. In J. Scott, J. Treas and M. Richards (eds), *The Blackwell Companion to the Sociology of Families*. Oxford: Blackwell, pp. 340–55.
Bunting, M. 2007 Family fortunes. *Guardian Online*, Saturday September 25. Available at: <http://www.guardian.co.uk/world/2004/sep/25/2020.madeleinebunting>.
Carers UK 2007 *Carers UK Reaction to Elder Abuse Report*, 14 June. Available at: <http://www.carersuk.org/Newsandcampaigns/News/1181828209>.
Carers UK 2011 *Unpaid Carers Save £119 Billion a Year*. Available at: <www.carersuk.org>.
Carers UK 2014 *State of Caring 2014*. Available at: <www.carersuk.org>.
Cheal, D. 2002 *Sociology of Family Life*. Basingstoke: Palgrave.
Department of Health (DH) 2008 *Carers at the Heart of the 21st-century Families and Communities: 'A caring system on your side. A life of your own'*. London: Department of Health.
Doane, G. H. and Varcoe, C. 2006 The 'hard spots' of family nursing – connecting across difference and diversity. *Journal of Family Nursing* 12/1: 7–21.
Doyal, L. 1995 *What Makes Women Sick: Gender and the Political Economy of Health*. Basingstoke: Macmillan.
Elliot, F. 1986 *The Family: Change or Continuity?* London: Macmillan Education.

Engels, F. [1845] 1999 *The Condition of the Working Class in England in 1844*, ed. D. McLellan. Oxford: Oxford University Press.

Fiese, B. H. 2008 Breathing life into family processes: introduction to the special issue on families and asthma. *Family Processes* 47/1: 1–5.

Giddens, A. 1989 *Sociology*. Cambridge: Polity.

GINA (Global Initiative for Asthma) 2007 *Global Strategy for Asthma Management and Prevention*. GINA, available at: <http://www.ginasthma.org>.

Graham, H. 1999 The informal sector of welfare: a crisis in caring? In G. Allen (ed.), *The Sociology of the Family*. Oxford: Blackwell, pp. 283–300.

Griffiths, R. 1988 *Community Care: Agenda for Action: A Report to the Secretary of State for Social Services*. London: HMSO.

Hall, C. 1982 The home turned upside down? The working-class family in cotton textiles 1780–1850. In E. Whitelegg, M. Arnott, V. Beechey, L. Birke, S. Himmelweit, D. Leonard, S. Ruehl and M. A. Speakman (eds), *The Changing Experience of Women*. Oxford: Martin Robertson, pp. 17–30.

Jackson, S. 1997 Women, marriage and family relationships. In V. Robinson and D. Richardson (eds), *Introducing Women's Studies*. Basingstoke: Macmillan, pp. 323–49.

Jary, D. and Jary, J. 1991 *Collins Dictionary of Sociology*. Glasgow: HarperCollins.

Jocham, H. R., Dassen, T. and Widdershoven, G. et al. 2006 Quality of life in palliative care cancer patients: a literature review. *Journal of Clinical Nursing* 15/9: 1188–95.

Laslett, P. 1972 Mean household size in England since the sixteenth century. In P. Laslett and R. Wall (eds), *Household and Family in Past Time*. Cambridge: Cambridge University Press, pp. 125–58.

Marchant, J. M., Newcombe, P. A. and Juniper, E. F. et al. 2008 What is the burden of chronic cough for families? *CHEST* 134/2: 303–9.

Morgan, S. 2001 Speech to the Women's Aid Federation of England, 26 September. Available at: <http://archive.cabinetoffice.gov.uk/ministers/2001/Speeches/Sally%20Morgan/WAFE%2026.9.htm>.

O'Keefe, M., Hills, A., Doyle, M., McCreadie, C., Scholes, S., Constantine, R., Tinker, A., Manthorpe, J., Biggs, S. and Erens, B. 2007 *UK Study of Abuse and Neglect of Older People Prevalence Survey Report*. London: Comic Relief/Department of Health. Available at: <http://www.natcen.ac.uk/media/308684/p2512-uk-elder-abuse-final-for-circulation.pdf>.

Office for National Statistics (ONS) 2014 *Statistical Bulletin*. Available at: <www.ong.gov.uk>.

Office for National Statistics (ONS) 2015 *2013/14 Crime Survey for England and Wales*. Available at: <www.crimesurvey.co.uk>.

Parsons, T. 1955 *Family Socialization and Interaction Process*. Glencoe, IL: Free Press.

Parton, N. 2010 'From dangerousness to risk': the growing importance of screening and surveillance systems for safeguarding and promoting the well-being of children in England. *Health, Risk & Society* 12: 51–64.

Parton, N. 2014 The changing politics and practice of child protection and safeguarding in England. In S. Wagg and J. Pilcher (eds), *Thatcher's Grandchildren?: Politics and Childhood in the Twenty-First Century*. Basingstoke: Palgrave Macmillan, pp. 45–68.

Princess Royal Trust for Carers 2008 *Key Facts about Carers*. London: The Princess Royal Trust for Carers. Available at: <http://www.carers.org/articles/information-for-press,2822,CA.html>.

Refuge 2005 *Refuge Assessment and Intervention for Pre-school Children Exposed to Domestic Violence, August 2005*. London: Refuge. Available at: <http://www.refuge.org.uk/cms_content_refuge/attachments/Effects%20of%20domestic%20violence%20on%20pre-school%20children.pdf>.

Refuge 2008 *Domestic Violence – the Facts*. Availale at: <http://www.refuge.org.uk/page_l1-2_l2-162_l3-175_.htm>.

Scott, J., Treas, J. and Richards, M. (eds) 2004 *The Blackwell Companion to the Sociology of Families*. Oxford: Blackwell.

Taket, A. 2004 *Tackling domestic violence – the role of health professionals*. London: Home Office.

Weeks, J., Heaphy, B. and Donovam, C. 2004 The lesbian and gay family. In J. Scott, J. Treas and M. Richards (eds), *The Blackwell Companion to the Sociology of Families*. Oxford: Blackwell, pp. 340–55.

World Health Organization (WHO) 1990 *Diet, Nutrition and the Prevention of Chronic Disease*. Geneva: World Health Organization.

7

Age and Ageing

Elaine Denny

KEY ISSUES IN THIS CHAPTER:

▶ The relevance of age and ageing to all nurses.
▶ Definitions of age.
▶ The social construction of age.
▶ Theoretical perspectives of age and ageing.
▶ Ageism, diversity, discrimination and anti-ageist nursing practice.

BY THE END OF THIS CHAPTER YOU SHOULD BE ABLE TO:

▶ Explore your own stereotypes of age.
▶ Consider the ways in which age is constructed in contemporary Western societies.
▶ Consider the impact of ageing on nursing practice.
▶ Develop your own guidelines to ensure your practice is anti-ageist.
▶ Reconsider the relevance of age for nurses.

1 Introduction

It is a truism to say that nurses work with patients of all ages, from pre-natal to very old. Indeed, pathways within nursing programmes are often delineated by 'age' either explicitly or implicitly, so before you have even commenced your nurse education you may have made decisions about the age range of the service users you wish to nurse. However, 'age' is often assumed to be 'neutral', an undeniable 'fact' on which we all agree. Sociologists often refer to this as making use of taken-for-granted knowledge. Surely 'age' is simply a useful way of summarizing the number of years we have been alive, and is manifested and celebrated via ceremonies such as birthdays, and symbols

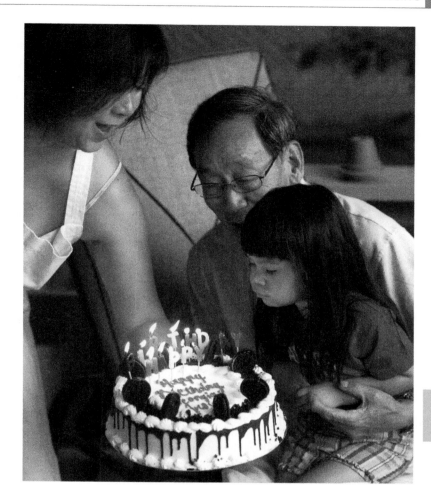

Figure 8.1 Birthdays are often important occasions, but chronological ageing is only one aspect of 'age'

8

social gerontology: the critical study of ageing

moral panic: media-inspired overreaction to certain groups or behaviour taken as signs of impending social disorder

such as birthday cards and presents. And yet, as this chapter seeks to demonstrate, chronological age is only one aspect of 'age'.

Rather, as the study of **social gerontology** demonstrates, the way in which 'age' is constructed and understood in any society is extremely complex, and has implications for practice. The image of working with older people created by well-worn phrases such as 'no previous experience needed' only serves to reinforce the 'age' hierarchy.

The first part of this chapter seeks to challenge some of these assumptions around age. For example, if you nurse in the field of child health, before you even meet them you may have expectations of a patient of ten years old that are different from your expectations of a teenager. Similarly, if you work in adult or mental health, the knowledge that a patient or service user referred to your service is aged eighty-five may conjure a picture in your mind of what that person will be capable of doing. A discussion follows of the way in which the age structure of societies is changing and how this has given rise to what might be described as a **moral panic** regarding the behaviour of policymakers and some professional groups.

life-course perspective: a view of a person's whole life, to better comprehend their present experiences and beliefs

Sociological theories of ageing, and their relevance to 'age' across the life course, will be explored, and a **life-course perspective** on 'age' that draws on current social gerontological thinking will be developed. In the final section of the chapter, we will consider the potential impact of 'ageism' on nursing practice. An opportunity will be provided to develop personal guidelines for anti-ageist practice in nursing.

---

2 Definitions of age

> ### Activity 8.1 What is 'age'?
>
> (a) Individually list five characteristics which you associate with the following age groups: 65+; 18–64; 12–17; 0–11.
> (b) Compare your answers with a colleague's and note similarities and differences in your lists. Are there differences between the ways in which you characterize the different age groups?
> (c) If yes, why do you think this is? Do you think there would be further differences if you were to consider the issue of learning disability in relation to these age groups?

Sociologists have found that more positive characteristics are often noted for under-65s than for over-65s. 'Growth and development', 'good health' and 'happiness', for example, are more likely to be listed as characteristics of the under-65s, whereas 'decline', 'ill health' and 'loneliness' are likely to be given for the over-65s. The Centre for Confidence and Wellbeing (<www.centreforconfidence.co.uk>) reports stereotypes of old people as being needy, unhappy, senile, inactive, unable to learn new things and less useful than their younger counterparts. The validity of these stereotypes has been refuted by research findings and yet they persist, even in nursing practice (Sarabio-Cobo and Pfeiffer 2015), and may influence the type and amount of care given, as will be explored later in this chapter.

Given that 'age' is clearly more than the sum total of a person's birthdays, we must beware of making assumptions or engaging with stereotypes based purely on chronology. Kagan and Melendez-Torres (2015) concur and argue that evidence to guide the care of older people is lacking because of age bias in systematic investigation. Although physiology, linked to chronology, is popularly (and sometimes professionally) assumed to be the most important component in defining 'age', it is only one factor among many. For example, evidence suggests that we do not all 'age' physiologically at the same rate: social, economic and cultural factors have a profound effect on this process (Fennell et al. 1989). Poverty, low educational attainment, poor diet, unhealthy social behaviours, such as smoking, and low levels of exercise all contribute to our physiological status.

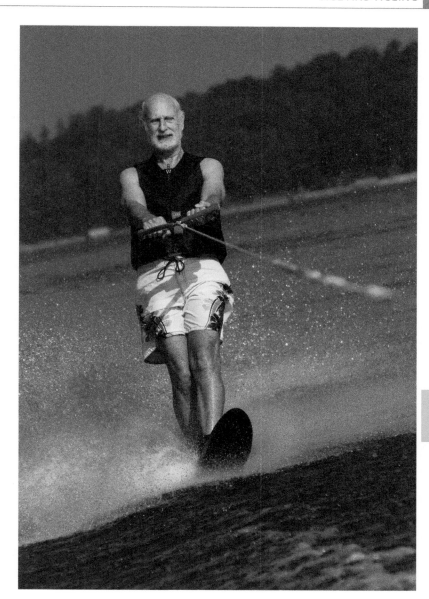

Figure 8.2 Does this conform to stereotypes of older people?

8

Let us consider two phenomena that emerged during the twentieth century, and their relationship to the changes in economics and social policy during that time, in order to understand the way in which society conceptualizes and organizes, sometimes through social policy, an age group to meet its perceived values, ideas or needs. First, the term 'pensioner', which did not exist in the earlier part of the last century before the introduction of a universal state pension, has since 1948 until recently applied collectively to all those who on reaching 'retirement age' were forced to retire from employment in order to create jobs for younger members of society. For some, retirement is a sentence to living on a vastly reduced income, whereas for others it is a time of choice and opportunity. However, this is fluid and dependent on the demographics and economy of a society, and a fixed retirement age has recently been phased out. State pension age has now been uncoupled from retirement age and is set to rise to sixty-six years in 2020; sixty-seven years by 2028; and sixty-eight years in 2044 for both sexes (<www.gov.uk/calculate-state-pension>). These changes have been introduced because increased life expectancy (see the section on 'Adulthood' below) means state pensions are now being paid for a much longer period of life than originally intended.

The second phenomenon is 'teenager', a term applied to those between the ages of thirteen and eighteen. Although originally conceived in the 1950s as a descriptor for the period between childhood and adulthood, a time of rebellion against adult values, and certainly during the 1960s encompassing young workers with disposable incomes, the term 'teenager' is now increasingly synonymous with extended full-time education and economic dependency on parents or the state.

History, that is, the period of time in which we live, and the cultural values of the society at that time in relation to normality and difference, also have a place in the construction of 'age'. Let us consider this briefly in relation first to childhood and then to adulthood.

Childhood

Social history accounts (see, for example, Pinchbeck and Hewitt 1973) remind us that childhood, like old age, has been constructed and defined differently across history and cultures. The separation of childhood was a result of the growth of the public-school system for the moral education of the wealthy in the eighteenth century. In nineteenth-century Britain, child labour was the norm (and remains so within some cultures), with education and health care only available for the privileged few; indeed, what we would now consider to be 'childhood' was a relatively short period prior to adulthood. 'Extended' childhood and state provision for children – financial support, education, health care – are all products of the post-war Welfare State, and reflect specific 'historical' values towards an 'age group'. The emergence of the child as 'dependent' on adults until achieving adult status was a phenomenon of the twentieth century, a process which Lee (2001: xiii) describes as 'child human becomings' moving through to 'adult human beings', with 'adulthood' as the desired state of stability and completion that constituted arrival at the 'journey's end' (p. 7). He goes on to argue that this image of the 'journey's end' has been crucial in maintaining the authority that adults have had over children and the right and duty to make decisions for them (p. 9). The international conferment of rights on 'children' in the United Nations Convention on the Rights of the Child (1989) has begun to shift this relationship, and, since the end of the twentieth century, the status of children as beings in their own right ('child human beings') has emerged. Childhood, then, although it has always existed, has been redefined and restructured and will continue to be so (see Hockey 1993). Our understanding of what constitutes the 'age of childhood' is both culturally and historically bound and is in a state of continual flux. An example of this is the right of children to consent to medical procedures and treatment, which used to be entirely a matter for parents. Young people between the ages of sixteen and eighteen years can now provide their own consent, and even younger children may do so if they are deemed '**Gillick competent**', that is, they 'can demonstrate sufficient maturity and intelligence to understand the nature and implications of the proposed treatment, including the risks and alternative courses of action' (Wheeler 2006: 807). We also view children as having their own needs in health care, and we employ specialist nurses, with their discrete programme of education, to care for them, usually in different settings from adults.

Gillick competence: ability to make own treatment decisions, based on mature understanding rather than chronological age

Adulthood

Legally, a person in the UK is an adult from the age of eighteen years, although some areas of life, such as joining the armed forces or getting married, are available with parental consent from the age of sixteen. A definition based on chronological age is, however, static and takes no account of the way in which adulthood, like childhood and old age, has been subject to redefinition and restructure. Even the term 'age of majority' is fluid and dependent on social policy and law. In the nineteenth century, 'adulthood', when construed in policy terms, encompassed what we now perceive to be adolescence and old age, although it must be acknowledged that chronologically 'old age' differed from today. Boys and girls born in 1901 could only expect to live to forty-five years and forty-nine years respectively. Figures from the Office for National Statistics (2014) demonstrate that these ages have changed dramatically in the course of just over 100 years: in 2012, life expectancy at birth was 79.0 for males and 82.7 for females.

8

Activity 8.2 Meet the Browns

Read the following case study about the Brown family.

John and Katie Brown are in their early forties and have two children, Mark (fifteen) and Rachel (ten). They live in a London suburb, although John spends a lot of time working abroad as a computer consultant. Katie works as a teacher in a nearby primary school, and during term time Rachel is cared for after school by John's parents, David and June, who are retired and live nearby. Mark also goes to his grandparents after school, particularly if he is hungry!

Mark is studying for GCSEs and is doing well at school, but struggles with maths, and often needs his mother's help with his homework. Rachel is very keen on gymnastics, and when her father is at home he spends weekends taking her to competitions. Katie says it is the only time she ever gets to herself.

David's mother, Joyce, lives nearer to London in a warden-controlled flat. She is becoming frail and sometimes forgetful but is fiercely independent. She receives visits from one of the family at least twice a week, and Mark will sometimes stay with her if he wants to go to see a band in the city.

David and June find it difficult to manage on their pension, and John pays the tax and insurance on their car in order for them to get around and to be able to visit Joyce and to do her shopping.

For each member of this family:

(a) What do you think the needs are for their particular stage in life?
(b) How is each one dependent on the others, and for what?
(c) Think of your own family structure. How do the different generations help and support each other?

3 The changing age structure of the population

Just as childhood and middle age have been redefined and restructured historically, so too has old age. In the 1980s fears about the ageing of the population, sometimes described as the 'greying' of the population, both contributed to and were a part of the negative stereotyping of older people, and have reinforced our notions of age structures. **Demography** can tell us the age structure of a particular population at a particular point in time. For example, in the UK, numbers of over-65s increased by 17.3 per cent between 2003 and 2013 to 11.1 million people, which was 17.4 per cent of the total (ONS 2014). This was an increase of 290,800 between mid-2012 and the end of 2013.

demography: the study of populations

The fastest-growing age group in the population is eighty years and over. This group has seen an increase of over 1.1 million between 1981 and 2007 (1,572,160 to 2,749,507), from 2.8 per cent to 4.5 per cent of the population (ONS 2014). The number of people over ninety went up from 384,800 in 2002 to 527,240 in 2013, and around a third of babies born in that year are projected to live to 100. Conversely, in 2004, there were 11.6 million people aged under sixteen in the UK, a decline of 2.6 million since 1971, and nearly one in five women is now childless at the age of forty-five. Projections suggest that the proportion of the population who are children will continue to fall.

Figure 8.3 shows that in 2013 there were more people over sixty-five than under sixteen, and it is projected that by 2025 there will be 1.6 million more people over the age of sixty-five than people under sixteen. These statistics have implications for the type of health care that needs to be provided and who provides it, and how this is managed is discussed in Part III of this volume.

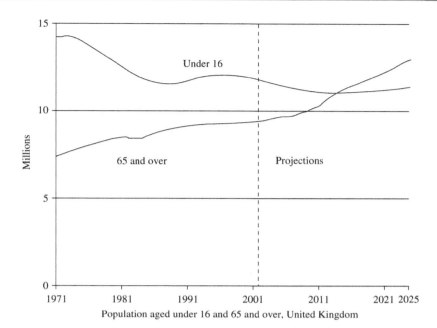

Figure 8.3 Age structure of the population

Why is the population ageing? The age structure is dependent on three variables: fertility, mortality and migration. Let us focus in this chapter on the first two.

Fertility and mortality

Before the end of the nineteenth century, fertility rates were high but life expectancy was low. High rates of infant mortality, epidemics and infections, poor working conditions and deaths in childbirth meant that those who survived to old age were in the minority. In the early part of the twenty-first century in the UK, as elsewhere, fertility rates are decreasing as a result of education, access to contraception, government policies and so on (Kagan and Melendez-Torres 2015). At the same time, we have seen improved mortality rates as a result of the massive public-health measures undertaken in the nineteenth and twentieth centuries. At a local level, migration can accelerate the greying of the population, by either an exodus (for employment) or an influx (for retirement) of one age group. This changing demography has caused alarm in some quarters, and, in the last part of the twentieth century, 'old age' became the source of a moral panic, and the ensuing debate only served to reinforce the ageist structure of British society. Rather than old age being celebrated and the prospect of a longer life span and a potentially fitter old age being welcomed, the ageing of the population was thought instead to be burdensome, and claims were made that younger adults would have to work for longer and pay higher taxes in order to support 'hordes' of frail, dependent older people. Gerontologists (such as Phillipson 1998) have challenged this perspective, pointing to the diversity of the ageing population, which includes older adults who contribute to the overall economy as volunteers and as family carers (of children and other adults), as well as those who continue in paid employment beyond the 'state' retirement age. Like all other 'age groups', old age is certainly not a homogeneous state; some older people will find themselves in need of more health and social care services than others, but for most older people 'old age' itself is not problematic. Although the dominant picture of old age is of poor health, conversely stereotyping leads to perceptions of older people as being asexual and therefore not at risk of contracting certain diseases associated with youth, such as sexually transmitted infections (STIs). Public-health messages have tended to ignore this age group, although the incidence of STIs is rising in older people (Mensforth et al. 2014).

4 Theories of ageing

Traditional theories

Traditional theories of human development and decline have also served to reinforce age difference and contribute to notions of the social construction of ageing. Until the 1980s, old age was theorized as a life stage, separate from childhood and adulthood. Cumming and Henry (1961) put forward a theory, disengagement theory, which suggested that in their sixties older people 'disengage' from society: they do this willingly and with the approval of successive generations who benefit via the enhanced employment opportunities which then become available. By contrast, activity theorists argued that the only way to resist disengagement was to maintain a 'middle-age' lifestyle (Fennell et al. 1989). Disengagement theory has been challenged as a convenient rationale for supporting the exclusion of older people from public life, and activity theory as taking no account of diversity. Critics argued that although many older people do withdraw from the public sphere, there is little evidence to suggest that they do so voluntarily; rather, ageist policies and practices (low retirement income and dependency-creating services) restrict their capacity to remain active citizens.

Contemporary theories

Contemporary theories have sought to challenge such rigid and uncritical perspectives on ageing, highlighting societal rather than individual responsibility for structuring ageing. First, the political economy perspective highlights the impact of an individual's location within the social and economic structure during the earlier part of their life course, on their financial status, their social location and the life choices available in old age (Phillipson 1998). This perspective, in particular, acknowledges the way in which advantages and disadvantages accrued earlier in the life course impact on an individual in old age. An example of this is the way in which many older women find themselves with reduced access to financial resources in later life as a result of working in part-time, low-paid and low-status employment or a lifetime's financial dependence on a spouse (Yin 2008). A political economy perspective on ageing also points to increasing polarity of the ageing experience, ranging from the social exclusion of those older people living in areas of extreme economic deprivation (Scharf et al. 2002) to those 'young-at-heart', fit and wealthy older people, who are a recent addition to 'niche' markets of the tourism and travel industry (Warnes et al. 1999; Ylanne-McEwen 1999).

Second, social gerontologists are increasingly acknowledging the importance of the subjective experience of ageing, as encapsulated in biographical studies, and the impact of this on ageing identities (Chambers 2005; Ray 2007). This cannot be understood in isolation from historical location or political economy. Ruth and Oberg (1996; 171), for example, in a quest to understand the experience of old age for Finns from the generation of 'the Wars and the Depression', argue that knowledge based solely on current circumstances is inadequate: 'Ageing must be seen as a continuation of an integrated process, starting with an earlier life, where the life lived gives meaning to old age.' In Chapter 1, we argued that sociology is multiparadigmatic; thus, experiences of ageing must be understood from the perspective of social structure as well as that of social action.

Age throughout the life course is characterized by and perhaps best understood in terms of 'diversity' of gender, ethnicity, social class, disability, geographical location and so on. Talking about 'age groups' is only useful as a marker, a shorthand term to describe those people who share a chronological age, and to provide some information relating to physiology. We would do better to try to understand an individual's experience of the life course, wherever she or he happens to be located at a particular point in time.

Activity 8.3 Biography and ageing

(a) Note down the major events or 'milestones' in your life so far in relation to your early years, family, relationships, school, work and so on.

(b) Interview a person who is much older than you, but the same gender, about the major milestones in their life. Note the differences and similarities.

(c) What does this tell you about individual (personal) and collective (sharing the same historical time) ageing, and the ways in which age, at different points of the life course, has been differentially constructed over time? How might this understanding help you in your nursing practice?

5 Ageism

ageism:
discrimination on the basis of age

Ageism exists throughout the life course (Bytheway 1995). Bytheway writes:

> Ageism generates and reinforces a fear and denigration of the ageing process, and the stereotyping assumptions regarding competence and need for protection. In particular ageism legitimates the use of chronological age to mark out classes of people who are systematically denied resources and opportunities that others enjoy, and who suffer the consequences of such denigration – ranging from well-meaning patronage to unambiguous vilification.

Ageism therefore is not simply a matter of personal prejudice but has its roots in the way society is organized and, unlike many other 'isms', will potentially be experienced by us all to some degree.

Ageism is manifested in a number of ways:

1　Negative judgements based on age, which may be linked to physical and emotional abuse.
2　Compassionate ageism by infantilizing or being overly protective.
3　Self-stereotyping when a person internalizes stereotypes about their own life stage and believes that these must be applicable to them (Kagan and Melendez-Torres 2015).

To this list may be added use of demeaning language, mockery and economic disadvantage. According to Thompson (1995), ageism occurs on a number of fronts, including: personal (individual experience); cultural (language, images, media); and structural (differential access to services and opportunities). He goes on to demonstrate that the impact of ageism on health and social-care practice with older people includes: dehumanization; ageist language; elder abuse; infantilization (treating older people as if they were children); denial of citizenship; welfarism; and medicalization. For example, in the modern world many people's views are influenced by social media, and Levy et al. (2013) found that of eighty-four Facebook groups that focused on older people 74 per cent excoriated them, 27 per cent infantilized them and 37 per cent advocated banning them from public activities.

The year 2012 was designated the European Year of Active Ageing and Solidarity between Generations, and it saw the publication of results from a European Union (EU) wide survey of 54,988 respondents on attitudes to age (Age UK 2012). It found that ageism is the most widely experienced form of discrimination, with 35 per cent reporting unfair treatment on the grounds of age, compared with gender (25 per cent) and race (17 per cent). The ways in which this manifested were through being ignored or patronized, being insulted, abused or denied services. Age discrimination in employment was a concern of 50 per cent of respondents, even though it is banned in the EU. Although ageism is commonly thought to be directed only against older people, Snowden (2012) reports a survey carried out by the ONS that showed perceptions towards workers over seventy as being more positive than towards those in their twenties. Older workers were perceived as more competent, friendly and possessing higher moral standards.

It would seem therefore that stereotypes of all ages abound in the world of employment. However, the term 'ageism' is usually used in relation to later life and is rooted in the 'social construction' of ageing highlighted at the beginning of this chapter.

As a result of living in an ageist society, many older people internalize ageist views, become ageist towards their peers, and try to distance themselves from other 'old people'. Furthermore, ageing women in particular feel coerced into 'passing' for middle-aged via strategies such as colouring their hair, dressing in 'younger' clothes and, more recently, cosmetic surgery.

However, in 2002, the Labour government made a commitment to rooting out ageism in health and social care services, and Standard One of the National Service Framework for Older People (Department of Health 2001) states that health services will be provided, regardless of age, on the basis of clinical need alone. Age discrimination was made illegal by the Age Discrimination Act 2006, which was much later than race or gender discrimination. Discrimination Acts were brought under the umbrella of the Equality Act in 2010.

Nursing and ageism

In 2013, in a response to the findings of the Francis Inquiry (see Chapter 14), NHS England stated that older people should be properly valued and listened to, and treated with compassion, dignity and respect at all times (NHS England 2013). However, Kagan and Melendez-Torres (2015) state that working with older patients is devalued nursing work, with poor social status and poor remuneration (see also Chapter 4 for a discussion on nursing student attitudes to working with people with dementia). This is particularly the case in long-term care settings. They go on to argue that the poor status of the care of older people, coupled with persistent patterns of poor care, underscores the presence of ageism in nursing. In a study with both nursing staff and patients in an acute medical setting, Maben et al. (2012) found that in clinical areas where high demand, low control and poor staffing levels were prevalent, nurses sought to alleviate these difficulties by gaining job satisfaction from caring for the elderly patients for whom they could make a difference. Other patients were regarded as 'parcels'. These were often patients who required more complex care, and yet they received less personalized care. Patients were aware of being thought of as difficult and tried to manage relationships with staff accordingly. Maben et al. (2012)

concluded that the work experience of nurses is an important factor in the quality of care for elderly patients.

In a study with Spanish nursing students, Sarabia-Cobo and Castanedo Pfeiffer (2015) analysed the modification of stereotypes and myths regarding ageing among third-year nursing students following an Ageing Nursing course. They administered the Questionnaire of Negative Stereotypes about Aging (*sic*) before and after the course. The pre-course results demonstrated that the students held the same stereotypes of older people as the general population, this being particularly true of the health and personality sections of the questionnaire. Older people were viewed as being dependent on others, as experiencing cognitive impairment, and being rigid and inflexible. Following the Ageing Nursing course, these stereotypical views had greatly reduced, leading the authors to conclude that specific training in gerontology and care of the elderly not only improves knowledge and skills, but also fosters a positive attitude to older people.

Similarly, in a study in the US, a simulation game played by nursing students was shown to improve empathy and attitudes towards the elderly. The students were required to role-play the part of an older person, experiencing physical, psychological and financial problems while also navigating the health-care system. They were randomly assigned disabilities; for example, sight loss, for which they were given petroleum jelly-coated goggles to simulate impaired vision. All students reported experiencing frustration, annoyance and impatience at not being able to carry out tasks or access services easily, or at losing an ability (Chen et al. 2015).

6 Anti-ageist practice

In working with older people we must recognize that our starting point is one of disadvantage and discrimination rather than equality. According to Hughes (1997), **anti-ageist practice** embodies the following three values:

anti-ageist practice: health and social care practice which does not discriminate on the basis of age

> *Personhood*: ascribes to all people of all ages the authenticity and worth of being alive and of having lived.
> *Citizenship*: relationship between the individual and society and how that relationship is defined; emphasizes rights of individual and reciprocal responsibilities of individual and society; validates membership of society; and is different from 'consumer'.
> *Celebration*: age to be celebrated as an achievement and as a period to be valued in its own right.

Although specifically addressing 'old age', these values should underpin practice with all age groups. Furthermore, such practice should be underpinned by the key principles set out in Box 8.1.

> ### Box 8.1 The principles of anti-ageist practice
>
> **Empowerment:** ensuring that the person has or acquires control over their own life and all that goes with power and control (freedom, autonomy, dignity and feelings of self-worth).
>
> **Participation:** meaningful sharing and involvement.
>
> **Choice:** important means of personal validation as well as a right in terms of personhood and citizenship.
>
> **Integration:** into mainstream of life at every level.
>
> **Normalization:** making available whatever is necessary to enable all people to live in the same way, with the same quality of life as other people in society.

Kagan and Melendez-Torres (2015) make specific recommendations for achieving anti-ageist practice in nursing.

1   Altering the language of age and ageing to positively reflect characteristics of age; for example, wisdom and experience.
2   Referring to chronological age only where it is relevant. No one is adequately represented by one characteristic, so calling someone a seventy-five-year-old man presents a very partial picture.
3   Conducting research to describe, interpret and recommend interventions to counter ageism.
4   Valuing the differential contribution to nursing work of varied care roles.

8

> ### Activity 8.4 Anti-ageist practice
>
> (a) With a colleague, think about how you can incorporate an anti-ageist stance into your practice.
> (b) Discuss your strategy with someone from a different field of nursing. What are the similarities and differences (if any)?
> (c) Do you think that different life stages require a different response?

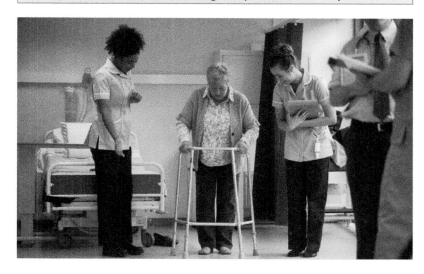

Figure 8.4 Anti-ageist practice involves supporting patients to achieve maximum quality of life regardless of age

Anti-ageist practice then requires that we do not discriminate on the basis of 'age'. This means, for example, that we do not assume that the early years of life are a period of development and the later years a period of decline. Nor do we assume that the 'voice' of a child is less important, or less believable, than that of an adult. Rather, for all those for whom we care, we should seek to maximize quality of life, and build in potential development, regardless of age. This idea will now be explored further in relation to three areas of practice: conceptualizing and responding to falls; understanding the patient's subjective experience; and working with grief and loss.

Falls and our response to them

First, let us consider the way in which we 'conceptualize' and respond to falls. Young children regularly fall over when they are learning to walk. The common response is to encourage the child to get back on its feet and try again. Imagine then another scenario, this time with an older person. She has already fallen a couple of times and has been deemed by family and professionals to be 'at risk of falling'. Nonetheless, the older person wishes to maintain her independence. However, in going to the toilet, a very private sphere of life and one in which she does not wish for support, she falls, and is told off for taking risks. Why the difference? According to Kingston (1998), falls are socially constructed on the basis of age, and risk-assessment tools are a manifestation of such a construction. Older people are not allowed to take risks and, if they do, they are chastised and considered to be 'reckless' and 'selfish'. Young children who fall, by contrast, are considered to be 'bold'. It would seem that 'age' is the determining factor.

An anti-ageist approach to practice ensures that a nurse using a risk-assessment tool with an older person does not use it mechanistically, but rather takes into account the key values of 'personhood', 'citizenship' and 'celebration' discussed above.

Patients' subjective experiences

Increasingly, the literature on childhood, learning disability, mental ill health and old age points to the importance of subjective experiences: 'how it feels' from the inside (patients' perspective), rather than 'how it is' from the outside (professionals' perspective). Fundamental to this approach is 'personhood' and listening to the 'voice' of patients rather than jumping to 'age-based assumptions'. Lee (2001) reminds us that, until fairly recently, children's voices were silent. Even today, although the failings of individual adults and adult institutions are acknowledged, there is still a tension between the need for children to speak and the traditional view that only adults are worth listening to (p. 91). He goes on to stress the importance of recognizing that policies and practices devised for children have often rested on assumptions that children are vulnerable 'becomings', 'investments to be cultivated and protected' (p. 100). Anti-ageist practice challenges this, and enables the nurse to work in partnership with the child or young adult and to value the patient's subjective experience; that is, 'what it feels like'. One way of accomplishing this is through the use of 'life-story' books, in which the patient is encouraged to share their understanding of their illness, in pictures or words, or both, in the context of personal autobiography. This is particularly helpful with children with chronic illness, or learning disability, and it can enable the nurse to gain an 'insider' perspective that can provide a useful counterbalance to so-called objective, often age-based, accounts of illness.

Eliciting the experience of older people in hospital was part of the study by Maben et al., discussed above, which found that not only did patients feel they did not always receive good care, but many had no expectations that they would. The most common complaint from patients was that staff would talk over them as if they were not there, followed by a lack of help with eating and drinking. Participants also noticed care deficits towards other patients; for example, observing someone being left in a chair without slippers so that their feet were on a cold floor (Maben et al. 2012).

Depression, grief and loss

Finally, let us consider the way in which anti-ageist practice can be used in relation to depression, grief and loss in work with older people and young children. Old age is commonly construed as 'a time of loss', and it therefore follows that depression in old age is an automatic consequence of the ageing process and does not need to be treated. The reality is that many older people adjust perfectly well to loss; after all, they expect to experience loss at that point in their life (Chamber 2000, 2002, 2005). However, they may need support and acknowledgement of their loss and must be allowed the time and space to give expression to their feelings. Some older people will suffer from depression; it may or may not be associated with loss, but without treatment they may not recover. Nurses who follow anti-ageist practices will be vigilant and will not assume that depression is an automatic consequence of the ageing process. Instead, they will seek appropriate interventions to enable the older person to return to maximum health. Nor will they ignore the older person who needs time and space to grieve in order to adjust to loss.

In a similar vein, the social construction of 'early childhood' often militates against the needs of very young children who experience loss being adequately addressed. Nurses who have an understanding of, and follow, anti-ageist practice are well placed to support children who are bereaved.

There is now general agreement, resulting primarily from the pioneering work of Stroebe et al. (1996), that the bereaved person, young or old, has to confront both the loss and the changes that result from that loss; this has come to be known as the dual-orientation approach; that is, to both loss and restoration.

Case Study: Older people and cancer treatment

In a *BMJ* editorial in 2014, Mark Lawler and colleagues posed the question: What has happened in the fifteen years since the *BMJ* suggested inadequacies in the treatment of cancer in elderly people? The answer was rather less than they would have hoped, and they gave the following examples in support of this view:

In the UK it is estimated that 76 per cent of cancer in men and 70 per cent in women will occur in people aged over sixty-five by 2030.

Yet the survival gap between older and younger people with cancer is widening in Europe and in other parts of the world.

They argued that the reason for this is twofold:

1. There is increasing evidence that older patients are undertreated and this leads to poorer outcomes. Prostate, colorectal and triple negative breast cancer are all examples where the majority of older patients receive less than optimal treatment

2. Clinicians may use chronological age as a proxy for other factors, such as co-morbidity or frailty, but these may not be relevant to individual patients.

(Adapted from Lawler et al. 2014)

In a systematic review of unmet need in older newly diagnosed cancer patients, a significant proportion of the studies reviewed reported unmet need following diagnosis and during treatment. These included psychological needs (particularly the fear of cancer spreading or returning), information needs (chances of cure, side effects of treatment) and physical needs (tiredness, low energy) *(Putts et al. 2012)*.

Activity 8.5 Levels of treatment available

(a) Why do you think that older people receive less than optimal treatment for cancer?

(b) Are there other groups in society who do not always receive the treatment they need?

(c) An argument that is often used to justify lower levels of care to older people is what is called the 'good innings' argument. The rationale here is that older people have had a long life and services should be concentrated on the young, whose lives are ahead of them. Discuss this in relation to the principles of the NHS.

Summary and Resources

Summary

▶ 'Age' is a complex process and state of being which is more than the sum total of birthdays a person has notched up. In addition to chronology, it encompasses physiology, psychology, law, social policy, culture and sociology.

▶ A society constructs its own meanings of 'childhood', 'adulthood' and 'old age', and these are constantly changing according to the social and economic needs of that society.

▶ Stereotypical assumptions are made on the basis of age, and nurses are no more nor less immune to such ageist assumptions than other members of society.

▶ A life-course perspective, rather than an 'age-based' perspective, is advocated.

▶ An understanding of ageism and anti-ageist practice is essential for nurses in all fields of nursing.

Questions for Discussion

1 What, in relation to 'age', informed your choice of nursing route? Consider the values and attitudes underpinning this choice.
2 How can an understanding of the social construction of 'age' inform nursing practice? Discuss this in relation to your chosen field of nursing.
3 Look at the way in which birthday cards and road signs depict different ages. What do you notice? What does it tell us about the way age is constructed in contemporary British society?
4 How and why is the latest generation of older people – 'the baby boomers' – challenging notions of ageism?

8

Glossary

ageism:	a negative view of a person based on their age; ageism is generally associated with older people, but can also affect the young, for example teenagers; myths and stereotypes are ascribed to all those within a certain age group
anti-ageist practice:	good practice in health and social care respects and values the individual, and does not make judgements about them based on age; optimal care should be provided on the basis of need, not chronological age

demography:	the statistical study of characteristics of human populations the science of vital and social statistics of populations, such as births, marriages, deaths, migration
Gillick competence:	Gillick competence is named after Victoria Gillick, who initiated a test case based on a parent's right to decide on the provision of contraception for under-sixteen-year-olds; the resulting guideline (Fraser guidelines) stated that a doctor could proceed with advice and treatment without parental consent based on the child's capability to give informed consent
life-course perspective:	a multidisciplinary approach which emphasizes time, context and meaning on human development over the lifespan; ageing is a continuous process seen through the prism of these concepts
moral panic:	a term first introduced in the work of Stan Cohen in the 1970s to describe the exaggerated social concern and reaction to a perceived threat to social order; it occurs when an event or condition emerges to become viewed as a threat to societal values, often fuelled by intense media attention
social gerontology:	a subfield of gerontology that is concerned with the social aspects of ageing; it focuses on issues such as ageism, gender in later life, and the financial implications of growing older

Further Reading

P. Higgs and C. Gilleard: *Rethinking Old Age*. Basingstoke: Palgrave Macmillan, 2015.
As people are living and staying healthy for longer, the idea of a fourth age that embodies the most feared and marginalized aspects of old age has emerged. This book provides a critical analysis of this stage of life, using sociological, medical and historical research.

C. Phillipson: *Ageing*. Cambridge: Polity, 2013.
This book considers a number of understandings of ageing and provides a critical assessment of attitudes and responses to the development of ageing societies. It looks at theories of social ageing, changing definitions of age, retirement trends, and poverty and inequality in old age.

M. Wyness: *Childhood*. Basingstoke: Palgrave Macmillan, 2014.
The changing ideas around the biological, social and psychological development of the early years of life are explored in this book. The author discusses competing theories and research that have emerged recently, and a range of contemporary issues that affect children.

A. James and A. L. James: *Constructing Childhood*. Basingstoke: Palgrave, 2004.
James and James look at the way in which childhood is constructed and the tensions between media representations and the vision of childhood in the law and social policy. Case studies include health and the family.

Also useful are the following online resources:

Age UK (<www.ageuk.org.uk>) This provides help and information for older people and also campaigns on issues such as dignity in hospital for older people, and ending loneliness and isolation.

Childline (<www.childline.org.uk>) This is a confidential service for young people up to the age of nineteen years. It provides a phone service and chatroom for discussion on any type of problem, including family relationships, bullying and female genital mutilation.

References

Age UK 2012 *Grey Matters – A Survey of Ageism Across Europe*. Available at: <www.ageuk.org.uk>.

Bytheway, B. 1995 *Ageism*. Buckingham: Open University Press.

Centre for Confidence and Wellbeing n.d. *The Detrimental Influence of Negative Stereotypes*. Available at: <centreforconfidence.co.uk/projects.php?p=cGlkPTk5>.

Chambers, P. 2000 Widowhood in later life. In M. Bernard, J. Phillips, L. Machin and V. Davies (eds), *Women Ageing: Changing Identities, Challenging Myths*. London: Routledge, pp. 127–47.

Chambers, P. 2002 The life stories of older widows: situating later life widowhood within the life course. In C. Horrocks, K. Milnes, B. Roberts and D. Robinson (eds), *Narrative, Memory and Life Transitions*. Huddersfield: Huddersfield University Press, pp. 23–41.

Chambers, P. 2005 *Older Widows and the Lifecourse: Multiple Narratives of Hidden Lives*. Abingdon: Ashgate.

Chen, A. M. H., Kiersma, M. E., Yehle, K. S. and Plake, K. S. 2015 Impact of the Generation Medication Game© on nursing students' empathy and attitudes to older adults. *Nurse Education Today* 35: 38–43.

Department for Work and Pensions (DWP) 2001 *Ageism: Attitudes and Experiences of Young People*. Nottingham: Department for Work and Pensions.

Department of Health (DH) 2001 *National Service Framework for Older People*. London: Department of Health.

Fennell, G., Phillipson, C. and Evers, H. (eds) 1989 *The Sociology of Old Age*. Milton Keynes: Open University Press.

Hockey, J. 1993 Constructing personhood: changing categories of the child. In J. Hockey and A. James (eds), *Growing Up and Growing Old*. London: Sage, pp. 45–72.

8

Kagan, S. H. and Melendez-Torres, G. J. 2015 Ageism in nursing. *Journal of Nursing Management* 23: 644–50.

Kingston, P. 1998 Older people and falls: a randomized control trial of Health Visitor intervention – a study of 108 older women who attended an Accident and Emergency Department after a fall. PhD thesis, Keele University.

Lawler, K. M., Selby, P., Aapro, M. S. and Duffy, S. 2014 Ageism in cancer. *British Medical Journal* 2014; 348: g1614.

Lee, N. 2001 *Childhood and Society.* Buckingham: Open University Press.

Levy, B. R., Chung, P., H., Bedford, T. and Navrazhina, K. 2013 Facebook as a site for negative age stereotypes. *The Gerontologist* 54: 172–6.

Maben J., Adams, M., Peccei, R., Murrels T. 2012 'Poppets and parcels': the links between staff experience of work and acutely ill older people's experience of hospital care. *International Journal of Older People Nursing* 7: 83–94.

Mensforth, S., Goodall, L., Bodasing, N. and Coultas J. 2014 Late diagnosis among our ageing HIV population: a cohort study. *Journal of the International AIDS Society* 17 (Suppl 3): 4.

NHS England 2013 *Hard Truths: the Journey to Putting Patients First.* Available at: <www.england.nhs.com>.

Office for National Statistics (ONS) 1991 Census. Available at: <www.statistics.gov.uk>.

Office for National Statistics (ONS) 2014 Statistical Bulletin. Available at: <www.ons.gov.uk>.

Phillipson, C. 1998 *Reconstructing Old Age.* London: Sage.

Pinchbeck, I. and Hewitt, M. 1973 *Children in English Society*, vols 1 and 2. London: Routledge and Kegan Paul.

Putts, M. T. E., Papoutsis, A., Springall, E. and Tourangeau A. E. 2012 A systematic review of unmet needs of newly diagnosed older cancer patients undergoing active cancer treatment. *Supportive Care in Cancer* 20: 1377–94.

Ray, M. 2007 Redressing the balance? The participation of older people in research. In M. Barnard and T. Scharf (eds), *Critical Perspectives on Ageing Societies*. Bristol: Policy Press, pp. 73–87.

Ruth, J.-E. and Oberg, P. 1996 Ways of life: old age in a life history perspective. In J. E. Birren et al. (eds), *Explorations in Adult Development*. New York: Springer, pp. 167–86.

Sarabia-Cobo C. M. and Castanedo Pfeiffer C. 2015 Changing negative attitudes regarding ageing in undergraduate nursing students. *Nurse Education Today*. Available at: <http://dx.doi.org/10.1016/j.nedt.2015.06.006>.

Scharf, T., Phillipson, C., Smith, A. E. and Kingston, P. 2002 *Growing Older in Socially Deprived Areas: Social Exclusion in Later Life.* London: Help the Aged.

Snowdon, P. 2012 Young and older people 'experience age discrimination at work'. *The Guardian*. Available at: <www.theguardian.com>.

Stroebe, M., Gergen, M. Gergen, K. and Stroebe, W. 1996 Broken hearts or broken bonds. In D. Klass, P. R. Silverman and S. L. Nickman (eds), *Continuing Bonds: New Understandings of Grief*. Washington, DC, and London: Taylor and Francis, pp. 31–44.

Thompson, N. 1995 *Age and Dignity.* Aldershot: Arena.

United Nations Convention on the Rights of the Child 1989. Available at: <www.unicef.org>.

Warnes, A. M., King, R., Williams, A. M. and Patterson, G. 1999 The well-being of British expatriate retirees in southern Europe. *Ageing and Society* 19/6: 717–40.

Wheeler, R. 2006 Gillick or Fraser? A plea for consistency over competence in children. *British Medical Journal* 332: 807.

Yinn, S. 2008 Older women, divorce and poverty. Available at: <www.pbr.org/Multimedia/Audio/2008/olderwomen.aspx>.

Ylanne-McEwen, V. 1999 Young at heart: discourses of age identity in travel agency interaction. *Ageing and Society* 19/4: 417–40.

8

Long-term Illness and Conditions

Elaine Denny

KEY ISSUES IN THIS CHAPTER:

▶ Sociological theories of chronic illness/long-term conditions.
▶ Interpretive and narrative accounts of long-term conditions.
▶ Long-term pain.
▶ Adherence to medical treatment.
▶ The role of nursing in long-term conditions.

BY THE END OF THIS CHAPTER YOU SHOULD BE ABLE TO:

▶ Understand different sociological theories and concepts in relation to long-term conditions.
▶ Explore the experience of long-term conditions.
▶ Understand the implications of living with long-term pain.
▶ Discuss issues around compliance, adherence and concordance with medical advice.
▶ Consider the role of the nurse in assisting people to live with long-term conditions.

1 Introduction

This chapter considers the growing importance both of long-term illness as a major challenge for twenty-first-century health-care systems, and of nurses in managing this challenge. Although for clarity the issues of disability and long-term illness are treated separately in this volume, it is acknowledged that people with long-term illness constitute a large proportion of those living with disability. Many conditions may fall into either category, or both, and how people view their situation may change over the lifetime and with various experiences, so the distinctions between long-term illness and disability may be fluid. For example, a teenage boy with Type 1 diabetes may be adept at managing diet and medication, and live what he considers a normal life with few restrictions. He may not recognize a label of 'disabled' as appropriate for his life experiences. Later in life diabetes may result in disabling complications, such as renal failure or a leg amputation which severely affects his mobility, leading him to reassess how he defines himself. His changed sense of identity may be influenced by policy that requires various assessments around activities of daily living in order to access state benefits or social services (see Chapter 15). You will find examples of the overlap between long-term illness and disability in this chapter and Chapter 10.

Before we consider sociological concepts and perspectives on long-term illness, it is useful to think about the terminology you will see used in publications and the broadcast media and also within sociology. In the past, the term 'chronic disease' was used to describe those illnesses that had no cure, but were not fatal in the short term. Institutions that cared for people with these diseases were sometimes called homes for incurables. However, this term was not very accurate in describing many diseases that were only problematic for some of the time, so 'long-term' gradually replaced 'chronic'. Disease was also thought to reflect a biomedical model, and to ignore a person's subjective experience, so 'illness' became more commonly used to incorporate this. More recently '**long-term condition**' is used in most government documents as this is seen to reflect the non-medical aspects of ill health. In this chapter, the term 'long-term conditions' will be employed, except when reporting literature in which a different term is used.

long-term condition:
incurable illness or condition, which may be controlled by treatment

Long-term conditions (LTCs) are the most common causes of death and disability in most developed countries, and increasingly in the rest of the world. Many people develop one or more LTC in later life, so an increase in life expectancy is associated with an increase in their incidence. In England, more than 15 million people have at least one LTC, accounting for 50 per cent of GP appointments, 64 per cent of outpatient appointments and 70 per cent of in-patient bed days (Coulter et al. 2013). At age fifty, 50 per cent of the population has at least one LTC; in those aged over sixty-five, the figure is 80 per cent. In absolute terms, more people under the age of fifty have an LTC, as they are a larger percentage of the population (Coulter et al. 2013), but the challenge for health systems is in caring for the frail elderly person in whom LTCs pose a greater problem for independent living. In Scotland, 42 per cent of the population has at least one LTC and 23 per cent has two or more (Barnett et al. 2012).

9

In this chapter we will consider sociological research on long-term conditions, and the implications for nursing. We will start with the early days of sociological interest in illness and medicine, and move on to more recent developments of the concepts around long-term illness and research into how those with LTCs, together with their carers, experience and make sense of their lives. Associated and relevant issues, such as pain and compliance with treatment, will follow. We will also think about persistent symptoms that remain unexplained, and the importance of diagnosis in Western medicine.

Although, as stated earlier, long-term conditions are often the cause of disability, there are important differences in the experience of each that affect the way in which we need to view them. For example, as we shall discuss later in this chapter, the importance of pain and reduced mobility for many people living with long-term conditions is identified as a crucial part of the experience. Yet for many disabled people who do not have a physical illness this may not be an issue, and such individuals would not even consider themselves as ill or unhealthy. Similarly, those with a long-term illness may actually want and seek out the medical labels and control of their condition that those within the disability movement reject.

2 Sociological theorists and long-term conditions

In Chapters 1 and 3, you were introduced to some of the major sociological theorists and their work. The sociologists whom we will be revisiting in this chapter are Parsons and Goffman, and you may want to remind yourself of their main theories before reading this section.

Talcott Parsons' work on the sick person within society was developed within the structural functionalist tradition, and was the first account to move beyond biomedical interpretations of sickness. His work has long been criticized for failing to account for people with long-term conditions, as the patient's responsibilities within the sick role, to want to get well, and to seek competent help and comply with treatment are not achievable or necessarily desirable in their situation. The notion of compliance with treatment will be discussed later in this chapter, but Parsons himself argued that the goal of wanting to get well or recover is an approximation, rather than an absolute (Parsons 1951). The importance of Parsons' work, however, is in categorizing illness as a **social phenomenon**, leading to the expansion of the field of sociology of health and illness in which subsequent sociological work on long-term conditions is located.

social phenomenon: the external influences on an individual

Goffman, stigma and long-term conditions

Goffman's work on stigma and the management of self has been influential in the understanding of how people make sense of and respond to living with a long-term condition. Goffman distinguished between discrediting (easily visible) and discreditable (less visible) conditions (Goffman 1968). For example, Jobling wrote about his experience of the stigma associated with both his experience of the skin disease psoriasis, characterized by scaly appearance of the skin which is highly visible, and the messy and ineffective treatments given to him (Jobling 1988).

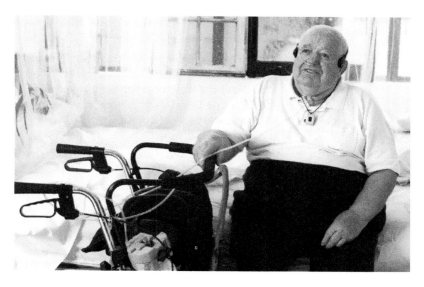

Figure 9.1 People suffering visible long-term illnesses may have little control over how and when their condition is disclosed, which can lead to stigma

Other conditions, such as certain heart problems, may be less visible and a choice can be made whether and how much to disclose to others. Participants in a study conducted by Kathy Charmaz with people who lived with long-term illness used their personal definition of 'illness' and an assessment of their own condition to help them make decisions about disclosure. One participant commented, 'I haven't been sick for a long time,' as for him 'sickness' meant being in hospital; everything else that occurred in connection with his illness was perceived as normal life (Charmaz 2010: 9). This view of his illness influenced decisions around who and when to tell about it. Discreditable conditions may become discrediting when disclosure becomes necessary, or when something occurs to make the condition visible. Whether this leads to stigma depends on the nature of that condition, and social and cultural perceptions of it. In Western societies, association with sexuality (for example, HIV), perceived responsibility for the condition (obesity) or lack of bodily control (incontinence), whether justified or not, are most likely to result in stigma, or the fear of it. So a person may not disclose that they have irritable bowel disease (the sixth most stigmatizing condition, according to *LiveScience*), fearing the reaction of friends, colleagues and family. However, an acute crisis in the condition may make it unavoidable. Disclosure may be partial and selective, and the balance between honesty and privacy causes a dilemma for people with long-term conditions, particularly in the workplace (Charmaz 2010).

9

Activity 9.1 Disclosing long-term illness

Mandy has lived with epilepsy since childhood. When she started work in the offices of a factory producing car components she decided to inform her employers and colleagues of her condition. Although she rarely experiences seizures, she needed to avoid certain triggers such as getting overtired. Mandy does not go out of her way to inform people of her epilepsy, but does so when she thinks they should know. Epilepsy is something that she lives with, but she does not feel that it is a big deal in her life.

George has had depression for many years and was recently diagnosed as having bipolar disorder. He has never told anyone at work about this, and has lied about absences when he has needed doctors' appointments. He has heard people in the garage where he works saying that people with mental health problems should pull themselves together, and he does not want to be the butt of criticism.

(a) Discuss with a colleague how these different decisions around disclosure reflect the individual's experience of living with a long-term condition.
(b) The two examples above are of a discreditable illness. How may each become discredited?
(c) How may disclosure of other illnesses/conditions cause problems for individuals and their families?

3 Interpretive and narrative accounts of long-term conditions

Interpretive perspectives seek to understand the impact that living with a long-term condition has on a person and their family and carers, and the meanings that they attach to it. Indeed, much of the interpretive work on long-term illness has arisen out of personal interest (see, for example, Jobling 1988, above). This work has been criticized as reinforcing a medical model, as many studies focus on specific diseases, but it does highlight the day-to-day experience of people's lives and the effects of living with illness over a long period. This is in sharp contrast to the perspectives of health practitioners whose views have dominated policy and practice. The chapters in Part III demonstrate how these patient experiences are now much more influential in shaping health and social care policy. Further, the use of the term 'long-term illness' as opposed to 'disease' reflects sociology's interest in these experiences as opposed to a paternalistic medical model, in which primacy is given to diagnosis and treatment.

narrative:
the stories people tell to give meaning to their suffering

Sociological work on 'lived experience' often uses **narrative** methods to discover what it is like to live with a particular illness over many years and the impact it has on one's life. The use of such methods allows the participant to impart the issues that are important to them, and gives voice to their interpretation of their condition and their life.

Kathy Charmaz has argued that the primacy of acute illness in Western health-care systems permeates thinking about chronic illness and influences policy and practice. She goes on to say that people with chronic illness lose the taken-for-granted continuity of their previous life, and from her qualitative studies with people with chronic illness and their carers identified three major problems they have to face. These involve the effort to make sense of bewildering symptoms, reconstruct order and maintain control over one's life (Charmaz 2000).

Others have also pointed out the uncertainties posed by the diagnosis of a disease for which there is no cure. Williams sums this up as '*diagnostic* uncertainty, *symptomatic* uncertainty and *trajectory* uncertainty' (Williams 2003: 97; original emphasis). People learn how to tolerate or 'put up with' the illness by normalizing, that is, bracketing off its impact, or regarding the illness or its treatment as normal (as in the example from Charmaz, above), in order to minimize the effects on self-identity and self-worth (Williams 2000). Simon Williams also writes about the ups and downs of chronic illness (Williams 1996), but 'ups and downs' occur in most people's daily life. We all face change throughout our lives (leaving school, ending a relationship, having children and so on), which challenges our sense of worth and identity and results in biographical disruption. Yet these changes are regarded as normal life events and are rarely used as a defining characteristic of an individual, in the same way as, for example, having bipolar disorder or epilepsy may be.

Typologies of narrative have been developed by Hydén (1997) and Frank (1995). Hydén argues that narrative is the most powerful way of expressing suffering, and has formulated three types of illness narrative. In the first type, illness as narrative, illness is articulated and expressed through narrative. This encompasses the person's story regarding the occurrence of the illness and the way in which it is accommodated into the totality of that person's life. Thus, it is possible to integrate symptoms and consequences of illness into the formulation of a new identity. The second type, narrative about illness, is primarily about the illness rather than the person, and constructs and conveys knowledge and ideas about illness. Health professionals use narratives about illness to gain information on a patient's illness, to reach a diagnosis and to formulate acceptable treatment regimes, but, as will be seen later in the chapter, health professionals' own interpretations of the patient's narrative may influence how this is interpreted. Hydén's third type, narrative as illness, reflects instances when the inability to narrate or to articulate is a crucial aspect of illness, as in the case of aphasia associated with a stroke (Hydén 1997).

Frank, too, discusses three forms of narrative, developed from his own experience. The restitution narrative exemplifies the acute, more short-lived, illness whereby an individual is ill, seeks medical help, or self-medicates, and recovers. The quest narrative is characterized by the belief that there is something to be gained from the illness experience, and is more relevant to long-term conditions. For example, following a diagnosis of breast cancer, the sociologist Barbara Ehrenreich found that many websites and blogs she encountered talked of the experience of cancer being a positive one, with one woman calling it a 'gift'. Even nurses spoke to her of the 'positives' of chemotherapy – tightened skin, weight loss, softer hair (Ehrenreich 2010). This positivity contrasted with Ehrenreich's own feelings of anger and outrage at the disease and its treatment. Frank's third narrative is chaos narrative, which is exemplified in the situations of those with unexplained pain, explored later in the chapter. Here there is no restitution and, as the name implies, the plot of the narrative is chaotic, unpredictable and random (Frank 1995).

Many of these works have taken as a starting point the notion that the experience of a long-term condition alters a person's current and expected biography, and it is this important idea within the sociology of health and illness on which the next section will focus.

Biographical disruption

The concept of biographical disruption has been very influential in the sociological analysis of long-term illness. It was developed by sociologist Mike Bury in the 1970s while researching people diagnosed with rheumatoid arthritis. He noted that the illness had interrupted the individual's life, and their future expectations, and caused her/him to re-evaluate themselves and their self-concept (Bury 1982). From this, Bury argued that previous sociological work had been concerned with the problems that people faced when living with a long-term illness, rather than their responses to such illness (Bury 1991). 'Biographical disruption', then, is the term Bury adopted to describe and explain the assault on identity and self-worth following the onset of a long-term illness. The 'taken-for-granted' life that had been lived is now altered, often irrevocably, and a new sense of 'normal' emerges. This may include the experience of pain, or the possibility of death, both of which were previously remote, or the change in a dependence relationship between a parent and child. However, the way in which this occurs and the impact on individual life expectation and achievement changes over time.

At the onset of the condition, the *consequences* and *significance* of the condition are paramount. That is, what is of most concern to a person is the impact that a condition has on a person's everyday roles and relationships and the **symbolic and cultural meanings** that surround different sorts of illnesses and impairments. Over time, biographical disruption can be overcome through individuals constructing explanations for their conditions and establishing their **legitimacy**. *The impact of treatment on everyday life* refers to the way in which individuals 'come to grips with treatment regimes and medical interventions, and with the bureaucracies from which they emanate' (Bury 1997: 126). It involves the person gaining an understanding of the official diagnosis and labelling, searching for information on their condition, making sense of this and incorporating it into their restructured social world. As discussed in Chapter 3 (see, in particular, Activity 3.1), people living with long-term illness are increasingly regarded as 'lay experts' on their own health and health-care needs. This expertise is in part experiential, in that they and their carers develop optimum ways of managing their condition and its treatments. Increasingly, though, people have access to the same resources as health professionals via

symbolic and cultural meanings: the way concepts and ideas are expressed through culture

legitimacy: general acceptance of an authority

the Internet, and also the knowledge and experience of others with the same condition through online self-help and advice sites. Activity 3.1 also points to the limitations of lay expertise.

Adaptation and management of illness and disability describes how individuals cope with an impairment, how they develop a strategy and a style to achieve 'the best quality of life possible' (Bury 1997: 129). It is the way that individuals achieve a 'normal' life, despite the presence of an impairment. The term 'coping', as Bury (1991, 1997) acknowledges, implies a moral framework against which an individual's ability to cope is judged. Despite claims by Bury and others that the notion of 'coping' is not judgemental, the very nature of the approach implies that there is something wrong with the individual in the first place. People with a long-term condition are presented as essentially different from their peers in that they have lost their sense of worth because of the presence of impairment. You may have seen people on your placements who are described as 'coping well' or 'not coping' with their illness or disability, and have noticed the expectation from health professionals that they will learn to 'cope'.

The *strategies* that disabled people adopt are the second element of the adaptation process (Bury 1991, 1997). These refer to actions or practices that people adopt in the face of chronic illness or impairment, rather than to meanings or attitudes. Through successful actions, the individual learns how to maintain hope and a sense of the future.

While this approach has provided useful avenues of research within sociology, the analysis does raise a number of issues. Bury, and others, have allowed for an exploration of the consequences of having a long-term condition in practical situations. The perspective of the person is taken seriously and credence is given to their views. However, despite the acknowledgement within this work of conditions of inequality, powerlessness and violence (see, for example, Bury 1997), these issues are rarely placed at the centre of the research or analysis (Williams 1996). Even where wider social issues are incorporated or acknowledged, the focus is still very much on individuals and their experiences. By focusing on the impact of treatment and care, this body of work presents an image of those with a long-term condition as inevitably being in need of long-term care, whereas in reality many develop their own strategies for living. It also fails to analyse how people who have a congenital condition, or develop a long-term illness early in life, perceive that condition and the impact it has on their lives.

A number of more recent studies have utilized the concept of biographical disruption in order to explore the experience of living with long-term conditions, and have moved on from the original thesis by utilizing different study populations, illnesses and place within the illness trajectory. For example, in their study of widespread pain, Richardson et al. (2006) suggest the need to add perceptions of life stage and life expectancy to the concept of biographical disruption, in order to obtain a fuller social and biographical context. These are not just predicated on biological age, but formulated from a person's history; for example, the premature death of parents may lead to a perceived lower personal life expectancy. In their Australian study with women who were diagnosed with breast cancer and were also mothers of dependent children, Fisher and O'Connor included the use of biographical disruption as an analytical framework. They found that for all of the women the diagnosis was entirely unexpected and a major disruption to their anticipated lives. However, this disruption had to incorporate a woman's ongoing role as a mother, and these two identities, cancer patient and mother, existed in constant tension, not least because of a woman's worries for her children's future well-being if the disease proved terminal. The women felt that health professionals did not always acknowledge the dual identities of mother and patient that they were continually having to construct and reconstruct throughout the course of the disease and its treatment (Fisher and O'Connor 2012).

A study which moves away from Bury's idea that biographical disruption starts with the sudden and unexpected nature of the onset of long-term illness is that of Larsson and Grassman, whose participants had lived with an early onset long-term illness. For people who, for example, are born with cerebral palsy or have had Type 1 diabetes diagnosed in childhood, or bipolar disorder in early adulthood, the experience is somewhat different. In their participants, Larsson and Grassman found that disruption was repeated over the lifespan and was not necessarily unexpected. 'These losses may have been unexpected, feared and expected at the same time, and may have disrupted a wished-for scenario for the future' (Larsson and Grassman 2012: 1167). They also challenge Williams' suggestion that people who have experienced illness from a young age normalize their situation, with the implication that disruptions in their lives are unproblematic. A case in point is Bjorn, born with a congenital eye problem, who said: 'I have lived all my life knowing that I might lose my eyesight . . . from the beginning. It was in the family. I focused my life planning on it. Yet when it happened, I lost my grip on life. I did not know what to do with myself or how to go on' (Larsson and Grassman 2012: 1164). Similarly, in a study with children with a long-term condition undergoing surgery to improve continence, and their parents, Bray et al. (2014) found that ongoing management of their condition involved 'diverse and changing biographical experiences, ongoing transitions and disruptions', and that 'time spent with their condition did not make it easier or harder to confront their life or complications after surgery' (Bray et al. 2014: 835).

The message for nurses from this body of work is that biographical disruption caused by the onset of a long-term condition must accommodate previous roles and identities, as well as disruptions to life caused by other events, such as bereavement. However, it cannot be assumed that a long history of illness, or illness from an early age, is normalized, and that expected disruptions are unproblematic.

Case Study: Cancer and biographical disruption

Gill Hubbard and Liz Forbat conducted a study with forty cancer survivors from Scotland, using written accounts. Seventeen had been diagnosed between one and five years prior to the research, and twenty-three over six years. Thirty reported themselves to be free of cancer, six reported that they were not, and four did not know. Participants were asked to write up to two pages about what had changed in their life that they attributed to cancer. The concept of biographical disruption guided the analysis of the accounts obtained.

For the participants cancer was constructed as:

Disruptive to everyday life many years after diagnosis and treatment

This was manifest in physical and psychosocial consequences of the disease and its treatment. So, for instance, radiotherapy had caused cystitis, abdominal pain and loss of libido for one woman; the inability to work as previously anticipated had led to a loss of power, influence and income for another.

A persistent and ongoing threat

For most people this was a constant fear of the disease, in particular a fear of recurrence, but also a vigilance concerning any bodily changes. One man reported being cautious or even paranoid over the smallest changes in his body or to his health.

A disease that heightens cancer survivors' sense of their own mortality

This was apparent in people diagnosed over six years ago as well as in those diagnosed more recently, so the association between cancer and death or shortened life expectancy persisted. One man compared his mother reaching her ninetieth birthday to his lesser chance of reaching seventy.

A disease that invokes a change to self, disrupting anticipated identity

A quarter of participants reported a change in themselves that can be construed as disrupting an anticipated identity. Mostly these were negative, but being stronger and more decisive were positive outcomes.

Hubbard and Forbat concluded that biographical disruption is useful for describing and explaining the impact of cancer in threatening one's sense of the taken-for-granted world and one's anticipated future. Cancer survivors' anticipated life expectancy, life course and identity are all disrupted. Yet, for some participants, there were also positive alterations to biography and identity following their cancer experience. *(Hubbard and Forbat 2012)*

9

Activity 9.2 Biographical disruption

(a) Biographical disruption has been influential in a sociological analysis of long-term conditions. Discuss with a colleague from a different branch of nursing how it can inform your practice.

(b) How can nurses work with patients/clients in order to incorporate people's multiple identities (e.g., parent, teacher, carer, student, sibling) into their care?

It is important for nurses to acknowledge all types of responses to illness from patients/clients and their carers. They need to consider individual biographies and life stage as they try to understand the impact of a long-term condition on patients, and help them to manage their illness.

4 Pain

One area where interpretive research on patient experience is frequently explored is the growing sociological work on chronic pain. Pain is generally accepted within the health field as a biopsychological phenomenon, but for sociologists it is an individual, embodied experience that needs to be understood within a structure, for example, as gendered and cultured. In her groundbreaking work on pain and gender, Gillian Bendelow (2000) argues that, although experimental research demonstrates that women possess a lower pain threshold, her study on beliefs and perceptions of pain, with men and women in an inner-city health centre, found that women were perceived as being more able to cope with pain. The reasons given for this were both biological and sociocultural: biological in that the reproductive role of women equips their bodies to endure pain, and sociocultural, as women's socialization and roles made it easier for them to admit to pain but harder for them to adopt the sick role and restrict their normal activities. The consequence is that women's pain is not taken as seriously as men's. Her respondents also felt that men would take longer to admit to pain or to seek treatment, but that when they did they would receive more attention and be taken more seriously. Bendelow argues that 'Being a gendered body in a hierarchical organized gender-differentiated world must have an impact on the ways in which different forms of pain are experienced and expressed' (Bendelow 2000: 132; see also Chapter 6). In their study of white cancer patients' perceptions of pain, Im et al. (2007) also found gender to be an issue raised by participants. The women all perceived gender differences in the experience of pain, with most feeling that they were treated differently from men in pain by family and friends, whereas none of the (admittedly small) sample of men mentioned gender. The participants also felt that predominant values within their personal culture influenced their experience of pain.

Patients with cancer tend to have their pain believed unquestioningly, but for some people, particularly those with unexplained pain, being believed by health professionals is a constant struggle. Richardson et al. (2006) have written about the 'power of the visible', by which they mean that a lesion or diseased organ that can be visualized by scan or X-ray gives credibility to a patient's story. Abnormal blood-test or biopsy results may also add to a patient's credibility with health professionals. In their study with women experiencing unexplained pain, Werner and Malterud (2003) describe how they saw their

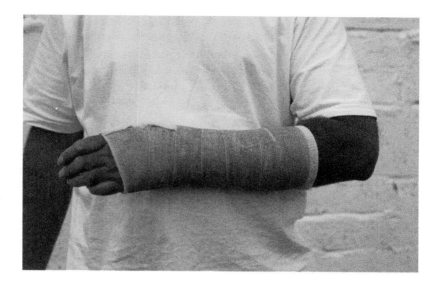

Figure 9.2 Patients with visible conditions which produce pain, such as broken bones, are more likely to have their experiences of pain believed than patients with invisible or silent conditions

attempts to be credible to health professionals as 'work'. They would act and dress in a way that they consider the doctor would think appropriate in an effort not to be thought of as 'wingeing' or time-wasting. In a review of the literature Clarke and Iphofen (2005) state that, although the importance to patients of having their pain believed is well documented, little research has been conducted on the impact for patients of not being believed.

In Western biomedical systems the main way for patients to be believed and seen to be authentic is through receiving a diagnosis. Where symptoms are short-lived or self-limiting this may not be important, but for those living with persistent and long-term conditions a diagnosis is what legitimizes them and allows access to the sick role. It also sets in train a set of structured interventions and treatments, rather than ad hoc responses to symptoms (Denny 2009). Participants in the study by Charmaz (2010), discussed in Section 2 above, were particularly reluctant to disclose illness when symptoms had been discounted by doctors in case they were considered to be hypochondriacs, and conversely they were more likely to disclose when a diagnosis had been given (Charmaz 2010). Studies also point to what Robinson (1988) has called the medical merry-go-round of people consulting various health specialists, trying to achieve a diagnosis or some kind of meaning or explanation for what is happening to them, and finding a treatment for the cause of their illness. The term 'medical merry-go-round' may be construed as pejorative in view of the desperation that some people feel in their interactions with health professionals.

One of the difficulties in being believed is that, as Bury has argued, some conditions 'may produce symptoms which because of their widespread occurrence in milder forms, among the normal (*sic*) population, make legitimation extremely difficult' (Bury 1991: 456). So, for example, people with low back pain, migraine or pelvic pain will often find themselves dismissed by friends and family as well as health professionals when their pain persists over a long period despite treatment, as similar pains are experienced over a short period by many people. Women in Denny's narrative study with a diagnosis of endometriosis told of being 'fobbed off' when repeatedly attending their GP with unexplained pelvic pain. As one reported, 'He brushes it off and says it's period pain and you can get on with it. That's his entire attitude, have some Ibuprofen and get on with it' (Denny 2009: 989).

Pain in children has long been underestimated and until fairly recently it was assumed, and even written into medical texts, that infants and children did not feel pain as adults did (Zisk 2003). This was thought to be due to their underdeveloped nervous system, and as young children cannot always adequately express how much pain they are in, so these beliefs prevailed. Doctors were also wary of administering powerful narcotics and anaesthetic agents to young children, so many procedures were conducted on them without adequate pain relief. It is only in recent years that attention has been paid to observing signs within a baby or child that indicate pain when they cannot express it.

Health professionals tend to see patients at a short consultation and may well rely on diagnostic tests and procedures to validate a patient's story. They may also use their previous experience with other patients to gauge a person's pain, and have ideas about the 'correct' level and duration of pain for a certain condition (Denny 2009). It is important for nurses to remember that a patient lives with his/her pain all of the time and that their interpretation of that pain may not be consistent with that of the nurse or doctor. It is only by listening to and respecting that interpretation that the impact and significance of pain on the lives of patients will be elicited.

Activity 9.3 Unexplained pain

Read the following case study and discuss the questions below with your colleagues.

Stan is a fifty-six-year-old man who has chronic back pain following an injury, but no cause has been found for his continuing pain. He has been unable to work for five years.

> When I first had the injury I thought the pain would go and that I would get back to work. I couldn't accept that I would not work again, and so I did not claim benefits. I lived on my savings after my sick pay ran out, rather than admit that this would be permanent.
>
> The problem with a condition like back pain is that it can't be seen, not like a broken leg or something. People don't understand that you can look normal but still be disabled. For instance when I go to the supermarket and park in a disabled parking bay, and then walk round without a stick or anything you can see people looking at you and thinking you are a fraud.
>
> People do get fed up with you after a while when you don't get better, and can't do things. They are sympathetic at first but as time goes on friends and

even family start to wonder whether you are putting it on, and not helping yourself. Being in pain is lonely.

Even health professionals don't understand. They see you for a few minutes at an appointment; they don't see what it is like day in day out. They see the part that's in pain, not the whole person. When I see the doctor he doesn't want to talk about anything other than my back.

(a) Do you think that Stan can be seen as having a stigmatized condition?
(b) With a colleague make a list of types of pain that are not always believed by health professionals or by the general public. What makes these pains different from pain that is believed?
(c) What can nurses do to understand and help people like Stan with unexplained pain?

5 Adherence to medical advice

People who live with long-term conditions often require medication or other treatments over a long period of time and so issues of compliance, adherence or concordance are very relevant to them and to the health professionals working with them. It is often claimed that people using long-term medication are more likely not to take it as prescribed than those using episodic drugs. The exception to this is antibiotic use. Estimates of non-compliance vary, and are difficult to substantiate, but literature reviews generally suggest that around a half of patients are non-compliant with medication (Donovan and Blake 1992). As we shall see below, what is meant by this is quite vague.

So what do we mean by compliance, adherence and concordance, and what is the difference between these terms? As we saw earlier in the chapter, the terminology that is used to describe or explain a phenomenon is often bound up with current perceptions of that phenomenon, and so it evolves over time. As health care moves from the paternalistic

9

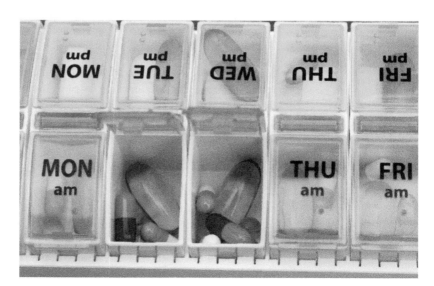

Figure 9.3 Pill holders are designed to help with compliance; can you think of other strategies which are used?

model adopted at the inception of the NHS (see Chapter 13) to one that is based on negotiation between health-care user and professional, so our use of language has changed. Health professionals used to talk about 'patient compliance', by which they meant the extent to which prescribed treatment was followed. Much importance to the success or otherwise of treatment was put on patients' responsibility to follow instructions, and indeed it is one of the facets of the sick role. 'Adherence' is the term currently in use (see, for example, Horne et al. 2013; Vrijens et al. 2012), which assumes a degree of patient/user agreement in treatment, but in a review of the literature Bissonette (2008) demonstrated that 'compliance' and 'adherence' are frequently used interchangeably. There is no real consensus as to a definition of either term, and within the literature they vary between passive notions of following instructions and more collaborative definitions. The term 'concordance' is a more recent construction, and implies a consultation between professional and health-care user as equals (Bissonette 2008). As yet, this term has not been widely adopted, perhaps because, as Vrijens et al. (2012) point out, it really describes the professional/patient relationship, rather than treatment taking. The rest of this section will refer to the more commonly used 'adherence', unless citing specific literature where the term 'compliance' is used.

Whichever term is used, the concept is constructed by health professionals within a biomedical framework, and research is focused upon improving adherence, particularly in stigmatized, vulnerable or hard-to-reach populations. As Britten (2001) has noted, the literature has concentrated on questions of how many people are non-compliant, and how they can be identified. This places the issue as a problem of patients, with consequences for them and for society in terms of costs and less than optimal management of disease (Sabaté 2003). Tools have been developed to measure non-adherence with a view to producing strategies aimed at increasing treatment adherence. So education of patients, telephone follow-up, electronic pill counters and more intrusively measuring either blood serum levels of the prescribed drug or urine for metabolites have all been suggested as ways of monitoring adherence. A study conducted by Fineman with health-care staff involved in a clinic used mainly by poor, white, single people in a large US city found that in addition to adhering to a treatment plan there were eighteen other areas of behaviour to which staff expected adherence. Non-compliance (the term used in the research) was 'socially constructed and subjectively defined by [health care] providers' (Fineman 1991: 371). One of the consequences was that future interactions with patients were based on these subjective understandings of non-compliance. Non-compliant patients were viewed by staff as deviant. Staff perceived themselves, however, to be moral and rational, with a role to counteract the irrational deviance of patients.

Whereas most of the literature appears to be concerned with improving patient care, it is in fact more to do with professional control of patients' treatments and non-compliance is viewed as a problem that needs to be solved (Russell et al. 2003). Playle and Keeley (1998) describe the introduction of depot injections for severe mental illness as a response to problems of non-compliance and further state that the rationale for community treatment orders is that non-compliance is a symptom of the illness that makes patients incompetent to make informed decisions. This, they argue, legitimizes an ideology of patient failure.

Adherence is, however, complex and dependent on many individual and structural factors, such as health beliefs, social support, and the financial and non-financial costs of health care (Sabaté 2003). For people with long-term conditions these change over time as their condition develops, and their position in the life course changes. Yet adherence is often couched in judgemental terms, labelling people and blaming a lack of improvement in their condition to problems of adherence. Missing from this narrative are the perspectives of healthcare users themselves and an understanding of how they make sense of their condition and its treatment, and use this to make decisions about their care. Pound et al. (2005), in a synthesis of qualitative studies on compliance that were mainly concerned with long-term illness, argue that health professionals do not always understand that lay people view medicine not as something to be taken only as prescribed, but as a resource to be used as they see fit.

As Britten (2001) argues, conflict between doctors and patients over medication-taking is not overt and occurs outside of the consultation. Similarly, Donovan and Blake (1992) point out that the setting for recommending treatment is remote from where implementation takes place. Many things impinge on decision-making around treatments. Their qualitative study on reactions to advice and medications prescribed in a rheumatology clinic found that, far from being ignorant or forgetful, patients were active in not complying with advice and medication. People's lay belief about health and illness, which emanate from their history, background, culture and previous experience, meant that they often had theories about their joint pains before they attended the rheumatology clinic. When offered advice and medication, they would weigh up the costs and the benefits of each within the context of their lives. So, for example, the stigma and inconvenience of wearing splints would be weighed against the improvement in pain. Drugs tended to be taken on a trial basis, and would be stopped or reduced if benefits were not experienced within what the patient considered a reasonable timeframe. This, argue Donovan and Blake, far from being deviant, amounted to reasoned decision-making. Patients complied with advice and treatment when it made sense to them, and coincided with their lay beliefs, and was perceived to be effective.

Russell states that nurses need to understand patients' lives and the context in which they make decisions regarding medication, and this sentiment also applies to other medical interventions. Discussions can

9

be had around people's hopes and expectations for prescribed medical treatments, and their acceptability. As a result of their relationship with patients, nurses are well placed to take leadership in this and in conveying decisions to other health-care professionals (Russell et al. 2003).

Activity 9.4 Adherence and long-term conditions

Healthtalk and *Youthhealthtalk* are online resources for patients with a range of health conditions (see resources below). One of the topics is 'Managing diabetes as a teenager'. Researchers interviewed thirty-nine young people with Type 1 diabetes and found:

> Most of the young people we talked to said that they had found it very difficult to control their diabetes when they were teenagers . . .
>
> Before they got their diabetes under good control, plenty of young people told us they had gone through times when they rebelled against their condition. They didn't want to think about diabetes and they didn't want diabetes to control them and stop them doing normal things with their friends.
>
> Rebelling could include eating too much or too little, not doing blood glucose tests, and eating the wrong kinds of foods.

Before discussing the questions below, it would be useful to go to <www.youthhealthtalk.org> and watch or listen to some of the teenagers' stories on the page 'Managing diabetes as a teenager'.

(a) Why do you think that teenagers in particular rebel against their treatment and medication?

(b) How can nurses help teenagers manage the tensions between what makes sense to them, and what makes sense to the health professionals caring for them?

(c) How can health professionals ensure that they understand the competing priorities of people with LTCs when recommending medication or other treatments?

Summary and Resources

Summary

▷ Many long-term conditions are stigmatizing, and disclosing to others may be problematic.

▷ Narratives of people's experience help us to understand what it is like for someone to live with an LTC, and the impact on them and their family.

▷ Being diagnosed with an LTC disrupts a person's identity, their present life and anticipated future.

▷ Many LTCs are characterized by pain, but much long-term pain remains undiagnosed, which may lead to problems of being believed and taken seriously.

▷ Adherence to medication and treatment regimes is seen as important by health professionals, but patients may make decisions on following advice within the context of their lives.

Questions for Discussion

1 What has an understanding of biographical disruption taught you that will help you in your clinical work?
2 Thinking about a patient/client with an LTC that you have met on placement, how was their own expert knowledge of their illness used in their treatment plan?
3 'Pain is what the patient says it is, not what the nurse thinks it is' has become a mantra in medical care. To what extent is the patient's story of their physical or emotional pain given credibility in clinical practice?
4 How can nurses avoid labelling people who do not comply with medical advice and treatment, and understand the decisions they make in managing their LTC?

Glossary

long-term condition:	an illness or condition which may be present from birth but more usually develops in later life, which may be amenable to medication or other therapy but as yet cannot be cured
social phenomenon:	illness is a social phenomenon because it is not a random biomedical event that occurs by chance; for example, many diseases are related to socioeconomic status and are seen more frequently in people living in poverty
narrative:	in qualitative research narratives are used in order for an individual to present real world events in a way that has meaning and significance to them; they narrate the story of their life or some aspect of it, rather than answer set questions
symbolic and cultural meanings:	concepts and ideas that individuals are socialized into, and that are reproduced in subsequent generations by a collective belief in them; for example, many cultures place meanings on different foods, either a taboo in the case of pork in Judaism or Islam, or celebration, as in eating turkey on American Thanksgiving Day
legitimacy:	in health and illness legitimacy is obtained by the person with a disease or condition and those around them accepting the condition is real; however, in Parsons' concept of the sick role, legitimacy comes from a doctor sanctioning the illness

9

Further Reading

C. E. Lloyd and T. Heller (eds): *Long Term Conditions: Challenges in Health and Social Care*. London: Sage, 2010.
This book explores the experience of living with long-term conditions, and the pressure this places on people and their families, carers and the health and social services. It does not just include contributions from academics, but from those with long-term conditions, carers and health and social care professionals.

L. Lynch: *The C Word*. London: Arrow, 2015.
Lisa Lynch began a blog on her experience of living with cancer, which was turned into this book and subsequently a TV play. It is a very honest account of the highs and lows, the good advice and the bad, and it shows the toll that the diagnosis and treatment of breast cancer had on Lisa and her family.

E. Denny and S. Earle (eds): *The Sociology of Long Term Conditions*. Basingstoke: Palgrave, 2009.
This book is written specifically for nurses and takes a sociological perspective on long-term illness. The first part considers theory, policy and research, while part 2 focuses on some of the specific diseases and conditions that are prevalent in society today.

Also useful are the following online resources:

<www.healthtalk.org and www.youthhealthtalk.org>
People's real-life experiences of a wide range of illnesses. There is also a section for health professionals.

<www.patients-association.org.uk>
This is a campaigning organization that receives accounts about care from health and social care services from patients, carers and relatives, which it uses to campaign for better service provision. There is also an advice service.

<www.carersuk.org>
Both a resource for carers through its website and local groups, and a campaigning organization for better services for carers.

There are many websites that provide help, support and advice for people with specific long-term conditions, and for health professionals. Examples include:

Diabetes <www.diabetes.org.uk>; Heart disease <www.bhf.org.uk>; Multiple sclerosis <www.mssociety.org.uk>.

References

Barnett, K., Mercer, S. W., Norbury, M., Watt, G., Wyke, S. and Guthrie, B. 2012. Epidemiology of multimorbidity and implications for healthcare and medical education: a cross sectional study. *The Lancet* 380: 37–43.

Bendelow, G. A. 2000 *Pain and Gender*. Harlow: Prentice Hall.

Bissonette, J. M. 2008 Adherence: a concept analysis. *Journal of Advanced Nursing* 63: 634–43.

Bray, L., Kirk, S. and Callery, P. 2014 Developing biographies: the experiences of children, young people and their parents of living with a long-term condition. *Sociology of Health & Illness* 36: 823–39.

Britten, N. 2001 Prescribing and the defence of clinical autonomy. *Sociology of Health & Illness* 23: 478–96.

Bury, M. 1982 Chronic illness as biographical disruption. *Sociology of Health & Illness* 4: 167–82.

Bury, M. 1991 The sociology of chronic illness: a review of research and prospects. *Sociology of Health & Illness* 13: 451–68.

Bury, M. 1997 *Health and Illness in a Changing Society*. London: Routledge.

Charmaz, K. 2000 Experiencing chronic illness. In G. L. Albrecht, R. Fitzpatrick and S. C. Scrimshaw (eds), *The Handbook in Social Studies in Health and Medicine*. London: Sage.

Charmaz, K. 2010 Disclosing illness and disability in the workplace. *Journal of International Education in Business* 3: 6–19.

Clarke, K. A. and Iphofen, R. 2005 Believing the patient with chronic pain: a review of the literature. *British Journal of Nursing* 14: 490–3.

Coulter A., Roberts, S. and Dixon, A. 2013 *Delivering Better Services for People with Long Term Conditions*. London: The King's Fund.

Denny, E. 2009 I never know from one day to another how I will feel: pain and uncertainty in women with endometriosis. *Qualitative Health Research* 19: 985–95.

Donovan, J. L. and Blake, R. 1992 Patient non-compliance: deviance or reasoned decision making? *Social Science & Medicine* 34: 507–13.

Ehrenreich, B. 2010 *Smile! You've Got Cancer* [Online]. London: *Guardian*.

Fineman, N. 1991 The social construction of non-compliance: a study of health care and social service providers in everyday practice. *Sociology of Health & Illness* 13: 354–74.

Fisher, C. and O'Connor, M. 2012 'Motherhood' in the context of living with breast cancer. *Cancer Nursing* 35: 157–63.

Frank, A. 1995 *The Wounded Storyteller: Body, Illness and Ethics*. Chicago, IL: University of Chicago Press.

Goffman, E. 1968 *Stigma: Notes on the Management of a Spoiled Identity*. Harmondsworth: Penguin.

Horne, R., Chapman, S. C. E., Parham, R., Freemantle, N., Forbes, A. and Cooper, V. 2013 Understanding patients' adherence-related beliefs about medicines prescribed for long-term conditions: a meta-analytic review of the necessity-concerns framework. *PLoS One*, 8, e80633.

Hubbard, G. and Forbat, L. 2012 Cancer as biographical disruption: constructions of living with cancer. *Supportive Care In Cancer: Official Journal Of The Multinational Association Of Supportive Care In Cancer* 20: 2033–40.

Hydén, L. C. 1997 Illness and narrative. *Sociology of Health & Illness* 19: 48–69.

Im, E.-O. et al. 2007 Gender and ethnic differences in cancer pain experience: a multiethnic survey in the United States. *Nursing Research September/October* 56: 296–306.

Jobling, R. 1988 The experience of psoriasis under treatment. In R. Anderson and M. Bury (eds), *Living with Chronic Illness: The Experience of Patients and their Families*. London: Unwin Hyman.

Larsson, A. T. and Grassman, E. J. 2012 Bodily changes among people living with physical impairments and chronic illnesses: biographical disruption or normal illness? *Sociology of Health & Illness* 34: 1156–69.

Parsons, T. 1951 *The Social System*. London: Routledge & Kegan Paul.

9

Playle, J. F. and Keeley, P. 1998 Non-compliance and professional power. *Journal of Advanced Nursing* 27: 304–11.

Pound, P. et al. 2005 Resisting medicines: a synthesis of qualitative studies of medicine taking. *Social Science & Medicine* 61: 13355.

Richardson, J. C., Ong, B. N. and Sim, J. 2006 Is chronic widespread pain biographically disruptive? *Social Science & Medicine (1982)* 63: 1573–85.

Russell, S., Daly, J., Hughes, E. and Op't Hoog, C. 2003 Nurses and 'difficult' patients: negotiating non-compliance. *Journal of Advanced Nursing* 43: 281–7.

Sabaté, E. 2003 *Adherence to Long-term Therapies: Evidence for Action*. Geneva: World Health Organization.

Vrijens, B. et al. 2012 A new taxonomy for describing and defining adherence to medications. *British Journal of Clinical Pharmacology* 73: 691–705.

Werner, A. and Malterud, K. 2003 It is hard work behaving as a credible patient: encounters between women with chronic pain and their doctors. *Social Science & Medicine* 57: 1409–19.

Williams, S. 1996 The vicissitudes of embodiment across the chronic illness trajectory. *Body and Society* 2: 23–47.

Williams, S. J. 2000 Chronic illness as biographical disruption or biographical disruption as chronic illness? Reflections on a core concept. *Sociology of Health and Illness* 22: 40–67.

Williams, S. J. 2003 *Medicine and the Body*, London: Sage.

Zisk, R. Y. 2003 Our youngest patients' pain – from disbelief to belief. *Pain Management Nursing* 4: 40–51.

10 Disability

Sue Ledger, Lindy Shufflebotham and Jan Walmsley

KEY ISSUES IN THIS CHAPTER:

▶ Definitions of disability.
▶ Disability and health inequality.
▶ Sociological approaches to disability.
▶ Models of disability.
▶ Disability and the role of nurses.

BY THE END OF THIS CHAPTER YOU SHOULD BE ABLE TO:

▶ Understand different approaches to defining disability.
▶ Recognize disabled people encounter barriers within society that lead to significant disadvantage.
▶ Identify barriers encountered by disabled people in obtaining good health care.
▶ Discuss medical, social and interactional models of disability and their relevance to nursing practice.
▶ Understand the significance of the social model of disability and the role of the disability movement in campaigning for change.

prejudice:
negative opinions regarding a particular social group

barriers:
factors which prevent full participation in society

discrimination:
often a result of prejudice, which disadvantages certain social groups

schema:
mental representation activated at the mention of a concept

1 Introduction

This chapter introduces sociological perspectives on disability. It draws upon sociological theory to show how **prejudice**, **barriers** and **discrimination** encountered by disabled people – often regarded as individual concerns – can be better understood when placed in a societal context. Sociology, with its multi-paradigmatic approach, provides a conceptual framework that explores connections between the roles of individual actors (through theories of social action such as **schema** theory) and wider social structures (through structural approaches such as functionalism and Marxism). C. Wright Mills (1959) developed the concept of the 'sociological imagination', arguing it is necessary to look beyond common sense to understand what is happening in society; that the personal is influenced by social, political and economic factors. In this way 'private troubles' are often, in fact, 'public issues'. This chapter shows how nursing practice can be informed by better understanding of the impact of disability at both individual and societal levels.

The 2011 World Health Organization (WHO) survey confirmed that disabled people are at higher risk of poor health-care treatment. People with learning disabilities are at particularly high risk of having their health-care needs neglected (Heslop et al. 2013). Chapter 1 explained how sociology has been particularly influential in identifying social inequalities in health. In this chapter we consider barriers within health systems that confront disabled people and encourage you to think about actions that you can take to overcome these.

Models introduced in the chapter enable you to reflect on what best nursing practice with disabled people might look like. There is strong emphasis on the need to listen, respect and understand the way each disabled person experiences their impairment. The chapter opens by exploring definitions of disability and changing demographics. This is followed by personal experiences and discussion of links between disability and health treatment. It then introduces sociological models of disability and considers their application to nursing practice. The chapter demonstrates how application of sociological knowledge assists nurses to recognize discriminatory barriers within health systems and so improve health-care outcomes for disabled people.

What do we mean by disability?

Within sociological literature the term 'disability' has been invested with different meanings (Thomas 2007: 10). This chapter will help you to understand that within sociological thinking the language of 'disability' is a key area of divergence and contestation.

substantial:
more than minor, e.g., taking longer than usual to dress

long-term:
twelve months or more

UK law defines a disabled person as 'someone with a physical or mental impairment that has a **substantial** and **long-term** effect on their ability to do normal, daily activities' (Equality Act, HMSO 2010; bold font added). Although the word 'disability' often evokes images of people using wheelchairs or guide dogs, the majority of disabled people are over sixty-five; many have invisible conditions like schizophrenia, or diabetes. Individuals diagnosed with HIV infection, cancer or multiple sclerosis are included in the category 'disabled'. The 2010 Equalities Act for the first time includes people with age-related conditions as disabled.

Prevalence of disability

It is estimated that one in five of the UK population has a disability (Department of Work and Pensions 2014). There are 11.6 million disabled people in Great Britain (Office for Disability Issues 2014). Prevalence of disability rises with age. Around 6 per cent of children are disabled, compared to 16 per cent of working-age adults and 45 per cent of adults over state pension age. The Mental Health Foundation (2014) reports that one in four British adults experiences at least one diagnosable mental health episode in any one year. Approximately a fifth of people with mental health problems are disabled by their condition (Office of the Deputy Prime Minister 2004). Depression and anxiety are the most common conditions.

> ### Box 10.1 Changing demographics
>
> Across wealthier countries, demographic changes suggest that numbers of disabled people will continue to increase. This will impact on the demand for health and social care. Additionally, advances in medicine are enabling more premature babies with complex health conditions to survive.
>
>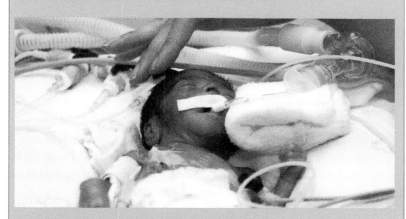
>
> **Figure 10.1** Survival rates for babies born at 22–25 weeks increased from 40 per cent in 1995 to 53 per cent in 2006; as the number of children surviving pre-term birth rises, so will the number who experience disability throughout their lives (Moore et al. 2012)

10

As Heslop et al. (2013) note:

- Medical advances have helped people with conditions such as cystic fibrosis and cancer to survive longer. Many experience associated long-term impairments.
- People are living longer, with associated increases in age-related conditions like dementia.
- As numbers of disabled people rise, ensuring that health-care professionals are skilled and confident in working with disabled people is critical.

Table 10.1 UK disability statistics 2014		
	Disabled people	**Non-disabled people**
Living in poverty	30%	15%
In paid employment	46.3%	76.4%
Victims of crime (16–34 years reporting being a victim of crime)	39%	28%
No qualifications	19.2%	6.5%
Degree-level qualifications	15%	28%
Access to car	40%	73%
Access to home Internet	61%	86%
Housing and independent living	Over a quarter of disabled people say that they do not have choice and control over their daily lives	

(*Adapted from the Office for Disability Issues 2014*)

Disability and societal disadvantage

Disabled people are more likely to be unemployed, living in poverty and be victims of crime: factors that impact on physical and mental health. Table 10.1 shows the extent to which disabled people continue to experience socioeconomic disadvantage compared with non-disabled people.

Living with disability

Whatever statistics tell us, every person's life and circumstances will be different. There is no short cut to listening to the experiences of individuals living with disability. Bearing this in mind, this section provides accounts from two disabled people.

Jane Campbell

Jane Campbell has campaigned and written extensively about disability issues. The life peer has spinal muscular atrophy, a degenerative condition. She uses a wheelchair and is increasingly reliant on a ventilator. She was the first Chief Executive of the Social Care Institute for Excellence and sits in the House of Lords, where she exerts a major influence on national disability policy.

> It's all about giving another perspective. Some of the debaters [House of Lords debate on assisted suicide] talked about how terrible it must be to have someone else take you to the toilet. That's my life, mate! And I hate the term 'vulnerable people'. It sets the image up before they find out what you're really like. Really I'm bossy, I'm ambitious and have ants in my pants, and am excited about things and people. I love ideas. I love life. (Birkett, D. (2009) Interview with Jane Campbell)

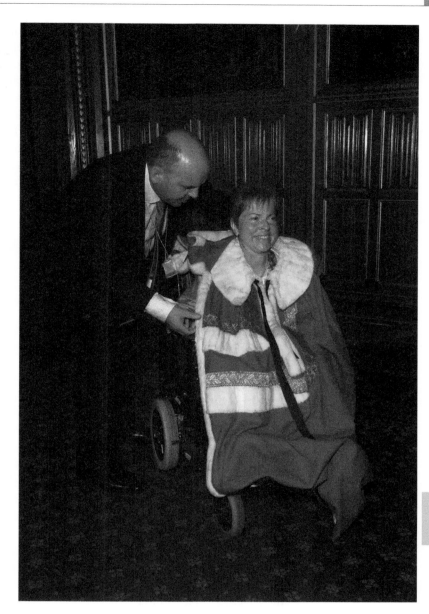

Figure 10.2
Jane Campbell

10

Graham's Story (not his real name)

I broke down in 2008. I couldn't have cared less about myself or anybody else. I went to see my GP. He told me that my weight, smoking and lifestyle had contributed to my poor health. He gave me one year to live and said that I would die of a stroke if things didn't improve. I was incapable of taking care of myself. For six months I continued to drink. I walked into the Adamson Road project in June 2013 – I thought it was the end of the world.

The project supported me to buy a swimming pass and I swam nine lengths, the first exercise I had done in three years. Day by day,

I increased my physical activity and changed my eating habits. Ten months on, with a great deal of application, I don't drink, I don't smoke, I'm four stone lighter and I have done something very rare . . .

I have reversed and eradicated my Type 2 diabetes.

When your life is chaotic, stability and care in any form is most welcome. Here is a humbling truth: what happened to me, can happen to anyone. I was at the height of my profession for twenty-two years. I had money, status and reputation. I lost it. It's life. Some of you reading this may say quietly to yourself, there by the grace of God go I. But the irony is, it is ME that says that well-worn phrase and I really mean it, because for whatever I have lost I am lucky. Lucky to be alive and grateful. (St Mungo's 2011)

Activity 10.1 The challenges of a disability

(a) Think about groups of people commonly described as disabled. List five examples.

(b) For each group, anticipate any problems an individual may encounter when going to the shops.

(c) Now for each group anticipate any problems an individual may encounter when accessing treatment in a health setting familiar to you.

Below are two examples of barriers encountered by disabled people in need of medical care – barriers that can all too easily lead to failure to provide the right treatment.

The first example is a man with learning disabilities who had always been lively. He became less and less active and was considered to be getting lazy. He started to lie in bed for much of each day and his staff team made plans to get him motivated. A visiting psychologist found him dead in his bed. A post-mortem discovered that he had died of leukaemia (adapted from Mee 2012: 44).

It is not possible to know if earlier medical intervention would have prolonged his life, but individuals who do not use words to communicate need to be listened to carefully and actively, to understand their feelings and to interpret what may be happening. Many people with learning disabilities find it harder to understand, remember and sequence information.

In this case, the man's learning disability had led staff to attribute the change in his behaviour to his disability rather than illness. Disabled people, perhaps most notably those who cannot communicate fluently, are often reliant on others to interpret their communication, including what changes in behaviour might mean. Disabled people are likely to experience 'diagnostic overshadowing' – where professionals assume a person's behaviour or symptoms are related to their disability, which results in ill health being missed and treatment being delayed.

The second example illustrates how in other situations powerful assumptions and **stereotypes** about disability may influence medical

stereotypes:
widely held but oversimplified ideas about a person or concept

decision-making. Another account from Jane Campbell describes what happened when she required urgent treatment for a chest infection:

> The consultant who was treating me commented: 'You are very ill. If you go into respiratory failure I am assuming that you do not want to be resuscitated with a ventilator.' I was taken aback by this and said, 'Well, why?' He replied that the chances of weaning me off the ventilator would be very remote – 'And you wouldn't want to live on a ventilator.' When I said that if the alternative meant I would die then of course I want to be ventilated, he looked (I thought) puzzled but appeared to let the matter drop. The next day I was in intensive care when another, more senior, consultant repeated the same message.[. . .] Again I protested but by now I was getting very scared. My husband tore home, grabbed a photograph of me in my doctoral graduation robes, and returned to the hospital shouting to the doctors: 'This is my wife, not what you think she is. She has everything to live for. You do everything for her just as you would for anybody in this situation.' Such extreme measures helped bring about a change of mind and I have lived to tell the story, albeit I kept myself awake for the next forty-eight hours, fearful that if I went to sleep I'd never wake up. (Campbell 2005)

These accounts demonstrate that while laws exist to ensure individuals are not disadvantaged by disability, in practice barriers in the form of negative stereotypes and insufficient understanding persist. In sociological terms, having a label of disability could be argued to act as a '**master status**' which negatively influences health-care treatment and expected outcomes. Hughes (1945) identified that, although people can have a variety of status categories, a master status is capable of overriding them. Jane Campbell is a life peer, a loved partner, well-known author and campaigner, yet what consultants saw was a severely disabled woman whose life might not be worth prolonging if it were dependent on a ventilator.

master status: label attributed to an individual and perceived as most important

During the twenty-first century evidence has mounted that people with disabilities consistently experience poorer health care in Britain. Blythe and White (2012) highlighted the association between mental illness and poor physical health. Mencap's report *Death by Indifference* (Mencap 2007) highlighted '**institutional discrimination**' within health-care settings, findings strongly supported by the 2008 Michael Report *Health Care for All* and the *Confidential Inquiry into Premature Deaths of People with Learning Disabilities* (Heslop et al. 2013). These investigations highlight how people with learning disabilities find it much harder than their non-disabled peers to access treatment for general health problems that have nothing directly to do with their disability. Recognizing their relevance to nursing practice, this chapter pays significant attention to health care for people with learning disabilities. These lessons, however, will apply equally to other impairment groups.

institutional discrimination: discrimination within the structures and procedures of organizations

10

Mee (2012), a sociologist and lecturer in learning-disability nursing, highlights that nurses are often required to do essentially practical things while thinking in an abstract theoretical way. In his book *Valuing People with a Learning Disability* Mee uses practice-based stories, including the story above, of the man with leukaemia, as a bridge to sociological theory. He argues theory is only of use if it enables improved understanding of everyday experiences of disabled people and can make a positive impact on the lives of the disabled people nurses are supporting.

reasonable adjustments: adapting physical structures or processes for ease of use

UK law requires all organizations, including the NHS and its contractors, to make **reasonable adjustments**. This might include flexible appointments for people with fluctuating mental health problems, accessible buildings for wheelchair users and allowing additional time to communicate with people with learning disabilities and their family or supporters to ensure their health needs have been fully understood and treated appropriately. Research with people with learning disabilities (Bell 2012) shows that small steps can make a huge difference. The flexibility demonstrated by one GP serves as an example. Margaret's GP noted that she was calmer in the surgery when accompanied by a particular carer. She suggested rearranging Margaret's annual health check to a time when this member of staff was available (Heslop et al. 2013: 64). This led to a better patient experience.

Activity 10.2 Breaking down barriers

(a) Think of your most recent nursing placement. List any adjustments that you noticed to support disabled people.

(b) List anything that could have presented a barrier to disabled people.

(c) How might these barriers be reduced or removed?

Progress but much further to go? Life opportunities and disability in the early twenty-first century

Earlier in the chapter we discussed how disability continues to be linked to socioeconomic disadvantage. Seeing the lives of disabled people in a historical context shows how ideas and norms from the past continue to exert influence on attitudes and health-care practice today (Chapman et al. 2014).

stigma: social disgrace attached to any condition

Notwithstanding serious problems with current welfare reform, Shakespeare (2014) asserts that conditions for disabled people have slowly improved over the last twenty years, largely as a result of campaigning by disabled people and their supporters. Until the 1960s and 1970s, throughout the Western world, thousands of children and adults with physical and mental disabilities were admitted to segregated long-stay hospitals, homes and boarding schools. People were separated from their families, local communities and their non-disabled peers. **Stigma** (Goffman 1963) was attached to people labelled as disabled, and many spent their lives in institutions (Mansell 2006). Disabled people were often assumed to be asexual and unsuitable to become parents. Many were sterilized without their knowledge (Tilley et al. 2012).

Disability today – life opportunities and equal treatment

Early twenty-first-century policy aims to promote inclusion of disabled people in society, and anti-discrimination legislation requires that disabled people are given the same opportunities as their non-disabled peers, including access to housing, education and health care. The principle underlying the policy is that disabled people are held back by social, economic and political factors, rather than simply individual impairment. Many people with disabilities live in their local community, in their own home, with or without support. Many disabled people are raising families independently or with support. Many, like Jane Campbell, are in leadership roles. But not everyone enjoys a good life.

Schema theory offers a way of understanding how stereotypes of disability continue to exert influence despite policy and legislation to promote human rights and equality (Oliver 2009). Augustinos and Walker (1995) describe a schema as a 'kind of mental shortcut that people use to simplify reality'. A schema is a mental representation of the world, which is activated at the mere mention of the object or concept represented. Human beings use these mental short cuts wherever possible. This has clear evolutionary potential as it is best to avoid expending unnecessary mental effort in order to leave spare capacity for dealing with unexpected events. Rumelhart and Ortony (1976) suggest that schemas have a double purpose: to enable understanding of the situation and to predict what will happen next. Earlier in the chapter, Jane Campbell described what happened to her at a hospital when she required urgent treatment. Revisiting this story, an interpretation could be that the overriding schema activated in the minds of the consultants was that of a person with a severe disability and therefore a poor quality of life. Evidence of Jane's role as a successful academic resulted in an alternative schema being activated, which may have influenced the treatment plan.

10

Activity 10.3 Schemas

Read the following list and consider each person in turn, being aware of the thoughts, images, feelings and judgements that come to mind for each one. This combination is your schema for this person:

- Conservative MP.
- Labour MP.
- Footballer.
- Priest.

(a) Write a sentence outlining your schema for each.

(b) Think about your schemas of individuals with physical disability, learning disability and mental health issues. Outline the key aspects of each schema as honestly as you can.

(c) After considering your own schemas, think about what may have informed their development. As a nurse, what steps could you take to make sure your own stereotypes do not negatively influence the care you provide?

(Adapted from Mee 2012: 68)

We all hold mental representations of disability, whether they are based on our own experiences, the experiences of others or representations in books, television and film. Inevitably these schema presuppose judgements. In relation to people with learning disabilities, Mee says 'it can be argued that the only way to genuinely value people is to become conscious of the negative cognitive representations we each own and to attempt to over-ride them with conscious thought' (2012: 84). In this respect, reflective practice is critical in delivering the best possible nursing care to disabled people.

Sociological concepts also enable you to reflect critically on system-wide aspects of health care; for example, the contracting out of and privatization of health care for disabled people. The shift of some health-care hospitals from NHS to private companies, where a primary aim is shareholder profit, has arguably contributed to the **commodification** of provision. Winterbourne View was a private hospital for adults with learning disabilities. It was set up by Castlebeck, a private company, in response to a perceived gap in provision for people with learning disabilities who had mental health needs and behavioural difficulties. The average weekly charge for each patient in 2011 was £3,500 per week. Statutory organizations referred people to it and funded their care. Many patients were placed far away from their families and home areas, echoing historical practices of sending people with disabilities away for institutional care. In 2011, a BBC Panorama documentary used hidden cameras to reveal a catalogue of repeated abuse of patients by hospital staff. Eleven staff eventually pleaded guilty to criminal offences of neglect or abuse, and six were jailed. Many former patients are still suffering with symptoms from the assaults (Mencap 2012). This raises important questions about whether delivering high-quality care or shareholder profit was the most important organizational outcome.

commodification: economic value given to something not previously viewed in this way

2 Sociological approaches to disability

Whatever the branch of nursing, thinking sociologically will enrich professional practice and enhance inter-professional working (Earle and Letherby 2008) by promoting appreciation of both individual and system-wide perspectives. The often highly charged debates within the sociology of disability centre on three major questions:

1 The extent to which physical or mental impairments determine the life chances of disabled people.
2 The actions we should take to improve the lives of disabled people: to cure, rehabilitate or change the individual, or to alter society so there are fewer barriers to disabled people enjoying a good quality of life.
3 The extent to which individual experience should be the subject of sociological enquiry.

Medical sociology

Sociological interest in the field of disability started in the 1950s with the work of Talcott Parsons (see Chapter 3). Parsons (1975) highlighted the role of medicine as a means of controlling a common form of deviance in society – illness. For medical sociologists, such as Parsons, it was the individual who must learn to adapt and cope. How this impacted upon people with disability was not initially explored – but may help to explain why disabled people were assigned to specialist segregated facilities, an acceptance that they were not going to conform to the productive life stereotype.

The medical or individual model of disability

Developing from Parsons' work, the conventional way of viewing disability was simply as a medical problem. For example, people might say 'he is disabled because he has a spinal injury' or 'she is disabled because she has Down's syndrome'. The focus is on medical treatment of individual physical or mental conditions.

Disability and associated inequalities are, with this approach, viewed as an inevitable function of 'deficits' located within individuals. Described by structural sociologist Mike Oliver as the 'medical' or 'individual' model (Oliver 2009), it formed the basis of the WHO's original *International Classification of Impairments, Disabilities and Handicaps (ICIDH)* (WHO 1980), and it continues to influence healthcare policy and treatment of disabled people today.

Although the term 'medical model' often has negative connotations, Shakespeare (2014) emphasizes that specialist medical knowledge can be really important to disabled people. Diagnosis for people with hidden impairments gives credibility and may lead to more effective medical, social or educational intervention. Medical treatment and rehabilitation can reduce pain and improve participation.

The social model of disability

In the late 1960s and 1970s, disabled people throughout the world began to organize, to demand equal rights and to challenge the medical model of disability. The social model emerged from the intellectual and political arguments of the Union of Physically Impaired Against

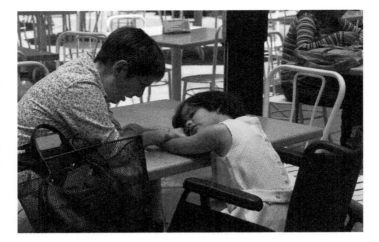

Figure 10.3 How might a disabled child's self-identity be affected by being treated as though they are fully dependent upon the help of others?

Segregation (UPIAS). UPIAS was a small group of disabled people, inspired by Marxist ideology, who argued for the closure of segregated facilities, and opportunities for disabled people to participate fully in society (Shakespeare 2014).

The social model makes a clear distinction between individual impairment and disability. It identifies social structures and political, economic and environmental factors as the cause of disability. These are beyond the control of the individual and Oliver argues that it is these societal factors that disable people and exclude them. He further argues that disability is a consequence of the individualizing nature of capitalism and the medicalization of everyday life. He contends that medicine determines who works, goes to school, who can marry, who has children. Medicine creates the notion of 'able-bodiedness' against which normality is judged. This ideology permeates society and determines how disabled people are viewed and treated. The social model rejection of any link between impairment and disability has been adopted by the majority of organizations of disabled people throughout the world, who call for political action to achieve change.

The Social Model as set out by Oliver (1990) was crucial to the Disability movement for two reasons. First, it identified a political strategy: barrier removal. If people with impairments are disabled by society, then the priority is to dismantle barriers, including barriers to health care. Second, replacing a traditional deficit approach with a social oppression understanding was, and remains, very liberating for disabled individuals (Shakespeare 2014). People were able to understand and articulate that it was society that was at fault, not them. They did not need to change; society needed to change.

Shakespeare argues that if disability is about social barriers, not individual impairment, then attempts to mitigate or cure medical problems may be regarded with suspicion by proponents of the social model. Morris (1991) emphasizes that while environmental and social attitudes do indeed disable people, to suggest that that is all there is, is to deny the personal experience of impairment, including pain, physical and intellectual restriction, progressive deterioration and the fear of dying. Shakespeare (2014) also argues that disability studies should be concerned with medical treatment of impairment.

The list below shows key elements of the social model.

- Impairment (physical limitation) is distinguished from disability (social exclusion) – the former is individual and private, the latter is structural and public.
- While doctors and professions allied to medicine seek to remedy impairment, the social model emphasizes that the real priority is to accept impairment and remove disability.
- The recognition of disabled people as an oppressed group.
- Often non-disabled people and organizations – such as professionals and charities – are the causes of or contributors to this oppression.
- Disability is culturally and historically specific, not a static universal and unchanging condition.
- Civil rights rather than charity or pity are the way to solve the disability problem.

Organizations and services controlled and run by disabled people provide the most appropriate solutions. Research accountable to and preferably done by disabled people offers the best insights.

Box 10.2 Barriers

The social model identifies barriers to full participation in society. The most obvious barriers are *physical*: the design of the environment which does not permit people whose mobility is impaired to move around; the absence of hearing loops in public buildings; buses/trains without wheelchair access or space; stairs; absence of dropped kerbs.

Structural barriers are the underlying norms and practices of a society, which are predicated upon a false concept of 'normal': practices which exclude people who cannot work or move at the same pace as young able-bodied adults; the amount of time allowed for crossing the road before traffic lights change; timescales for work or study which do not take account of mental health problems; care pathways which assume everyone can read hospital letters or drink when they are thirsty.

Attitudinal barriers are beliefs that because someone has an impairment they are unable to do things: the practice of talking to a carer rather than to a disabled person in a consultation is an example of the assumption that people with disabilities will not be able to understand.

10

- An inability to read is an impairment.
- An inability to understand because the information is not in a format that is accessible or because it is not adequately explained is a disability.

- An inability to move one's body is an impairment, but an inability to get out of bed because appropriate physical help is not available is a disability. (*Adapted from Morris 1993*)

The biopsychosocial model

Various attempts have been made to reconcile medical and social models, one of the most influential being the International Classification of Functioning, Disability and Health (ICF), developed by the World Health Organization. The ICF adopts a 'biopsychosocial' model (WHO 2002: 9), which aims to integrate the two conflicting frameworks. The model describes disability as an interaction between features of the person and features of the overall context in which the person lives. However, some aspects of disability are almost entirely internal to the person, while other aspects are almost entirely external. In other words, both medical and social model responses are appropriate to the problems associated with disability; we cannot wholly reject either kind of model.

The biopsychosocial model is consistent with a more holistic conception of health. Health is seen as a state of complete physical, mental and social well-being and not merely as the absence of disease or infirmity (WHO 1946). This definition emphasizes health as positive well-being within a broad social context, rather than health as being the absence of disease within an individual. Shakespeare argues that impairment and disability – the biological and the social – are always entwined and that relational accounts of disability, such as the biopsychosocial model, provide the best way of understanding the complex and multidimensional experience of disablement. Shakespeare's own 'interactional' (2014: 80) approach acknowledges the importance of environments and context, prejudice and discrimination, while arguing that the priority is to engage with impairment, not ignore it.

The social and biopsychosocial models promote understanding of how discrimination and prejudice can impact on a person's mental and physical health, and quality of life.

Activity 10.4 Working with disabled people

(a) Reflecting on medical, social and biopsychosocial models, what do you think are the most important issues for nurses working with disabled people?

(b) Should nurses concentrate on helping people to manage individual impairment or on helping disabled patients to overcome barriers that may impede recovery?

(c) Is the latter too political for nurses? Should nurses concentrate on medical issues?

The medical model emphasizes the need to attend to the best possible individual medical care. The social and biopsychosocial models remind us how external factors impact negatively on health and may need to be addressed if treatment outcomes are to be the best.

3 Listening to lived experience?

A strong tradition in medical sociology has been to uncover the impact of living with impairment and disability by conducting interviews with disabled people (Plummer 2001). Critics of this approach point out that negativity is often the hallmark of such papers, with disabled people portrayed as victims. Oliver (1996) argues that experiential accounts often fail to explore the way a disabling society impacts on individuals. However, more recently, some disability theorists (Goodley et al. 2004) have acknowledged that lived-history accounts provide insights into experiences of disability that otherwise may remain unnoticed.

At first sight, the divide is between medical sociologists and disability studies advocates. However, feminists in particular, like Liz Crow (1996), have insisted that attention needs to be paid both to people's personal experiences and to the impact of disablism. Shah and Priestley (2011) used the stories of fifty people born since the 1940s to illuminate how policy changes have impacted on people's lives. The value, the authors argue, is that life stories enable the reader to consider the personal as political, to challenge assumptions, for example that the earliest generations experienced the most segregated childhoods. Mindful of the disabled people's movement's well-documented suspicion of using personal tragedy to elicit charitable sympathy, the authors contend that personal narratives must be read with a focus on social relations and institutional practices rather than as ends in themselves.

Disability studies researchers have begun to explore the tensions in supporting disabled people to share personal accounts, while at the same time ensuring that people are not exploited and that myths about disability are not inadvertently perpetuated (Goodley et al. 2004). In the field of intellectual disability, individual life stories have been used to uncover insider stories of life inside long-stay institutions. Former residents (Atkinson and Cooper 2000) have told stories about incarceration which act as a powerful antidote to the tales told by historians and professionals and others in positions of power.

10

> **Activity 10.5 Understanding individual life stories**
>
> (a) Think about disabled people you have met in your nursing placements. Have you listened to first-hand accounts from people with disabilities and their families?
> (b) Make a list of the things you learned from listening to experiential accounts.
> (c) As a nurse, how might you find out about the experiences of people with complex disabilities, who cannot speak and find it hard to communicate with strangers?

necessary reasonable adjustments in relation to her disability. However, the medical model was still important – the pain in her hip could not have been addressed through removal of access barriers alone (Shakespeare 2014). Jessica's impairments were multidimensional and her learning disability contributed to the disadvantage or barrier she encountered with communicating her need to drink.

Part 2

Prior to readmission for hip surgery, Jessica became very distressed. The community learning-disability nurse and GP requested a meeting to plan the readmission. The aim was to ensure lessons had been learned from the earlier stay and that reasonable adjustments would be made.

The hospital team were receptive. Jessica, her family and the community nurse completed a Hospital Traffic Light passport. This contained information about the support Jessica needed, including reminders and physical help to drink. It also included personal details such as favourite music that helped Jessica relax. The hospital team suggested a lightweight notice board to display photos of her family, friends and pets. Prior to the operation the surgeon explained the procedure to Jessica, using simple language. This time, at the suggestion of the family, the nursing staff used gestures and photographs to support their communication. The second admission was a great success. Jessica had a named nurse and was well supported. The operation went well and she was discharged home according to plan.

Comment – social and biopsychosocial approaches: The social model focuses on removing disabling systems and structures. In Jessica's second admission there is evidence of social model thinking in the steps taken to anticipate and overcome barriers.

In part 2 of Box 10.3, there is clear evidence of this approach through provision of music and photographs to reduce stress and promote well-being. Relational models of disability, including the biopsychosocial, adopt a more holistic approach by addressing medical and social aspects of disability. This approach seems appropriate to the complexity and diversity of disabled people entering hospital, and a helpful basis for future practice and research.

In relation to health and social care, Carr (2012) emphasizes that all staff, systems, processes and services need to put people at the centre. In this respect the personalization of health care requires an approach that could perhaps be argued to be most consistent with an interactional or biopsychosocial approach (Shakespeare 2014).

Conclusion

The 2011 World Health Survey revealed that disabled people consistently experience poorer standards of health care. Reducing health inequality is a key nursing responsibility: one that will enable disabled individuals to experience better lives. This chapter set out to explore the practical relevance of sociology to nurses working with disabled people. It provides new ways of understanding and responding to the needs of disabled patients.

Within health-care systems it is essential that the 'problem of disability' is located in the right place – the problem of disability is not located in an individual but in prejudicial attitudes and societal systems that impact on the lives, and more specifically the health care, of disabled people.

The chapter has considered the contribution of sociology to understanding the complexity of disability. The importance of factors such as environment, social and economic policies, cultural and individual attitudes, in disabling people and influencing their treatment, cannot be denied. The biopsychosocial (interactional) model shows how post-social model thinking has developed. In this way we see how the sociological imagination can enable nursing practice to be improved by a multifactorial account of disability. Like Tom Shakespeare (2014: 72), in this chapter we have been 'unashamedly eclectic and pragmatic' in our approach, finding a plurality of sociological approaches beneficial in the analysis of disability and its application to best nursing practice.

Summary and Resources

Summary

- Prevalence figures indicate one in five of the UK population has a disability.
- Disabled people are at higher risk of receiving poor health-care treatment.
- Disabled people continue to experience socioeconomic disadvantage when compared to their non-disabled peers. Examples include higher numbers of disabled people living in poverty and experiencing unemployment. This will also have an impact on health.
- The traditional sociological approach to disability focuses on the experience and impact of impairment on an individual (medical model).
- The social model of disability argues that disability arises as the consequence of the way society is organized. There is no link between disability and impairment.
- The social model of disability states that, to improve the life chances of disabled people, we should focus on changing society rather than changing the individual.
- Critiques of the social model argue that the experience of impairment can also be disabling and that this has been downplayed.
- There is a need to listen to, respect and understand the way each disabled person experiences their impairment.

10

Application of sociological knowledge can assist nurses working with disabled people to recognize discriminatory barriers within health-care systems and so improve individual health-care outcomes.

Questions for Discussion

1 Consider the points raised in the extract below:

> The claim that people are disabled by society, not by their bodies, has been effective in highlighting the human-created obstacles to participation in society. Yet outside the city, the social model seems harder to implement. Wheelchair users are disabled by sandy beaches and rocky mountains. People with visual impairments may be unable to see a sunset, people with hearing impairments will miss out on the birds, wind and waves. It is hard to blame the natural environment on social arrangements. (Shakespeare 2014: 36)

Discuss this idea in relation to the social, medical and biopsychosocial or relational models. What do you feel the different perspectives can offer? How is this relevant to nursing?

2 How can nurses provide individual care and yet still adopt the social model of disability within their practice?

3 Nursing has often been said to predominantly offer a medical approach to disabled people. How can nurses provide person-centred care and still draw upon the social model of disability in their practice?

Glossary

barriers:	factors which prevent disabled people participating fully in society; the social model defines disability in terms of oppression and barriers, and breaks the link between disability and impairment
commodification:	when economic value is given to something not previously considered profitable; the shift of some hospitals from NHS to private companies, where a primary aim is shareholder profit, could be considered an example of commodification
institutional discrimination:	is concerned with discrimination that has been incorporated into the structures, processes and procedures of organizations, either because of prejudice or because of failure to take into account the particular needs of different social identities
master status:	term used to describe the status of greatest importance in a person's life; 'disability' is often a master status, and Everett Hughes introduced this term

to indicate a characteristic that, from the perspective of other people, floods out other aspects of a person's identity; since status is a social label and not a personal choice, the individual has little control over his or her master status in any given social interaction

schema: mental representation of the world, which is activated at the mention of the object or concept

stereotypes: widely held but fixed and oversimplified images or ideas about a particular type of person or thing

stigma: an attribute, behaviour or status which is socially discrediting in a particular way: it causes an individual or group to be classified and often rejected as undesirable rather than being readily accepted

Further Reading

S. Mee: *Valuing People with a Learning Disability*. Cumbria: M&K Publishing, 2012.
In this book sociologist Steve Mee draws on his experience as a practitioner and lecturer on a learning-disability nursing course. Each chapter introduces a particular area of theory and uses stories to apply academic concepts to everyday practice.

T. Shakespeare: *Disability Rights and Wrongs Revisited*. London: Routledge, 2014.
Tom Shakespeare, a leading disability scholar, provides a highly informative and readable overview of current arguments and concerns within disability studies. The book explores the contemporary relevance of social, cultural and biomedical aspects of disability.

H. Thomas: *Sociologies of Disability and Illness*. Basingstoke: Palgrave, 2007.
An analysis of the competing and conflicting perspectives on disability, the book explores debates between interpretive and structuralist approaches within sociology, and looks at disability studies from historical traditions to recent shifts in theoretical positions.

Also useful are the following online resources:

<http://www.scie.org.uk/health-social-integrated-care/>
The Social Care Institute for Excellence (SCIE) provides practical support and resources to help health and social care practitioners and other partner agencies to coordinate services based around a disabled person's needs. This integrated approach is essential to improve outcomes for disabled people who use health and social care services.

<https://www.mencap.org.uk/get-involved/campaigns/what-we-campaign-about/ health>
National UK charity Mencap is running a campaign to address the premature deaths of people with learning disabilities by improving health-care practice.

This site provides many useful resources and personal accounts of good and poor practice from people with learning disabilities and their families.

<http://www.open.ac.uk/health-and-social-care/research/shld/>
The Social History of Learning Disability (SHLD) Research Group, based in the Faculty of Health and Social Care at The Open University, UK, researches and disseminates learning disability history in ways which are inclusive of people with learning disabilities, their families, relatives and advocates. This website provides access to a short film *No Longer Shut Up*, which shares the story of Mabel Cooper, a woman with learning disabilities who spent many years in a long-stay hospital. The research group promotes recognition that people with learning disabilities are experts on their own lives, and have historical knowledge, viewpoints and skills to contribute that are key to improving future support.

<www.Mind.org.uk>
Mental Health charity Mind provides advice and support to empower anyone experiencing a mental health problem. It also provides information to support families and health-care practitioners, including good practice guidance and legal information. The organization campaigns to improve mental health support and promote understanding.

References

Abraham, J. 2014 Personal communication.

Anderson, R., Shah, R. S. and Priestley, M. 2012 *Disability and Social Change*. Bristol: Policy Press.

Atkinson, D. and Cooper, M. 2000 Parallel stories. In L. Brigham, D. Atkinson, M. Jackson, S. Rolph and J. Walmsley (eds), *Crossing Boundaries: Change and Continuity in the History of Learning Disability*. Kidderminster: BILD.

Augustinos, M. and Walker, I. 1995 *Social Cognition: An Integrated Introduction*. London: Sage.

Bell, R. 2012 Does he have sugar in his tea? Communication between people with learning disabilities, their carers and hospital staff. *Tizard Learning Disability Review* 17/2: 57–63.

Birkett, D. 2009 I'm bossy. I'm ambitious. I love ideas. And I love life. Interview with Jane Campbell, *Guardian*, 11 July 2009. http://www.theguardian.com/society/2009/jul/11/lady-campbell-disability-peer

Blythe, J. and White, J. 2012 Role of the mental health nurse towards physical health care in serious mental illness: an integrative review of 10 years of UK literature. In *International Journal of Mental Health Nursing* (June) 21/3: 193–201. doi: 10.1111/j.1447-0349.2011.00792.x.

Campbell, J. 2005 Select Committee on Assisted Dying for the Terminally Ill Bill. Available at: <http://www.publications.parliament.uk/pa/ld200405/ldselect/ldasdy/86/86we05.htm>.

Carr, S. 2012 *Personalization: A Rough Guide*. London: SCIE.

Chapman R., Ledger, S. and Townsend, L. with Docherty, D. (eds) 2014 *Sexuality and Relationships in the Lives of People with Intellectual Disabilities: Standing in My Shoes*. London: Jessica Kingsley.

Crow, L. 1996 Including all our lives. In J. Morris (ed.), *Encounters with Strangers: Feminism and Disability*. London: Women's Press.

Department of Work and Pensions (DWP) 2014 *Disability Prevalence Estimates* 2011/12. Available at: <https://www.gov.uk/government/uploads/system/uploads/attachment_data/file/321594/disability-prevalence.pdf>.

Earle, S. and Letherby, G. 2008 *The Sociology of Healthcare*. London: Palgrave Macmillan.

Goffman, E. 1963 *Stigma*. London: Simon and Schuster.

Goodley, D., Lawthom, R., Clough, P. and Moore, M. 2004 *Researching Life Stories: Method, Theory and Analyses in a Biographical Age*. London: Routledge Falmer.

Heslop, P., Blair, P., Femining, P., Houghton, M., Marriot, A. and Russ, L. 2013 *Confidential Inquiry into Premature Deaths of People with Learning Disabilities (CIPOLD)*. Bristol: Norah Fry Research Centre.

HMSO 2010 *Equality Act*. London: HMSO. Available at: <http://www.legislation.gov.uk/browse>.

Hreinsdottir, E., Stefansdottir, G., Lewthwaite, A., Ledger, S. and Shufflebotham, L. 2006 Is my story so different from yours? Comparing life stories, experiences of institutionalization and self-advocacy in England and Iceland. *British Journal of Learning Disabilities* 34/3: 157–66.

Hughes, E. 1945 Dilemmas and contradictions of status. *American Journal of Sociology* 50/5: 353–9.

Manley, K., Hill, V. and Marriot, S. 2011 Person-centred care: principle of nursing practice. *Nursing Standard* 25/31: 35–7.

Mansell, J. 2006 Deinstitutionalization and community living: progress, problems and priorities, *Journal of Intellectual and Development Disability* 31/2: 65–76.

Mee, S. 2012 *Valuing People with a Learning Disability*. Cumbria: M&K Publishing.

Mencap 2007 *Death by Indifference*. London: Mencap.

Mencap 2012 *Out of Sight*. London: Mencap.

Mental Health Foundation 2014 *Mental Health Statistics UK and World Wide*. Available at: <http://www.mentalhealth.org.uk/help-information/mental-health-statistics/uk-worldwide/>.

Michael, J., Richardson, A. 2008 Healthcare for All: Report of the Independent Inquiry into Access to Healthcare for people with learning disabilities. *Tizzard Learning Disability Review* 13/4: 28–34.

Moore, T., Hennessy, E. M., Myles, J., Johnson, S. J., Draperm, E. S., Costeloe, K. L. and Marlow, N. 2012 Neurological and developmental outcome in extremely preterm children born in England in 1995 and 2006: the EPICure studies, in *British Medical Journal*. Online, 4 December; 345:e7961. doi: . 1136/bmj.e7961.

Morris, J. 1991 *Pride Against Prejudice*. London: Women's Press.

Morris, J. 1993 *Independent Lives? Community Care and Disabled People*. London: Macmillan.

Office for Disability Issues, The 2014 *Disability Prevalence Estimates*. Available at: <https://www.gov.uk/government/uploads/system/uploads/attachment_data/file/321594/disability-prevalence.pdf>.

Office of the Deputy Prime Minister 2004 *Mental Health and Social Exclusion Unit, Social Inclusion Unit Report*. London: ODPM.

Oliver, M. 1990 *The Politics of Disablement*. Basingstoke: Macmillan.

10

Oliver, M. 1996 Defining impairment and disability: issues at stake. In C. Barnes and G. Mercer (eds), *Exploring the Divide: Illness and Disability*. Leeds: The Disability Press.

Oliver, M. 2009 *Understanding Disability from Theory to Practice*, 2nd edn. London: Palgrave Macmillan.

Parsons, T. 1975 The sick role and the role of the physician reconsidered. *The Milbank Memorial Fund Quarterly. Health and Society*: 257–78.

Plummer, K. 2001 *Documents of Life 2*. London: Allen and Unwin.

Rumelhart, D. and Ortony, A. 1977 The representation of knowledge in memory. In R. Anderson, S. Shah and M. Priestley 2012, *Disability and Social Change*. Bristol: Policy Press.

St Mungo's Broadway 2011 *Graham's Story: St Mungo's 2011: Oral History Project*. Available at: http://www.mungosbroadway.org.uk/streetstories(last <www.mungosbroadway.org.uk>.

Shah, S. and Priestley, M. 2011 *Disability and Social Change: Private Lives and Public Policies*. Bristol: Policy Press.

Shakespeare, T. 2014 *Disability Rights and Wrongs Revisited*. London: Routledge.

Thomas, C. 2007 *Sociologies of Disability and Illness*. Basingstoke: Palgrave.

Tilley, E., Walmsley, J., Earle, S. and Atkinson, D. 2012 'The Silence is Roaring': Sterilization, reproductive rights and women with intellectual disabilities. *Disability and Society* 27/3: 412–36.

World Health Organization 1946 *Constitution of the World Health Organization*. Geneva: World Health Organization.

World Health Organization 2002 *International Classification of Functioning, Disability and Health*. Geneva: World Health Organization.

World Health Organization 2011 *World Report on Disability*. Geneva: World Health Organization.

Wright Mills, C. 1959 *The Sociological Imagination*. London: Oxford University Press.

Yarrow Housing 2014 *Thoughts about Healthcare and Hospitals*. Session recorded at The Gate, Hammersmith, December 2014.

Social Class and Health

Sarah Earle

KEY ISSUES IN THIS CHAPTER:

▶ A historical overview of the relationship between class and health.

▶ Class and the measurement of socioeconomic difference.

▶ The extent and causes of health inequalities.

▶ The policies adopted to tackle health inequalities.

▶ Contemporary nursing, class and health.

BY THE END OF THIS CHAPTER YOU SHOULD BE ABLE TO:

▶ Map the history of the relationship between class and health.

▶ Explain the concepts of class and understand the measurement of socioeconomic difference.

▶ Discuss the evidence relating to class inequalities in health.

▶ Explore some of the policies used to tackle health inequalities.

▶ Understand the significance of class and health for nursing practice.

1 Introduction

Low incomes, poor environments and social deprivation are all associated with earlier death, and poorer health at all ages during life. The association between ill health and material deprivation was first made in the early nineteenth century. During the last two decades of the twentieth century, the gaps between both the incomes, and the health, of the richest and poorest in our society actually widened (Acheson 1998; NAO 2010). Box 11.1 outlines some of the key health inequalities in Britain today.

Box 11.1 Health inequality in Britain

- Health inequalities associated with class, income or deprivation are pervasive and can be found in all aspects of health, from infant death to the risk of mental ill health. The limited information on progress over time (infant death, low birth weight) shows no sign that they are shrinking.
- Men aged twenty-five to sixty-four from routine or manual backgrounds are twice as likely to die early as those from managerial or professional backgrounds, and there are also sizeable differences for women. Scotland has by far the highest proportion of premature deaths for both men and women.
- Adults in the poorest fifth of the income distribution are much more likely to be at risk of developing a mental illness than those on average incomes.
- Two-fifths of adults aged forty-five to sixty-four on below-average incomes have a limiting long-standing illness or disability, more than twice the rate for those on above-average incomes.
- Babies from manual social backgrounds are somewhat more likely to be of low birth weight than those from non-manual social backgrounds.
- Teenage motherhood is eight times more common amongst those from manual social backgrounds than for those from professional backgrounds.
- Five-year-olds in Wales and Scotland have, on average, more than twice as many missing, decayed or filled teeth as five-year-olds in the West Midlands.

(Poverty Site)

In over two centuries of gathering hard evidence showing that disease and death are related to deprivation and disadvantage, we have often encountered political dispute about the validity of the research findings, how they should be interpreted and whether, and how, governments should act to improve the people's health. It is only since the very end of the twentieth century that we have had concerted efforts by a British government both to tackle health inequalities, and to do so using strategies clearly informed by the full range of research findings, rather than just selecting those findings that it found acceptable.

This chapter begins with a brief historical overview of the relationship between class and health. It will explore the sociological concept of 'class' and discuss the ways in which socioeconomic difference has been measured. Drawing on current research evidence, it will examine the extent and the causes of health inequalities and review some of the policies adopted to tackle health inequalities. Lastly, this chapter will explore how class and health inequalities are relevant to contemporary nursing practice.

2 Modernization, class and health

modern:

type of society beginning in eighteenth-century Europe, valuing scientific and technological progress

As the nineteenth century opened, Britain was already on an increasingly fast track towards becoming a new kind of social formation – a **modern** society in which wealth was increasingly created through industrial manufacture. The population of England and Wales doubled from 9 million to 18 million between 1801 and 1851, by which time more than half of these people lived in towns and cities (Mathias 1983). It is during this early period of modernization and industrial growth that the term and concept of '**class**' came into increasingly common usage.

class:

the major form of social stratification in modern societies

Class

'Working class' came to describe the masses who depended on working for either a capitalist manufacturer, or a member of the aristocracy. Very long hours were worked for wages that were often inadequate to meet even the most basic necessities of rent and food. The aristocracy were the main landowners, although some also invested in the new industry, and were considered to be the upper class. The capitalists owned the new forms, or means, of industrial production, including factories, workshops, raw materials and transport; they were considered to be middle class. This class also included owners of shops, farmers and the members of the growing professions such as doctors, lawyers, accountants and clergymen.

The earliest theoretical account of this new class society was provided by Marx – a structural theorist – in 1848, and the relationship between what he called the bourgeoisie and the proletariat is discussed in Chapter 1.

Health

11

The main causes of death in the nineteenth century were infectious diseases such as respiratory tuberculosis, typhoid and cholera. For much of that century, it was believed that these diseases were caused by bad air coming from the filth generated by the living and working conditions. This polluted air was called miasma and its presence was detected by bad smells.

A growing number of studies showed that the killer diseases infected the working class in greater numbers, and killed them more often, than the middle and upper classes. The studies varied in their explanations of why this was so, and what should be done. Chadwick's report (1842), the *Inquiry into the Sanitary Condition of the Labouring Population of Great Britain*, was the result of a national statistical survey that showed:

- Mortality rates were highest for the poorest.
- Urban dwellers were more adversely affected than those living in rural areas.
- The poorer classes lived in the most unsanitary areas.

Chadwick, who believed in miasma theory, argued for schemes to safely dispose of the filth he believed to be an inevitable consequence of modernization. Most social reformers in this time focused only on the environmental impact of the Industrial Revolution and sought to improve the physical condition of homes and workplaces.

Engels, a close collaborator of Marx, took a different perspective. His study of working-class life and death, mainly in the Manchester area, was published as *The Condition of the Working Class in England* in 1845. He used several sources, including official reports from the Registrar-General for England and Wales, to document working-class mortality. He observed appalling living and working conditions and argued that they were the result of actions by the propertied classes. Engels argued that the propertied classes failed to deal with the pollution they caused in their workplaces, imposed hazardous working conditions for which they paid very low wages, and provided poor housing that lacked appropriate basic services, and for which they charged high rents. Furthermore, Engels argued that these actions, driven by profit, were directly responsible for the patterns of disease and early death in the working class and that they amounted to what he termed 'social murder'.

It was not until the last two decades of the nineteenth century that the full extent and causes of poverty were fully explored. Charles Booth (Fried and Elman 1971) and Seebohm Rowntree (1902) showed that poverty was mainly caused by incomes below subsistence levels, either from low wages or from inadequate provision for when people could not work. They also showed that poverty undermined individual efforts to struggle for respectability, health and well-being. Nonetheless, governments tended more heavily towards the view that poverty was caused by the personal shortcomings of poor people and how they chose to live.

3 Understanding class

By the early twentieth century, it was evident that, far from polarizing into just two classes as Marx predicted, we had moved instead to a complex of groups ranked in relation to ideas about their social and economic differences; this is also known as **social stratification**. Both the working class and the middle class contained subgroups reflecting significant differences in relation to such matters as size and security of income, housing circumstances, schooling experiences and their perceived social prestige. Weber (1958) (see also

social stratification: division of society into levels that form a hierarchy

Chapter 1) provided a theoretical basis for understanding this growing complexity by distinguishing between class situation and status situation. Like Marx, he viewed a person's class situation as determined by her or his position in the markets for capital and labour. Those owning property, such as shares and land, are placed on the capital side of the main economic divide, while the possession of more, or less, valued skills, or educational credentials, puts the majority on the labour side of the main economic divide. According to Weber, we also have a status situation that groups us with similar others according to the social value placed on our styles of life, which includes our tastes, our social networks, and our consumption practices, both for goods, such as cars, and for services, such as education. Weber took the view that our life chances are shaped not only by our class situation, but also by our status situation, which has an important impact on our well-being.

Various schemes of social and occupational classification, described in the rest of this chapter, have been developed in order to allocate us to a place in these socioeconomic hierarchies.

Social and occupational classifications

Rose and Pevalin (2001) identify two major traditions of socioeconomic classification in Britain. The dominant one, in terms of its use in the analysis of official data, especially in relation to life, health and death, comes from successive generations of government statisticians. This tradition produced the Registrar-General's Social Classification (RGSC) in 1911. This classification was modified in 1921 and in 1980, and renamed in 1990 (see Box 11.2). The other tradition was formed by British sociology as it analysed the various expressions of class identity, and changes in the British class structure, from 1945 onwards.

Contemporary sociological analysis of class

The early compilers of the RGSC believed that society consisted of a definite social hierarchy that ranked people according to their inherited and innate abilities. These beliefs about the social structure have increasingly limited its validity as a measure of socioeconomic difference for sociologists today. Sociology is interested in the relations between the classes, and has developed sociological classifications to study social mobility, in particular. In doing so, it has identified many limitations of the RGSC. Concern about these limitations, combined with the impact of ongoing class analysis within sociology, led to a thorough review of the RGSC in 1994 and its replacement by a new scheme, the National Statistics Socioeconomic Classification (NS-SEC), from 2001 (see Box 11.3).

11

Box 11.2 Registrar-General's social class based on occupation

Class	Description of occupations
I	Professional: accountants, doctors, lawyers
II	Managerial and technical/intermediate: managers, senior technicians, school teachers, police officers, nurses
IIIN	Skilled non-manual: clerk, secretary, waiter, shop assistant
IIIM	Skilled manual: HGV and PSV drivers, fitters, electricians
IV	Partly skilled: warehouse workers, machine tool operators
V	Unskilled: labourers (e.g., building, roads, tunnels construction), cleaners

Important notes

* People are assigned to a class on the basis of what they state as their occupation.
* Each job is assigned to a specific class, but if, within an occupation, persons are supervisors or managers, they are placed in a higher class than the others holding that job.
* People in the armed forces are treated separately and put in an additional group: Occupied – other.
* People known to be employed, but who have provided inadequate details, are also placed in Occupied – other.
* People who say they have never worked or who give no information are put in an additional group: 'Unoccupied'.

The NS-SEC classification was developed from the Goldthorpe schema (Goldthorpe 1980, 1997) produced by sociologists in the 1980s and revised in the 1990s. This schema separates employers who buy and direct the work of others, and the self-employed who work for themselves, from employees who account for up to 90 per cent of the economically active population. Employees clearly have only the fact that they work for someone else in common. They otherwise differ with regard to:

* Stability of their job and income.
* Size of that income.
* Prospects for advancement and promotion.
* Pension provisions and other indirect elements of remuneration.
* Specialized knowledge and expertise and how these are valued.
* Relative importance of educational qualifications compared with competences acquired in organizations.
* Authority over others.
* Personal autonomy and control over the job.

Box 11.3 National Statistics Socioeconomic Classification (NS-SEC)

1 Higher managerial and professional occupations
   1.1 Large employers and higher managerial occupations: health service managers, company directors
   1.2 Higher professional occupations: doctors, teachers, social workers, university lecturers
2 Lower managerial and professional occupations: nurses and midwives, journalists, police officers, laboratory technicians
3 Intermediate occupations: dental nurses, secretaries
4 Small employers and own account workers: publicans, farmers, restaurateurs
5 Lower supervisory and technical occupations: train drivers, plumbers, electricians
6 Semi-routine occupations: hairdressers, shop assistants, security guards
7 Routine occupations: waiters, cleaners, labourers, couriers
8 Never worked and long-term unemployed

By seeking to take account of these crucial lines of difference, the NS-SEC reflects contemporary socioeconomic differences in the labour market and work situations. It may be useful to identify the class position of nurses and to consider some of the differences identified above.

The research discussed below also shows that these differential experiences of employment markets and job characteristics influence our experiences of health and disease, both directly and indirectly.

Case Study: The Black Report

The value of the RGSC scheme for identifying and tracking health differentials is most clearly shown in the *Inequalities in Health Report*, commissioned by a Labour government and published in 1980. It is popularly known as the Black Report and gives a detailed analysis of official statistics showing that a clear gradient of inequality runs all the way from the richest to the poorest (Townsend et al. 1988). Class V had worse health and died sooner, and in greater numbers, from the major causes of death – heart disease, cancers and strokes – than Class IV, and so on in a straight line up to Class I, which had the lowest death rates, the longest life expectancy, and the best health. Death from skin cancer was the only clear exception to this pattern. The health gap between Classes I and II combined and Classes IV and V combined widened between 1948 and the mid-1970s. The gap was particularly wide for infant death (under one year) and child death (under fifteen years).

11

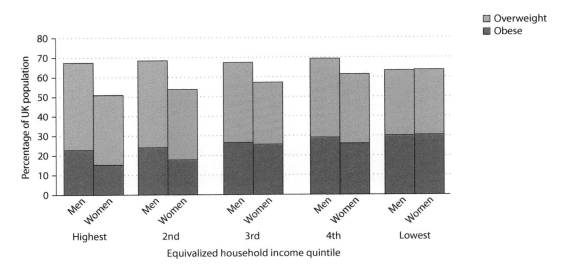

Figure 11.1 Obesity and social class

Activity 11.1 Obesity and social class

Look at the chart in Figure 11.1, then answer the following questions.

(a) What social classification is being used in this chart and how does obesity and being overweight vary by social class?
(b) Explain how food poverty contributes to obesity.
(c) Are there other factors that might help to explain the connections between obesity and social class?
(d) What role can nurses place in reducing obesity and alleviating food poverty?

Box 11.4 The Black Report: explaining the findings

Artefact explanation

The difference between classes was unintentionally enlarged by the techniques used to measure class and the methods of managing the statistics.

Evaluation There are some technical problems, but the findings are likely to be real. The Longitudinal Study and the Whitehall Studies subsequently endorsed the reality of widespread health inequalities.

Social selection explanation

People's class is determined by their health, not the other way round. It is all part of a natural pattern whereby the least able occupy the least demanding and rewarding jobs.

Evaluation Only an insignificant amount of downward mobility is caused by illness. A range of subsequent studies point to a complex interaction between individual biology, psychosocial stresses and material disadvantage that accumulates across the life course.

Behavioural/cultural explanation

Poor health is caused by individual behaviours within personally chosen lifestyles. Middle-class culture tends to embrace health-enhancing behaviours while working-class culture seems to value health-detracting behaviours, such as smoking and unhealthy dietary choices.

Evaluation Individual health-detracting behaviours are involved and feature more heavily amongst working-class people. However, they were produced in an impoverished socioeconomic environment that makes daily life a constant struggle to make ends meet. The behaviours should be understood as coping mechanisms, and as efforts to obtain some pleasure and enjoyment within generally adverse circumstances. However, some health-detracting behaviours are not only more common in the lower RGSC and NS-SEC classes, but also do more damage to them. For example, Whitehall II showed smokers in the highest Civil Service job grades had less heart disease and longer life expectancy than smokers in the lowest Messenger grades.

Materialist/structuralist explanation

Poor health and earlier death are dimensions of marked socioeconomic inequalities in society as a whole. In particular, they stem from low and insecure incomes, unemployment and unstable employment, poor working conditions, and poor housing in materially and culturally under-resourced neighbourhoods.

Evaluation The Black Report identified this as the dominant explanation. The Acheson Report, drawing on data from the 1990s, validated this analysis. There is no serious, empirical basis for questioning its central thesis that tackling health inequalities means tackling social inequalities. This perspective has informed wide-ranging government policy since 1999.

11

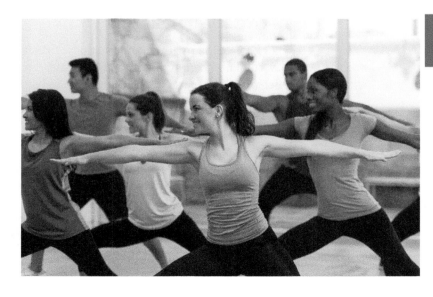

Figure 11.2 Middle-class people are more likely to engage in health behaviours such as yoga which promote health and well-being

Table 11.1 Prevalence of mental health problems amongst 5–15-year-olds by family social class

Family social class								
	I	II	IIIN	IIIM	IV	V	Never worked	All
Percentage of children								
Emotional disorders	1.8	3.4	5.3	4.5	5.5	5.8	8.4	4.3
Conduct disorders	2.5	3.4	6.1	5.0	7.8	10.1	15.5	4.3
Any disorder	5.2	7.0	11.6	9.4	12.4	14.5	21.1	9.5

(*Adapted from London Health Observatory online: Table 1*)

Activity 11.2 Mental disorders in childhood and social class

Look at Table 11.1, then answer the questions below.

(a) How much more likely are children in unskilled families (V) to have a mental disorder than children in professional families (I)?

(b) How much more likely than the national average are children in families where the head of the household has never worked to have a mental disorder?

(c) What factors should you take into account when trying to explain these patterns, and how do these factors influence nursing practice?

The Black Report concluded that Britain's health inequalities were determined by inequalities in the distribution of wealth, power and status. The report evaluated four possible approaches to explaining its findings (see Box 11.4), but was neither welcomed nor implemented, even partially, by the Conservative government to which it reported in 1980.

---

4 Tackling health inequalities in the twenty-first century

The 1990s ended with a combination of research developments and governmental commitment to act on research evidence that together offered real prospects of achieving some reductions in health inequalities by the end of the first decade of the new century. These key developments are outlined in Box 11.6, although it is worth noting that, in the main, health inequalities were not reduced and in some instances increased.

Acknowledging the fact that there was still much work to be done to eradicate health inequalities, the Acheson Report, headed by Donald Acheson and published in 1998, observed that average mortality had fallen in the last fifty years, but that unacceptable health inequalities still existed and, in some instances, had widened. Indeed, Acheson pointed out that some populations in the UK had the same levels of early death as the national average during the 1950s. The report supported the view that health inequalities are a dimension of wider social inequalities. These shape neighbourhood and community environments as well as patterns of work, and they influence individual lives from conception onwards. The Acheson Report drew on a now well-known model developed by Dahlgren and Whitehead (1992), which set out the determinants of health (see Box 11.5).

Box 11.5 The social determinants of health

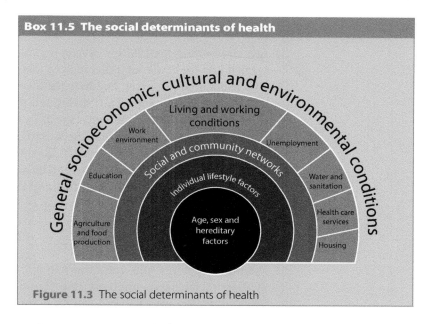

Figure 11.3 The social determinants of health

More recently, the independent Marmot Review (2010), led by Professor Sir Michael Marmot, again highlighted the importance of reducing health inequalities, arguing that it is a matter of social justice and that action is required across all of the social determinants of health. The review specifically concluded that in order to reduce health inequalities, action is required on six policy objectives:

1 Give every child the best start in life
2 Enable all children, young people and adults to maximize their capabilities and have control over their lives.
3 Create fair employment and good work for all.
4 Ensure a healthy standard of living for all.
5 Create and develop healthy and sustainable places and communities.
6 Strengthen the role and impact of ill-health prevention.

11

Activity 11.3 The social gradient in health

One of the key messages of the Marmot Review is on the health gap between different social groups:

In England, the many people who are currently dying prematurely each year as a result of health inequalities would otherwise have enjoyed, in total, between

1.3 and 2.5 million extra years of life . . . There is a social gradient in health – the lower a person's social position, the worse his or her health.

(a) Why is life expectancy a significant measure of health inequalities? What other measures of health inequalities should there be?

(b) What do you think can account for the continuing health gap?

(c) Why do you think nurses should know about these inequalities?

Contemporary explanations of health inequalities

Research begun in the 1990s is developing our knowledge of the pathways that link the bodies of individuals to their life experiences, including their material resources, and how these are all shaped by the social structure (see also Chapter 1). It is through these complex, connected mechanisms that the less affluent, especially the poor, become sicker, at an earlier age, than the more affluent. Bartley (2004) gives a detailed account of the psychosocial explanation, the life-course explanation (discussed in Chapter 8) and the neo-materialist explanation, and discusses how these can inform each other and thus provide the potential for deepening our understanding.

Psychosocial explanation

Contemporary ways and conditions of life produce social stresses that affect social classes unevenly, and members of these groups have uneven access to material and personal resources to manage these stresses. Such stresses do not only affect mental well-being. They also affect the body through the cardiovascular, endocrine and immune systems. Siegrist et al. (1990) argue that *socioemotional distress* occurs when a high workload is matched with job insecurity, poor promotion prospects and low control. They suggest such effort–reward imbalance at work predicts heart disease and its precursors, such as raised blood pressure and high fibrinogen levels. Psychoneuroendocrine and psychoneuroimmune mechanisms may thus contribute to diseases such as cancers and, especially, heart disease. Additionally, negative experience of hard-to-manage stress, for example, ever-increasing debt, often induces harmful coping mechanisms like smoking, high levels of alcohol consumption and unhealthy eating patterns. Ability to change these health-damaging behaviours is restricted by access to important resources of money, time and supportive outlets such as gyms, health clubs and community networks. Kaplan et al. (1996) argue that high levels of psychosocial stress not only reflect exposure to antisocial behaviour, violent crime and reduced **social cohesion**, but also help to produce and maintain patterns of reduced social participation. However, these stresses occur in poor neighbourhoods. They are *ecological* experiences, which means they characterize places rather than individuals.

social cohesion:
a sense of belonging to wider society

> **Box 11.6 Key developments on health inequalities:**
> **1990s–present**
>
> - Wilkinson analysed mortality and morbidity data from several countries and found that the widest gaps in health inequalities were to be found in those countries that had the widest gaps in incomes (Wilkinson 1996).
> - The Office for National Statistics published a Health Inequalities Decennial Supplement in 1997 containing evidence-based accounts of health and mortality in children, unemployment and mortality, illness and health behaviours in adults and data from the Longitudinal Study (Drever and Whitehead 1997).
> - The Independent Report into Inequalities in Health (The Acheson Report 1998) concluded that, although overall mortality had fallen over the past fifty years, unacceptable inequalities existed.
> - A new public-health strategy, *Saving Lives: Our Healthier Nation*, was published in July 1999, which accepted the recommendations of the Acheson Report and identified some immediate strategies to reduce health inequalities, for example Health Action Zones (HAZs) and Healthy Living Centres.
> - In 2002, the Cross-Cutting Review identified a long-term strategy to reduce health inequalities involving all areas of government and calculated its costs (HM Treasury and Department of Health 2002).
> - The government published *Tackling Health Inequalities – A Programme for Action* in 2003. It is a three-year plan to lay the foundations for achieving various challenging targets for reducing health disadvantage in key areas such as infant mortality and deaths from heart disease, cancers and suicide by 2010 (Department of Health 2003).
> - In 2008, *Tackling Health Inequalities: Progress and Next Steps* (Department of Health) reported that many of these targets have been met and, beyond 2010, the goal is to focus on wider inequalities that are the root of health inequalities. The key areas are investing in early years and parenting; using work to improve health and well-being; promoting equality; developing mental health services further; and coordinating action – both nationally and locally.
> - In 2010, *Fair Society, Healthy Lives* was published, also known as the Marmot Review. This report proposed evidence-based strategies for reducing health inequalities in England from 2010 onwards.

11

Lynch et al. (2000) use an airline travel metaphor to illustrate the shortcomings of the psychosocial explanation. They point out that first-class passengers on long-haul flights have more space, better food and seats that recline into beds, and so tend to arrive relatively refreshed. Economy-class passengers lack these advantages and are likely to arrive feeling a bit rough. The problem is more likely to be that they could not sleep in cramped conditions than that knowledge of the better provisions in first class kept them awake.

Nurses and other health-care professionals can contribute to projects in deprived areas that aim to empower communities as well as to address some of the direct effects of poverty. Such projects involve the members of the community as decision-makers and include setting up

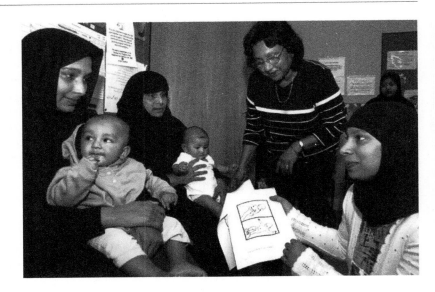

Figure 11.4 Nurses play a key role in empowering communities

credit unions and food cooperatives that provide access to cheaper, healthy foods, training people to run health and fitness courses in their neighbourhoods, and providing free community transport to social events as well as to clinics and hospitals. In addition, nurses and their colleagues can avoid contributing to disempowerment by ensuring that service users from all communities across the lifespan are fully informed, active participants rather than passive recipients.

Life-course explanation

The health effects of adverse socioeconomic circumstances accumulate from conception, through childhood and adolescence, to adulthood and life in later years. Early work by Barker et al. (1989) led to the concept of *foetal programming*, which argues that poor maternal nutrition, and the generally poor health associated with living in poverty, affect the developing baby during pregnancy. Material and social disadvantage for adults are thus reflected in the lower birth weight and poor health of their children, for example in higher levels of asthma. Bartley et al. (1994) found that **longitudinal** study data showed low birth weight itself predicted socioeconomic disadvantage through childhood and adolescence. Additionally, poor socioeconomic conditions in childhood have been shown to have an independent effect on both adult health and adult socioeconomic status. Indeed, the highest health risks have been found in those who both grow up in, and remain in, disadvantaged material circumstances (van de Mheen et al. 1998).

longitudinal: a research study that follows the same group of people over time

Health problems in adult life do not result in downward mobility, but poor health in childhood and youth, combined with poor socioeconomic circumstances, can produce a downward spiral. Health care is delivered at specific points in time. However, the life-course perspective asks those working in health care to recognize that illness and health-damaging behaviours occur in social contexts to people who are living their lives in good or poor circumstances, and with varying degrees of control over their lifestyles. Nurses are especially well placed to take account of the whole person with an ongoing life story and to challenge **victim-blaming** within their practice. Victim-blaming oversimplifies the pathways through which major diseases such as coronary heart disease, diabetes and cancers occur in particular individuals and may lead to low self-esteem, which can further detract from health. The Marmot Review (2010) is strongly influenced by the view that health inequalities can be tackled using a life-course perspective.

victim-blaming: considering people individually responsible for their own ill health

Neo-materialist explanation

Adverse socioeconomic and psychosocial environments and the risky exposures and experiences associated with them are the material productions of social formations. These social formations have historically produced an unequal distribution of personal income and wealth, which in turn shapes unequal access to the infrastructure of markets for food, transport, housing, health care, education and lifestyle consumption. In Britain, for example, the poorest tenth of the population receives around 1.5 per cent of the country's total income; the second poorest tenth around 4 per cent. More than 3 million children live in households whose income is less than 60 per cent of the average (**median**) income. By contrast, the richest 10 per cent of the population receive 30 per cent of total income, and the second-richest tenth 15 per cent (Palmer, MacInnes and Kenway 2007). It is these structured inequalities that produce **social exclusion** and low levels of **social capital**.

median: midpoint, e.g., median income is the point where half of all incomes lie above, and half below

Researchers working within this explanatory approach warn against putting too much emphasis on social cohesion, social participation and self-esteem, so that the consequences of inequality become the focus of attention rather than the need for structural change (Lynch et al. 2000). They point out that losing sight of the unequal social structure while working on what socially excluded and materially deprived communities can do for themselves may be a subtle form of victim-blaming. From a neo-materialist perspective, it is income inequality together with inequitable distribution of public resources such as health services, schooling and social welfare provisions that produce health inequalities. These wider inequalities are themselves produced by economic and political processes operating at a macro-level and as such require major social interventions to create effective change. Professional organizations, such as the Royal College of Nursing and the British Medical Association, recognize the importance of the neo-materialist perspective, study evidence in its support and debate the impact of economic structures on health. All individual members of such organizations may follow and participate in these activities.

social exclusion: impact of poverty and low income on involvement in mainstream social life

social capital: community spirit, belonging to and supported by social networks

11

Activity 11.4 Learning disability and economic disadvantage

A study based in three day centres in Northern Ireland by McConkey and Mezza (2001) looked at the views of both care workers and people with learning disabilities about possibilities for types of, and benefits from, paid employment. Some of their key findings are outlined below.

Experience of work or training for work

- 42 per cent of the 275 day-centre attendees had previously had an unpaid job or done work experience.
- 33 per cent had previously had a vocational training placement provided by a voluntary organization.
- 17 per cent had previously had some other placement set up by a day centre.
- 25 per cent were currently doing a specific job in a day centre.
- 22 per cent were currently on a further-education college course.
- Only 1.5 per cent (four people) had ever had paid employment.

Aspirations of people with learning difficulties

- Significantly more people who had done two or more placements wanted a paid job compared with those who had no, or limited, work experience.
- Twice as many people who were on an FE course, or had been in the last year, wanted a paid job compared with those who had not been to college.
- Those who wanted a paid job were significantly younger than those who didn't.
- Overall, eighty-five of the day-centre attendees said they wanted a paid job.

Key workers' perceptions about suitability of clients for paid employment

- Staff rated 38 per cent of those who wanted a job as being capable of doing one, 29 per cent as unlikely to cope, and said they were unsure about the prospects of the rest.
- Staff preferred the chances of those whom they rated as above average in self-care skills, those who had been on three or more work experiences, and those who had above-average skills in reading, writing, and time- and money-management skills.
- Staff thought the main obstacles to clients holding down jobs were poor concentration, poor communication skills and understanding, and lack of motivation.
- Staff also identified instances where they thought parents might be a negative force in their adult child's work prospects.

(a) In what ways might current patterns of attendance at day centres be unhelpful for clients' prospects of holding down paid work?

(b) Consider the roles that work-derived income and social contacts from work might play in relation to both the well-being and the socioeconomic position of people with learning disabilities. You might want to think about this for both those living with their parents and those living in supported independent settings. You may also find it helpful to think about applying the concepts of social exclusion and social capital to your analysis.

Health care and the inverse care law

The 'inverse care law' is a phrase first used by Julian Tudor Hart to describe how those who have most need of NHS care health services actually obtain them later, and in smaller amounts, while those who have less need use more, and often better, health services (Hart 1971). Hart did not carry out a systematic review of evidence but rather observed his working environment as a GP and coined the phrase to make a political point. However, subsequent research has shown the description of an inverse pattern within health care to be largely accurate. Gainsbury (2008) reports that budgets allocated to GPs to pay for drugs and hospital care for their patients show that the wealthiest tenth of the population are, on average, more than 2 per cent overfunded, while the poorest tenth are 2 per cent underfunded. The National Audit Office (2010) also shows that there are fewer GPs in the areas that are the most socially deprived.

For example, a detailed review by Dixon et al. (2003) has shown that hip replacements are 20 per cent less frequent among lower socioeconomic groups, despite around 30 per cent higher need, and that a one-point move down a seven-point deprivation scale resulted in GPs spending 3.4 per cent less time with the individual concerned. The review shows that these inequities result from two sorts of disadvantage: those that make access to services difficult, such as lack of transport and available time away from work, and those that make consultations less productive, such as patients being less assertive about demanding information, participation in treatment decisions, and appropriate referrals for further treatment. Similar examples of the inverse care law in practice have been found across different areas of health. For example, in a study focusing on the provision of cardiac services (Langham et al. 2003), researchers found that there is considerable inequity in service provision between areas that could not just be explained by differences in demand for services. These authors argued that the 'inverse care law is alive and well. Substantial proactive work is required to ensure that health-care provision acts to alleviate rather than exacerbate inequalities in wealth and health' (2003: 207). Nurses have an important role to play in helping to restore patients' 'voice' by listening, and by encouraging more talk and self-expression. They may also act as mediators and advocates for patients in encounters with other health-care professionals.

11

Activity 11.5 Heart disease and social class

Deaths from cardiovascular disease (CVD) have declined but, according to a report published by Heart UK (2013), between 1982 and 2006 CVD inequalities between rich and poor have increased across nearly 8,000 wards in England:

- The decline in rates for men and women aged sixty-five or over was smaller in the poorest communities – so that the gap between the richest and most deprived areas is wider.

the least access to resources, and the least power, at the bottom of the hierarchy

victim-blaming: considering people to be individually responsible for their own ill health; looking to the actions of individuals to explain their ill health rather than looking at the wider range of social factors within society that constrain or encourage them and provide the context for overall health and well-being within a population

Further Reading

H. Graham: *Unequal Lives: Health and Socioeconomic Inequalities*. Maidenhead: McGraw-Hill, 2007.
Graham is one of the most respected writers in the field of inequality and health, and this book looks at contemporary evidence on the persistence of inequality and the ways in which we can understand it.

C. Pantazis, D. Gordon and R. Levitas: *Poverty and Social Exclusion in Britain*. Bristol: Policy Press, 2006.
This book reports on the most comprehensive survey of poverty and social exclusion to be undertaken in Britain. It contains chapters on mental health, children, youth, single mothers and pensioners.

S. E. Curtis: *Health Inequality: Geographical Perspectives*. London: Sage, 2004.
This volume considers health and well-being, as well as disease, from a geographical perspective, which is not widely used within health care. It shows how space and location can advantage or disadvantage the health of individuals and communities.

M. Bartley: *Health Inequality: An Introduction to Theories, Concepts and Methods*. Cambridge: Polity, 2004.
This is a detailed exploration of research methods and findings on health inequality at the beginning of the twenty-first century. It is a difficult, but thorough, account and will be useful to those who wish to probe further.

H. Sutherland, T. Sefton and D. Piachaud: *Poverty in Britain: The Impact of Government Policy since 1997*. York: Joseph Rowntree Foundation, 2003.
This review examines many sources of evidence in its assessment of government policies aimed at reducing inequalities.

References

Acheson, D. 1998 *Independent Inquiry into Inequalities in Health Report*. London: Stationery Office. At: <www.archive.official-documents.co.uk/document/doh/ih/ih.htm>.

Barker, D. J. P., Martyn, C. N., Osmond, C., Hales, C. N. and Fall, C. H. D. 1989 Growth in utero, blood pressure in childhood and adult life, and mortality from cardiovascular disease. *British Medical Journal* 298: 564–7.

Bartley, M. 2004 *Health Inequality: An Introduction to Theories, Concepts and Methods*. Cambridge: Polity.

Bartley, M., Power, C., Blane, D., Smith, G. D. and Shipley, M. 1994: Birth weight and later socio-economic disadvantage: evidence from the 1958 British cohort study. *British Medical Journal* 309: 1475–8.

Benzeval, M., Judge, K. and Whitehead, M. (eds) 1995 *Tackling Inequalities in Health: An Agenda for Action*. London: King's Fund.

Black Report 1980 *Inequalities in Health: Report of a Research Working Group*, chair Sir Douglas Black. London: Department of Health and Social Security.

Chadwick, E. 1842 *Inquiry into the Sanitary Conditions of the Labouring Population of Great Britain*. London: W. Clowes and Sons.

Dahlgren, G. and Whitehead, M. 1992 Policies and strategies to promote equity in health. Copenhagen, WHO Regional Office for Europe (document number: EUR/ ICP/RPD 414 (2). At: <http://whqlibdoc.who.int/euro/-1993/EUR_ICP_RPD414(2).pdf>.

Department of Health 1999 *Saving Lives: Our Healthier Nation*. London: Stationery Office.

Department of Health 2003 *Tackling Health Inequalities – A Programme for Action*. London: Department of Health. At: <http://www.dh.gov.uk/en/Publicationsandstatistics/Publications/PublicationsPolicyAndGuidance/DH_4008268>.

Department of Health 2007 *Tackling Health Inequalities: 2007 Status Report on the Programme for Action*. London: Department of Health. At: <http://www.dh.gov.uk/en/Publicationsandstatistics/Publications/DH_083471>.

Department of Health 2008 *Tackling Health Inequalities: Progress and Next Steps*. London: Department of Health. At: <http://www.dh.gov.uk/en/Publicationsandstatistics/Publications/PublicationsPolicyAndGuidance/DH_085307>.

Department of Health 2013 *Health Survey for England 2013. Volume 1*. London: Department of Health. At: <http://www.hscic.gov.uk/catalogue/PUB16076/HSE2013-Ch10-Adult-anth-meas.pdf>.

Dixon, A., Le Grand, J., Henderson, J., Murray, R. and Poteliakhoff, E. 2003 Is the NHS equitable? A review of the evidence. *LSE Health and Social Care Discussion Paper 11*. London: London School of Economics.

Drever, F. and Whitehead, M. 1997 *Health Inequalities Decennial Supplement 15*. London: Stationery Office.

Drever, F., Fisher, K., Brown, J. and Clark, J. 2000 *Social Inequalities*. London: Stationery Office. At: <www.statistics.gov.uk/statbase/Product.asp?vlnk=5771>.

Engels, F. 1999 *The Condition of the Working Class in England*, ed. D. McLellan. Oxford: Oxford University Press. First published 1845.

Fried, A. and Elman, R. M. (eds) 1971 *Charles Booth's London*. Harmondsworth: Penguin.

Gainsbury, S. 2008 Health inequalities: Wealthiest overfunded as poor lose out. *Health Service Journal* (30 October): 4–5.

Goldthorpe, J. H. 1980 *Social Mobility and Class Structure in Modern Britain*. Oxford: Clarendon.

Goldthorpe, J. H. 1997 The 'Goldthorpe' class schema: some observations on conceptual and operational issues in relation to the ESRC review of

11

governmental and social classifications. In D. Rose and K. O'Reilly (eds), *Constructing Classes: Towards a New Social Classification for the UK*. Swindon: ESRC and ONS, pp. 40–8.

Hart, J. T. 1971 The inverse care law. *The Lancet* 1: 405–12.

Heart UK 2013 *Bridging the Gaps: Tackling Inequaities in Cardiovascular Disease*. Berkshire: Heart UK. At: <http://heartuk.org.uk/files/uploads/Bridging_the_Gaps_Tackling_inequalities_in_cardiovascular_disease.pdf>.

HM Treasury and Department of Health 2002 *Tackling Health Inequalities – Summary of the Cross-Cutting Review* 29854. London: Department of Health. At: <http://www.hm-treasury.gov.uk/d/exec_sum_tacklinghealth.txt>.

Kaplan, G. A., Pamuk, E., Lynch, J. W., Cohen, R. D. and Balfour, J. L. 1996 Income inequality and mortality in the United States: analysis of mortality and potential pathways. *British Medical Journal* 312: 999–1003.

Langham, S., Basnett, I., McCartney, P., Normand, C., Pickering, J., Sheers, D. and Thorogood, M. 2003 Addressing the inverse care law in cardiac services. *Journal of Public Health Medicine* 25/3: 202–7.

London Health Observatory, online 2005 Prevalence of mental health problems amongst children and young people aged 5-to-15 years. At: <http://www.lho.org.uk/viewResource.aspx?id=9338>.

Lynch, J. W., Smith, G. D., Kaplan, G. A. and House, J. S. 2000 Income inequality and mortality: importance to health of individual income, psychosocial environment, or material conditions. *British Medical Journal* 320: 1200–4.

Marmot Review, The 2010 *Fair Society, Healthy Lives: Strategic Review of Health Inequalities in England post-2010*. At: <www.ucl.ac.uk/marmotreview>.

Mathias, P. 1983: *The First Industrial Nation: An Economic History of Britain 1700–1914*. London: Routledge.

McConkey, R. 2001 Book reviews. *Journal of Learning Disabilities* 5/4: 369–74.

McConkey, R. and Mezza, F. 2001 Employment aspirations of people with learning disabilities attending day centres. *Journal of Learning Disabilities* 5/4: 309–18.

National Audit Office (NAO) 2001 *Tackling Obesity in England*. London: Stationery Office. At: <www.nao.gov.uk/publications/nao_reports/00-01/0001220.pdf>.

National Audit Office (NAO) 2010 *Department of Health: Tackling Inequalities in Life Expectancy in Areas with the Worst Health and Deprivation*. London: Stationery Office. At: <http://www.nao.org.uk/wp-content/uploads/2010/07/1011186.pdf>.

Palmer, G., MacInnes T. and Kenway, P. 2007 *Monitoring Poverty and Social Exclusion 2007*. York: Joseph Rowntree Foundation. At: <http://www.poverty.org.uk/reports/mpse%202007.pdf>.

Poverty Site, The (undated) *Key Facts: Health* Online At: <http://www.poverty.org.uk/summary/key%20facts.shtml#health>.

Rose, D. and Pevalin, D. J. 2001 *The National Statistics Socio-economic Classification: Unifying Official and Sociological Approaches to the Conceptualization and Measurement of Social Class*, ISER Working Papers 2001–4. Colchester: University of Essex.

Rowntree, B. S. 1902 *Poverty: A Study of Town Life*. London: Macmillan.

Siegrist, J., Peter, R., Junge, A., Cremer, P. and Seidel, D. 1990 Low status control, high effort at work and ischemic heart disease: prospective evidence from blue-collar men. *Social Science and Medicine* 31/10: 1127–34.

Townsend, P., Davidson, N. and Whitehead, M. 1988 *Inequalities in Health: The Black Report and the Health Divide*. Harmondsworth: Penguin.

van de Mheen, H., Stronks, K. and Mackenbach, J. P. 1998 A lifecourse perspective on socio-economic inequalities in health: the influence of childhood socio-economic conditions and selection processes. *Sociology of Health and Illness* 20/5: 754–77.

Weber, M. 1958 *The Protestant Ethic and the Spirit of Capitalism*. New York: Charles Scribner's Sons.

Wilkinson, R. 1996 *Unhealthy Societies: The Afflictions of Inequality*. London: Routledge.

11

Paula McGee

KEY ISSUES IN THIS CHAPTER:
▶ Concepts of race and ethnicity.
▶ Ethnicity and health inequalities.
▶ Ethnicity and health.
▶ Implications for nursing.

BY THE END OF THIS CHAPTER YOU SHOULD BE ABLE TO:
▶ Discuss concepts of race, ethnicity and culture.
▶ Describe ethnic differences in health status and some of the possible reasons for them.
▶ Explain the concept of cultural competence and why it is important in nursing.

1 Introduction

The estimated population of the UK is currently 64.1 million; 53.9 million live in England; 5.3 million in Scotland, 3.1 million in Wales and 1.8 million in Northern Ireland. According to the 2011 census, 86 per cent of the population of England and Wales is composed of people who describe themselves as white British or white Other; similar majorities are evident in Scotland and Northern Ireland. The remaining 14 per cent of the population is comprised of people who describe themselves as belonging to a **minority ethnic group**. Indians (1.4 million in England and Wales) form the largest minority, followed by Pakistanis, black Africans, African-Caribbeans, Bangladeshis and Chinese (393,000). There are many other numerically smaller minority ethnic groups; an increasing number of people identify themselves as having mixed ethnicity (Office for National Statistics 2011a).

minority ethnic group:
differing in ethnicity and culture from the dominant population

ethnicity:
a social group with shared origins

race:
distinction between people based on specified characteristics

The **ethnicity** of local populations varies considerably across the UK. In cities, such as London, Leicester and Birmingham, members of minority ethnic groups make up a larger proportion of the population, over 40 per cent, whereas in towns such as Norwich and Chester they form less than 10 per cent. It is, therefore, useful to begin any consideration of **race** and ethnicity in the UK by finding out about the population in the places in which we live and work (Activity 12.1). It is very easy to make assumptions and generalizations; examining the profiles of places we think we know may challenge some of our preconceptions.

Activity 12.1 Exploring your locality

Your city/town/area:

(a) What is the total population of the city/town/area in which you live?

(b) Which are the largest minority ethnic groups?

Where you live:

(a) How many people live in your electoral ward?

(b) Which are the largest minority ethnic groups?

Where you work:

(a) How many people live in the area?

(b) Which are the largest minority ethnic groups?

Resources that will help you:

Office for National Statistics (<http://www.ons.gov.uk>) provides information based on census data.

Local council websites provide information about the areas in which you live and work.

---

2 Race, ethnicity and culture

The term 'race' originally referred to an individual's lineage, their family and shared ancestry. However, in late eighteenth-century Europe, it was argued that human beings could be classified into distinct groups or races based on certain observable characteristics such as skin colour, hair texture and perceived variations in 'ability, temperament and moral qualities', which were considered fixed and unchanging (Fenton 2010: 18). Science and religion were harnessed to justify these ideas, and races came to be seen as fixed, immutable groups, some of which were deemed inherently superior to others (Meer 2014). Evidence to support these ideas is conspicuous by its absence. The observable characteristics on which classification relied are not consistent or dependable. Skin colour varies widely; the texture of hair may or may not match a particular skin colour; people intermingle; their children add to the many variations of humanity (Fenton 2010). Moreover, there has never been any agreement about how many human races there are. For example, in Europe race is frequently associated with colour – black or white – but the United States has five official categories: White;

12

Black American; American Indian; Asian; and Native Hawaiian or Other Pacific Islander (Baer et al. 2012; United States Census Bureau at <http://www.census.gov>). Brazil also has five categories but these are based on skin colour; Canada uses a different system that focuses on ethnicity (Bradby 2012). In biological terms race does not exist. Rather, it is a social construct based on beliefs and perceptions that are used to create and sustain exclusive groups of people, separating group members, insiders, from non-members, outsiders.

The term 'race' is frequently conflated with *ethnicity*, a poorly defined concept that incorporates notions of social groupings based on shared history, culture, language, beliefs, myths, place of origin and many other elements (Ahmad and Bradby 2008). According to Platt (2011: 69), ethnicity may be 'adopted by people themselves to establish a shared **identity**', a sense of uniqueness. It may be an indicator of how individuals see themselves, particularly in Western cultures which place a high value on individual identity. Alternatively, ethnicity may be used to determine insider and outsider status, affording privilege to insiders in terms of access to resources while limiting that of others (Karlsen and Nazroo 2006). Ethnicity is not the same as **nationality**, which is a legal status which confers certain rights such as being allowed to vote in elections.

Ethnicity is dynamic because people's sense of themselves and who they are changes over time in response to both internal and external forces associated with each minority ethnic group (Hariri 2014). In the 2011 census, 4 per cent of Bangladeshi and 26 per cent of Irish respondents changed their ethnic group; 43 per cent of people with mixed ethnicity changed their ethnic group (Centre on Dynamics of Ethnicity 2014). People may opt to change their ethnic group for a number of reasons. They may be at a stage in life in which they view themselves differently, which in turn affects how they define their ethnicity. How people are asked about their ethnicity may also influence their decision. This may certainly be the case as far as census data are concerned. Questions about ethnicity were first added to the census in 1991 and were expanded to include more categories in 2001 and 2011. Some respondents may have switched to a category that better reflected their ethnicity or they may have felt that they now belonged in more than one. Others may have changed their ethnicity for political reasons. For example, the 2001 census was the first in which the Irish were identified as a separate category from the overall white population. While some respondents may have found it easy to change their recorded ethnicity and describe themselves as 'white Irish' rather than 'white British', others may have felt uncertain about which category they should choose because either they or one of their parents were born in Britain rather than in Ireland, or because one of their parents was English. Moreover, given the long history of **prejudice** and **discrimination** against Irish people in the UK, some respondents may have preferred to opt for a 'white British' ethnic identity. In addition, given the political situation

identity:
a person's sense of self

nationality:
legal status of belonging to a specific country

prejudice:
preconceived, negative and hostile beliefs about others

discrimination:
unjust treatment of individuals because of perceived characteristics

with regard to Northern Ireland at that time, some respondents may have learned not to draw attention to their Irishness in any way for fear of attracting reprisals. If, as time passed, they felt more secure, some respondents may have felt confident in defining themselves as 'white Irish' in 2011. The Irish are not alone in experiencing these dilemmas. Migrants fleeing from areas of conflict or persecution may also be reluctant to identify overtly with particular ethnic groups. With increasing intermingling, more people may see themselves as having mixed ethnicity that is not compatible with census classifications. Experiences of **racism** and discrimination may militate against some options. Thus choices about ethnicity can be influenced by political and social factors that are outside the individual's control.

Ethnicity is broader than but incorporates **culture**, which is described as 'a set of guidelines that individuals inherit as members of a particular society, and that tell them how to view the world, how to experience it emotionally and how to behave in relation to other people, to supernatural forces or gods and to the natural environment' (Helman 2007: 2). Cultures are not homogeneous or static. There is more variation within than between cultures, and changes occur over time in response to both internal and external influences (Helman 2007).

Everyone has a culture. As children we are socialized into our culture as a way of enabling us to feel that we belong, learn about values and beliefs and how to function appropriately in many different social roles: as a man, a woman, a worker, a husband or a student in school or college. Culture is, therefore, initially associated with family, but daily life also requires us to function in other types of culture. The schools we attend and the settings in which we work will each have their own **organizational culture** which can be summed up as 'the way we do things around here'. Student nurses are socialized into a **professional culture** based around a code of professional conduct which encapsulates the values and behaviours to which they are expected to adhere (Nursing and Midwifery Council 2015). Thus, as individuals,

racism:
beliefs and behaviours that discriminate against people deemed inferior

culture:
a way of life practised by a group

organizational culture:
shared values, norms and practices of an organization

professional culture:
shared values, norms and practices of a profession

12

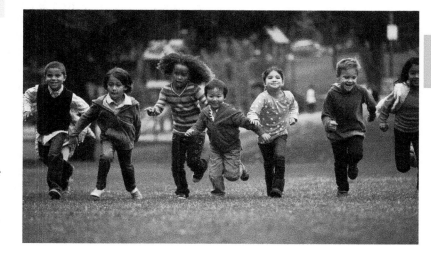

Figure 12.1 Everyone has an ethnicity and a culture, which informs and forms part of their identity

professionals and employees, people balance multiple ideas about their ethnicity, culture, identity and work roles. Most of the time this requires very little effort, but we may become more conscious of these factors when we encounter someone we think is different.

Activity 12.2 Exploring your ethnicity and culture

Imagine you have been asked to describe your ethnicity and culture to someone from another country.

(a) What do you think would be the most important points to mention?
(b) How would you describe yourself?
(c) Has your ethnicity or culture changed since you were a child? If so, in what way?
(d) How do you think the other person might react to your descriptions?
(e) If a patient was described to you as 'South Asian' would this influence the nursing care you provide?

Trying to describe our own ethnicity and culture can be quite challenging. It reveals enormous diversity which cannot be easily captured or explained regardless of which culture or ethnic group we think we belong to. People described as African-Caribbean may have origins in any one of thousands of islands, each of which has its own culture; their first language may be English, French, Dutch, Spanish or Papiamento. Similarly, the term 'South Asian' refers to people whose origins lie in a subcontinent comprised of several countries. India alone has over 1.2 billion inhabitants, more than twenty official languages and many different cultures and religions. Some English people may describe themselves in terms of the county in which they were born or their membership of one of the surviving indigenous minority groups. Cornish people, for example, were formally recognized as a minority ethnic group in 2014; Cornish and Gaelic are two indigenous minority languages in the UK. Recognition of indigenous minorities in the UK represented a significant step because much of the discourse about ethnicity and culture is couched in terms of people who are not white. The study of whiteness and white cultures is a fairly recent phenomenon. Whiteness has been associated with being 'Western' and 'modern' and thus as a yardstick against which others are judged. Just as the concept of race created a hierarchy in which some races were considered superior to others, cultures, when viewed in relation to colour, may be regarded in terms of how 'advanced' or Westernized they are thought to be (Fernando 2010).

In summary, race, ethnicity and culture are labels that may be used interchangeably, which 'makes it difficult to use the terms as if they were distinct' (Bradby 2012: 955). These labels are essentially social constructs rather than scientifically based facts, but they are used to differentiate social groups, to define insider and outsider status and as a basis for allowing or restricting access to resources.

3 Race, ethnicity, culture and health inequalities

Ethnicity and *culture* do not of themselves cause health problems, but there is considerable evidence to show that some members of minority ethnic groups experience much poorer health than the rest of the population. This section examines some of the possible explanations for these differences, but it is important to consider them within the wider context of factors that affect health in all sections of society: poverty, social class, gender, age, disability and chronic illness.

Reporting poor health

Attempting to measure health inequalities is not straightforward. Two methods are currently in use: mortality (deaths) and morbidity (self-reported health status). Death certificates state the immediate and underlying causes of death, age at death, sex, address and occupation. This information may be incomplete for members of some minority ethnic groups such as Somalis, who do not regard age and date of birth as important; occupation in the UK may be very different from that in the country of origin. The practice of changing a woman's family name on marriage may also contribute to inaccurate data. Consequently, at least four factors in measuring mortality cannot be relied upon. Furthermore, mortality rates for those born outside the UK may not adequately reflect rates among the large numbers of British-born members of minority ethnic groups (Nazroo 2006).

> **Activity 12.3 Reporting poor health**
>
> Look at Tables 12.1 and 12.2, and consider what possible explanations there might be for differences in reporting poor health.

Table 12.1 Percentages of people reporting poor health per ethnic group 2011

White British	20%	White Irish	28%	Gypsy and travellers	30%
Black African-Caribbean	22.9%	Arab	14%	Mixed white & black African-Caribbean	11.9%
Bangladeshi	17%	Chinese	10.4%	Black African	8.4%
Other black	13.3%	Indian	15%	Mixed white & Asian	8.8%

(Office for National Statistics 2011b)

Table 12.2 Percentages of women aged over sixty-five reporting limiting long-term illness

	All	Pakistani	Bangladeshi	White Gypsy or Irish Traveller	Arab	Indian
Women	56%	70%	70%	70%	66%	68%

(Centre on Dynamics of Ethnicity 2013)

12

Measuring self-reported health status is also unreliable because it depends on respondents who understand their health and the symptoms of illness in the terms used in the questions asked. It also depends on their ability to recall and report those symptoms accurately on request. Culturally based differences in beliefs about the causes of illness and the significance of symptoms are well documented (Helman 2007); certain illnesses such as mental health problems, HIV/AIDS and, currently, ebola are heavily stigmatized, and so people may not wish to disclose information because they fear repercussions. Nevertheless, minority ethnic older adults, gypsy and traveller people, and women of Bangladeshi and Pakistani origin are all known to have higher rates of illness than their counterparts in the majority population (Centre on Dynamics of Ethnicity 2013). However, information about the health of some other minority ethnic groups is limited; for example, Chinese, Polish and other Eastern Europeans.

ethnic monitoring: collecting and using data about an ethnic group

Alongside these two measurements is **ethnic monitoring**. The 2010 Equality Act requires all public services to take active steps to eliminate inequalities and discrimination. Ethnic monitoring forms a part of this. Patients, service users and staff should be asked to identify their ethnicity. However, in reality, data collection is patchy; whether and how data are used is not always clear. Moreover, some people may not wish to draw attention to their ethnicity because of past experiences of discrimination (Bradby 2012).

Genetics

While the concept of race has been rejected, there are some differences in the genetic profiles of ethnic groups and, in some instances, these are associated with particular diseases. A brief examination of diabetes helps to illustrate this point. Diabetes is a condition in which the pancreas cannot produce a hormone called insulin which promotes the uptake of glucose by cells throughout the body. It is estimated that 387 million people worldwide have this condition; the highest incidence occurs in Southeast Asia (8.3 per cent) and in countries bordering the Pacific Ocean (8.5 per cent) (International Diabetes Federation 2014). Many more may not be diagnosed until complications arise. These include peripheral neuropathy, cardiovascular disease, retinopathy, stroke, depression, sexual dysfunction and multi-organ failure. The World Health Organization (2015) estimates that diabetes will be the seventh leading cause of death worldwide by 2030.

There are several types of diabetes, but the most common is Type 2 in which a previously normal pancreas becomes unable to produce enough insulin for the body's needs; associated factors include obesity, lack of exercise and ageing. In the UK 3,208,014 adults (6 per cent of the population) have a diagnosis of diabetes; of these, 90 per cent have Type 2 (Diabetes UK 2014). They are mainly older adults, aged over fifty years, but the incidence is increasing among younger people, especially those who are overweight.

There is no doubt that Type 2 diabetes is a disease of increasing affluence but it seems to be particularly prevalent among certain groups of people. South Asian and African-Caribbean people are more likely to develop diabetes and to do so at an earlier age than their white counterparts (Diabetes UK 2014). In India, an estimated 62 million people have been diagnosed with diabetes, the highest figures in the world. Indian people are more likely to develop the disease in their twenties and thirties and to experience cardiovascular and neuropathic complications (Kaveeshwar and Cornwall 2014). The reasons for this are still not clear. Genetic factors may play a part; Kooner, Saleheen, Sim et al. (2011) surveyed 5,561 South Asian people with Type 2 diabetes in three countries and identified six genes that do not occur in non-South Asians. However, all this shows is that there is an association between certain genes and the onset of diabetes; it does not follow that the genes cause diabetes, although they may in some instances contribute to a predisposition to its development. Presumably the six genes have been present in South Asian people for generations without there being what amounts to an epidemic of diabetes, and so other factors must have occurred for this to happen. Moreover, millions of people around the world who are not South Asians also develop diabetes, so we need to be wary of placing too much emphasis on genetic factors at present.

Health beliefs

Every culture has a system of beliefs about the nature of health and the causes of illness and disease. These beliefs are complemented by ideas about how illness should be treated, by whom and the expected outcomes. Health professionals are taught to regard illness and disease in terms of scientific knowledge about how the body works; normal and disordered physiology, body chemistry, microbiology and other scientific disciplines inform their work. People who are not health professionals, regardless of whether they are members of minority ethnic groups or not, do not necessarily share the same perspectives. They may want to know why a particular illness is happening to them and what can be done about it. Ideas about illness, disease and what goes on inside the body vary widely, but are frequently understood in terms of one or more of the following beliefs.

1   The 'faulty' body. In this context some part of the body is not functioning as it should and requires 'fixing'. Western societies tend to favour this belief. They emphasize personal responsibility for health and see it as up to the individual to do something about it. Western ideas about the 'faulty' body may go beyond the absence of illness or disease because it is a major part of the presentation of the self to the world, a 'project to be worked on',

12

altered or even partially reconstructed to fit prevailing fashions and desires (Helman 2007).

2 The environment. Here illness is attributed to the weather or other natural phenomena. The English, for example, frequently believe that damp miserable weather causes 'chills', a condition that has no equivalent anywhere else; they treat the weather much like an awkward and difficult relative. There is nothing that can be done about it, except to have a good moan (Fox 2004).

3 Breakdowns in relationships with others. Where illness cannot be adequately accounted for by medical science, individuals will often look for other explanations. Thus the cause of illness may be attributed to a punishment or test from God or the harmful actions of others; the use of witchcraft, the **evil eye** or a curse, perhaps as a result of envy, dislike, a falling out or malice. Such beliefs are very common in developing societies; they are not necessarily related to lack of education (Helman 2007).

evil eye:
a form of witchcraft

These beliefs call for diverse courses of action, which may include religious practices and rituals to promote healing or to counteract the harm incurred by breakdowns in relationships. For example, Rastafarians may use marijuana to cleanse the body and mind and promote well-being.

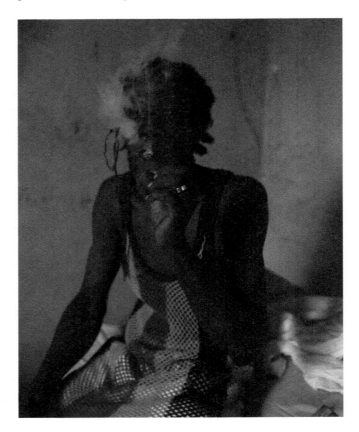

Figure 12.2 It is important to consider cultural factors which may have an effect on health; in Rastafarian culture smoking cannabis is part of spiritual worship

Most societies also have traditional remedies such as herbal preparations to relieve symptoms or modify disease. For example, people of African-Caribbean origin have a high risk of developing hypertension and stroke, but some people are fearful of Western medication, arguing that it is too strong. They may substitute or combine Western medication with herbal remedies made from breadfruit plant leaves, fever grass, lime juice mixed with garlic or other ingredients (Higginbottom and Mathers 2006). Considering these beliefs highlights the importance of understanding and respecting the patient's point of view. It is not always enough to treat and care for people using modern, Western paradigms. Competence in nursing practice can sometimes require the nurse to provide care that acknowledges beliefs and, where possible, incorporates factors that the patient believes will help.

Racism

Racism is an attitude of mind arising from ideas about race and refers to the behaviour of individuals, organizations and society towards those deemed to be outsiders and inferiors. Racism involves value judgements about the worth of outsiders and the subsequent exercise of power to assert superiority over them through psychological, social, spiritual, economic, physical or any other means (Fernando 2010). Jokes, threats, harassment, discrimination and violence are all forms of behaviour associated with the enactment of racism. One of the many problems with these behaviours is that, even though racist behaviours are illegal, they are often subtle and difficult to substantiate, especially if there are no witnesses. Complaints about offensive jokes, for example, are frequently countered by accusations that the complainant lacks a sense of humour. In this way racist behaviour is used to both consciously and unconsciously structure hierarchical social relations and justify discrimination on the grounds that both are 'natural' and recipients have no right to complain (Hariri 2014: 136).

Exposure to racist behaviour has a negative effect on people's self-worth. It creates a constant sense of threat, which in turn affects both mental and physical well-being. Exposure to stress triggers physiological changes; levels of cortisol rise, causing changes in the cardiovascular and the immune systems. Difficulties in trying to manage feelings and deal with the emotional distress add to the situation. Until fairly recently it was believed that these responses occurred only when an individual perceived themselves to be the object of racist behaviour. However, it is now evident that physiological changes may occur independently of conscious awareness (Harrell, Burford, Cage, Nelson et al. 2011). For members of minority ethnic groups, encounters with racist behaviour are not occasional events that can be shrugged off; racism is a daily experience, and even when it does not actually occur, it remains a possibility. Consequently the effects of stress accumulate over time, causing physical changes that affect health.

12

4 Access to health care

Activity 12.4 Accessing care

Mr Singh is an elderly South Asian man who lives with his son and daughter-in-law. Mr Singh was diagnosed with Type 2 diabetes three years ago, after he complained to his GP that he could not feel the foot pedals when driving. Mr Singh attends the diabetes centre regularly for check-ups and tries hard to follow the advice given by the staff. He speaks some English as his fifth language and always comes to the clinic alone; he does not want to bother his son and daughter-in-law as they both have busy jobs and young children.

His condition was fairly stable until recently, but oral medication became less and less effective and two months ago he commenced insulin injections. The diabetes nurse specialist explained why this was necessary and taught Mr Singh how to inject himself. She impressed on him the importance of taking his insulin half an hour before meals at 7 a.m., 12 noon and 6 p.m.

Mr Singh has been admitted to hospital with hypoglycaemia for the fifth time this month, but insists that he is following the instructions he was given by the nurse specialist and always takes his insulin on time. Mr Singh is very upset by these frequent admissions, which usually occur in the evenings. Now, as he arrives on the ward, the nurse in charge is heard to say 'Not him again!' Mr Singh is accompanied today by his son and daughter-in-law.

(a) What factors may be contributing to Mr Singh's frequent admissions?

(b) What assumptions might the nurse in charge be making about Mr Singh?

(c) How might this situation be resolved?

(d) What aspects of the self, the patient and the context are relevant here?

(e) What factors do you think members of minority ethnic groups might encounter as barriers to accessing treatment and care, and why?

The following resource may be helpful:

Zeh, P., Sandhu, H., Cannaby, A. and Sturt, J. 2014 Cultural barriers impeding ethnic minority groups from accessing effective diabetes care services: a systematic review. *Diversity and Equality in Health and Care* 11/1: 9–33.

Access to health care depends first on knowing what is available and how to make use of services effectively. Language is one of the most important issues in achieving access. Patients and professionals need to be able to communicate clearly and effectively. Lack of understanding can lead to incorrect or missed diagnoses, inappropriate prescriptions, poor compliance with treatment, continued illness and frustration for both parties. Relying on relatives or colleagues who may speak the same language as the patient is not a satisfactory solution. They may not have the vocabulary to explain complex health issues or convey to the professionals what a patient really means when she says, 'I have a pain in my heart' (I am unhappy and depressed) (McGee and Johnson 2008).

In the United States, the Office of Minority Health (2014; at: <http://minorityhealth.hhs.gov/omh>) is responsible for leading 'activities that improve the health of racial and ethnic minority populations and eliminate health disparities' in a number of departments, providing standards for working with patients and service users who do not speak English. These are part of the National Standards for Culturally and Linguistically Appropriate Services in Health and Health Care (The National CLAS Standards) and are generally regarded as the gold standard for health care, although it is not clear whether all American health-care providers implement them.

In the UK, language is construed as a minority problem. Viewed through the lens of ethnicity, inability to converse in and read English may be construed as a sign of cultural deficiency that incurs blame. Neither the NHS Constitution (Department of Health 2013a) nor the accompanying handbook (Department of Health 2013b) make any reference to interpreting or language other than to say that people are entitled to be treated with respect and dignity and to be involved in all decisions about their treatment and care. Many patient rights and staff responsibilities in the Constitution depend on communication but, it seems, only for those who speak English. While most NHS Trusts have engaged interpreting services, there is still no national requirement that individual interpreters receive formal training to prepare them for working in health care, although courses are available via the Institute of Linguists (<https://www.ciol.org.uk>). Moreover, interpreting services can be difficult to access for any number of reasons: staff may not know in advance whether a patient can communicate, interpreters may not be booked, or there may not be enough of them, and delays in treatment while an interpreter is located may not be feasible. Financial problems in NHS Trusts may lead to reductions in interpreting services. Thus, it may appear that something is being done while pushing the problem back to members of minority groups.

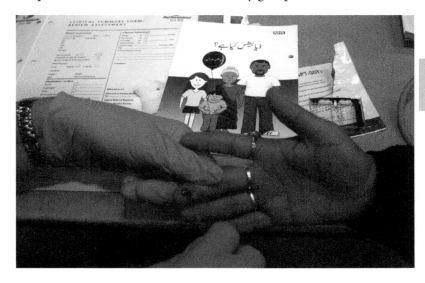

12

Figure 12.3
Language can be a significant barrier to accessing health care

Additional barriers to accessing health services include lack of knowledge. Nurses who lack knowledge and understanding of the cultural backgrounds of their patients and, even worse, are unaware of their shortcomings, cannot be regarded as safe practitioners. In the case of Mr Singh, it seems that no attention has been paid to family circumstances. There is no evidence of engagement with whoever prepares food and the times at which meals are taken. It is very easy to lay the blame on culture and ethnicity, but the real reason for Mr Singh's hypoglycaemia may be that the evening meal is not served until 8.30 p.m. A glass of milk and biscuit after his insulin at 6 p.m. might well prevent hypoglycaemia and allow Mr Singh and his family to enjoy their evening meal.

This is not to imply that lack of knowledge does not also occur among members of minority groups. Investigation of the low uptake of palliative care among black and South Asian people in Leicester, a city which has one of the most diverse populations in England, revealed a different picture which challenged previously held assumptions. Lack of knowledge about the service was a major obstacle because there were no sources of reliable information except health professionals. Disclosure of need to anyone outside the family might incur stigma, and so, unless GPs or other professionals took the initiative to inform patients and families about the service, families did not know about palliative care and so could not access this. Even if they had heard about the service, many were worried that they would have to pay for it and so did not seek referrals (Markham et al. 2014). Thus, knowledge about services may not of itself lead to service use. Much may also depend on who has the power to allow or facilitate access. Power structures and decision-making within families may have a profound influence on service uptake (Row et al. 2013). Other barriers to accessing effective diabetes care may include paternalistic attitudes, gender issues, cultural norms about food, religious beliefs and practices, language and communication, health beliefs, low literacy and lack of confidence in professionals (Lowe et al. 2007; Zeh et al. 2014).

5 Migration

Just over half a million people, 583,000, immigrated to the UK in 2014; most came to work (247,000) or to study (176,000); 24,300 applied for asylum. In the same period, approximately 323,000 people emigrated (ONS 2014). If they have migrated for work or study, most migrants are quite healthy when they arrive but are often employed in low-paid jobs. The ensuing combination of low wages, poverty and poor nutrition may have a negative effect on health. The health of refugee migrants claiming asylum may be further compromised by trauma arising from war or persecution in their home countries and compounded by the risky business of escape. Thus, individuals may arrive with health problems for which they have been unable to obtain treatment: communicable diseases, long-term conditions such as diabetes, injuries sustained as a result of conflict or torture and mental health problems arising from experiences of severe trauma. Women and children are particularly likely to have suffered physical and/or sexual abuse (Jayaweera 2014). All these problems may be exacerbated by UK policies, which require those seeking asylum to be detained and dispersed around the country.

For all migrants, and even for those who believe that they are well prepared, the experience of moving to another country can cause immense stress, a state of '**culture shock**', in which they feel disorientated, homesick, exhausted and unable to cope, and dislike the new, host culture (Andrews and Boyle 2011). To some extent, 'culture shock' follows naturally after the excitement of travel and arrival, but it can be profound and debilitating, particularly if people feel socially isolated or already have poor health. Adapting to life in the new country may also involve changes in behaviour that affect health: smoking, encounters with racism and discrimination, lack of exercise, changes in diet, alcohol or drug use.

Changing patterns in migration may also play a part. In the past, migration, particularly to countries far away, was often a one-way journey, but in the modern world this is far less likely. Mobile phones, the Internet and the availability of cheap air fares mean that migrants can now 'forge and sustain multi-stranded social relations that link together their societies of origin and settlement' (Faist, Fauser and Reisenauer 2013: 8). Previous migrants may also have done this, but what is new is the immediacy. Instead of waiting months for a letter or saving for years for a trip home, communication and travel can now take place instantly, in real time. Understanding of these changes has led to the development of **transnationalism** as a new area of study. Modern communication and travel mean that ties with the country of origin, and indeed a widespread diaspora, can be better sustained and may be much closer than in the past. This connectedness transcends national boundaries and geography to facilitate family and friendship networks that can now be a global enterprise in which values, norms, new ideas and social and financial help can be transmitted back and forth. While this may be helpful in maintaining family ties, it can also mean extra worry and pressure for people in both settings, as they are more closely involved in each other's lives, and perhaps militate against settlement in the new country. Transnationalism has implications for health and health care in several ways. Positive influences include two-way emotional support and remittances but there might be continued reliance on the health-care systems, practices and medicines from home, which may be problematic if migrants are also using the health-care system in their host country.

culture shock: fear and uncertainty when in an unfamiliar culture

transnationalism: interconnectedness across national borders between migrants and non-migrants

12

6 Implications for nursing

Caring for patients requires nurses to think consciously about three factors: *the self, the patient* and *the context*. Thinking about *the self* means developing self-awareness about personal values and beliefs and how these may impact on interaction with patients. Everyone has likes, dislikes and prejudices of one sort or another, which may influence how they behave. In caring for people, nurses need to be aware of how their behaviour impacts on patients and their relatives; they will remember more about how nurses behaved towards them, their attitudes and manners than about what they did (Papadopoulos, Tilki and Taylor 1998). Technical and clinical brilliance are not enough; interpersonal skills are just as important.

Thinking about *the patient* means treating that person as an individual, with respect and dignity. This involves being open to the possibility of difference and willing to accept people as they are without blaming them or looking down on them. Nurses have a responsibility to develop their knowledge of the patients' backgrounds, their values and beliefs. In doing so, they need to consider not only what they know already but also how they know. Unreliable and biased knowledge may be generated through hearsay and prejudice. Patients and relatives possess valuable knowledge about their health, health beliefs and practices, but this may not be couched in terms that are valued by professionals or academics (Papadopoulos 2006). Taking time to listen to members of minority ethnic groups is therefore important in ensuring that knowledge about them is accurate.

Thinking about *the context* refers to the environment in which nursing care takes place and how this setting may affect the type of care activities that can safely take place (Nursing and Midwifery Council 2015). Caring for people of diverse ethnicities and cultures also requires some adaptation of nursing knowledge and skills to provide safe, competent care. The term 'cultural competence' refers to nursing care that takes account of and appropriately incorporates the patient's cultural values and beliefs, religion, ethnicity, health beliefs and individual preferences (Papadopoulos 2006).

cultural competence: incorporation of cultural values and beliefs into patient care

---

Activity 12.5 Understanding diabetes within high-risk communities

Mrs Dhillon is a middle-aged South Asian woman who has recently returned from holiday in India. While she was there she felt very well and so she stopped taking the medication for her Type 2 diabetes. On her return home she has suffered a stroke. The right side of her body is weak and is receiving therapy to help improve her balance, mobility and coordination.

(a) What aspects of *the self, the patient* and *the context* are relevant in providing care for Mrs Dhillon after her stroke?

(b) What strategies could be used to promote understanding about diabetes among high-risk communities?

Summary and Resources

Summary

▶ The concepts of race, ethnicity and culture are universal issues that influence experiences of health, illness and health care in the UK.

▶ The experience of racism, discrimination, migration and lack of access to services can adversely affect the health of members of minority ethnic groups.

▶ Nurses, who may themselves also be members of diverse ethnic and cultural groups, have a legal and professional responsibility to provide culturally competent care for all patients irrespective of any distinguishing characteristic.

Questions for Discussion

1 Compare and contrast the data you collected in Activity 12.1 with a different town or city. What are the main differences in the population?

2 Discuss the ways in which nurses in your field of practice could access the views and experiences of patients/service users who are members of minority ethnic groups.

3 Take a copy of the nursing assessment tool used in one of your placements and ask a patient/service user who is a member of a minority ethnic group about how questions relate to their culture. What other points would they like to see included?

Glossary

community:	a term often used to denote minority groups that are perceived by outsiders to be homogeneous, but whose members may have little in common
community leader:	a person who is deemed by outsiders to lead and speak for a community, but who may or may not hold a formal mandate to do so
cultural competence:	nursing care that takes account of and appropriately incorporates the patient's cultural values and beliefs, religion, ethnicity, health beliefs and individual preferences; becoming culturally competent is a process through which the nurse progresses over time
culture:	an inherited and shared way of life which encompasses traditions, beliefs, food, clothing, values, social systems, language and behaviour

12

culture shock:	a sense of fear, distress and uncertainty that may occur after moving to live in an unfamiliar culture
discrimination:	unfavourable and unjust treatment of individuals because of perceived characteristics such as race, gender or disability
ethnicity:	a socially constructed grouping of people who perceive themselves to share or who are perceived by others to share common origins, ancestry, language, religion and other attributes; the term 'ethnicity' is often used synonymously with 'race' and sometimes with 'nationality'
ethnic monitoring:	the processes of collecting and using data about members of an ethnic group
evil eye:	a form of witchcraft based on the belief that misfortune is caused by looking at someone in a particular way
identity:	a person's sense of self as a separate person; individuals may have multiple identities depending on their family, work and social roles and their cultural and ethnic backgrounds; Western notions of identity value and emphasize individuality, and the individual is deemed capable of taking responsibility for the self and making decisions; non-Western notions of identity emphasize a more collective view in which identity is community and family based
institutional racism:	the tendency within an organization to discriminate against individuals because of perceived differences, such as colour, and the failure of the organization to treat individuals equitably
minority ethnic group:	a social group which differs in terms of ethnicity, culture and sometimes nationality from the dominant population which exercises and controls the state
nationality:	an individual's legal status in relation to a specific country as a result of birth or naturalization; the term 'nationality' is sometimes used synonymously with 'race' and 'ethnicity'
organizational culture:	characteristic values, norms and practices which determine how staff relate both to each other and to external parties

prejudice:	preconceived, negative and hostile beliefs about members of a minority ethnic group
professional culture:	characteristic values, norms and practices which determine how members of the profession relate both to each other and to external parties
race:	an artificial and discredited distinction between groups of people based on specified unchangeable characteristics; the term 'race' is often used synonymously with 'ethnicity' and sometimes with 'nationality'
racism:	refers to beliefs and behaviours by individuals and groups towards those whom they judge to be inferior on the grounds of racial characteristics such as skin colour; racism may also occur as an expression and outcome of organizational policies and procedures
transnationalism:	the increasing interconnectedness between family members and friends who migrate and those who do not, which transcends national boundaries and geographical distance

Further Reading

C. Helman: *Culture, Health and Illness*, 5th edn. London: Hodder Arnold, 2007.
Written by a medical anthropologist and former GP, this text is used throughout the world to enable health professionals to develop insight into the impact of culture on health and illness. It is particularly helpful in explaining the differences between professionals' understanding of illness and how it should be treated and that of patients and their families. Additional topics include influences on and the behaviours associated with pain in different societies, cultural aspects of stress and suffering, and the impact of the Internet and World Wide Web on health care.

Nursing and Midwifery Council: *The Code. Professional Standards of Practice and Behaviour for Nurses and Midwives*. London: NMC, 2015.
This document sets out the standards required for professional nursing and midwifery practice in the UK. Of particular relevance to this chapter are requirements to 'avoid making assumptions and recognise diversity and individual choice' (section 1.3) and to 'take reasonable steps to meet people's language and communication needs' (section 7) and to practise safely.

P. Zeh, H. Sandhu, A. Cannaby and J. Sturt; Cultural barriers impeding ethnic minority groups from accessing effective diabetes care services: a systematic review. *Diversity and Equality in Health and Care* 11/1 (2014): 9–33.

12

This review provides easy access to a wide range of literature about the ways in which members of minority ethnic groups may be deterred or prevented from accessing and using health services.

References

Ahmad, W. and Bradby, H. (eds) 2008 *Ethnicity, Health and Healthcare: Understanding Diversity, Tackling Disadvantage.* Oxford: Wiley Blackwell.

Andrews, M. and Boyle, J. 2011 *Transcultural Concepts in Nursing Care*, 6th edn. Philadelphia: Lippincott, Williams and Wilkins.

Baer, R., Arteaga, E., Dyer, K., Eden, A., Gross, R., Helmy, H., Karnyski, M., Papadopoulos, A. and Reeser, D. 2012 Concepts of race and ethnicity among health researchers: patterns and implications. *Ethnicity and Health* 17: 1–15.

Bradby, H. 2012 Race, ethnicity and health: the costs and benefits of conceptualizing racism and ethnicity. *Social Science and Medicine* 75: 955–8.

Centre for Mental Health 2013 *The Bradley Commission: Black and Minority Ethnic Communities, Mental Health and Criminal Justice.* London: Centre for Mental Health.

Centre on Dynamics of Ethnicity 2013 *Which Ethnic Groups Have the Poorest Health? Ethnic Health Inequalities 1991 to 2011.* At: <http://www.ethnicity.ac.uk>.

Centre on Dynamics of Ethnicity 2014 *How Have People's Ethnic Identities Changed in England and Wales?* At: <http://www.ethnicity.ac.uk>.

Curtis, L. P. 1971 *Apes and Angels. The Irishman in Victorian Caricature.* Newton Abbot: David Charles.

Department of Health 2013a *National Health Service Constitution.* London: Department of Health.

Department of Health 2013b *The Handbook to the NHS Constitution.* London: Department of Health.

Diabetes UK 2014 *Diabetes: Facts and Stats.* Diabetes UK. At: <www.diabetesuk.org>.

Faist, T. Fauser, M. and Reisenaur, E. 2013 *Transnational Migration.* Cambridge: Polity.

Fenton, S. 2010 *Ethnicity.* Cambridge: Polity.

Fernando, S. 2010 *Mental Health, Race and Culture*, 3rd edn. Basingstoke: Palgrave Macmillan.

Fox, K. 2004 *Watching the English. The Hidden Rules of English Behaviour.* London: Hodder.

Hariri, Y. N. 2014 *Sapiens. A Brief History of Humankind.* London: Harvill Secker.

Harrell, C. J. P., Burford, T., Cage, B., Nelson, T. M., Shearon, S. Thompson, A. and Green, S. 2011 Multiple pathways linking racism to health outcomes. *Du Bois Review* (15 April) 8/1: 143–57.

Helman. C. 2007 *Culture, Health and Illness*, 5th edn. London: Hodder Arnold.

Higginbottom, G. and Mathers, N. 2006 The use of herbal remedies to promote general wellbeing by individuals of African-Caribbean origin in England. *Diversity in Health and Social Care* 3/2: 99–110.

International Diabetes Federation 2014 *IDF Atlas*, 6th edn. At: <http://www.idf.org>.

Jayaweera, H. 2014 *Health of Migrants in the UK: What Do We Know?* Oxford: Migration Observatory.

Karlsen, S. and Nazroo, J. 2006 Defining and measuring ethnicity and 'race'. In J. Nazroo (ed.), *Health and Social Research in Multiethnic Societies.* London: Routledge.

Kaveeshwar, S. A. and Cornwall, J. 2014 The current state of diabetes mellitus in India. *Australian Medical Journal* 7/1: 45–8.

Kooner, J., Saleheen, D., Sim, X., Sehmi, J., Zhang, W. et al. 2011 Genome-wide association study in individuals of South Asian ancestry identifies six new Type 2 diabetes susceptibility loci. *Nature Genetics* 43: 984–9.

Lowe, P., Griffiths, F. and Sidhu, R. 2007 'I got pregnant, I was so like crying inside . . .' experiences of women of Pakistani ancestry seeking contraception in the UK. *Diversity in Health and Social Care* 4/1: 69–76.

McGee, P. 2008 *Irish Mental Health. What is Appropriate and Culturally Competent Primary Care?* Birmingham: Centre for Community Mental Health, Birmingham City University.

McGee, P. and Johnson, M. 2008 I never needed to know the word for diabetes till I took this job. *Diversity in Health and Social Care* 5/1: 1–3.

McGhee, D. 2005 *Intolerant Britain? Hate, Citizenship and Difference.* Maidenhead: Open University Press.

MacPherson, W. 1999 *The Stephen Lawrence Inquiry: Report of an Inquiry by Sir William MacPherson,* Cm4262-1. London: Home Office.

Markham, S., Islam, Z. and Faull, C. 2014 I never knew that! Why do people from Black and Asian minority ethnic groups in Leicester access hospice services less than other groups? A discussion with community groups. *Diversity and Equality in Health and Care* 11/3–4: 237–45.

Meer, N. 2014 *Key Concepts in Race and Ethnicity.* 3rd edn. London: Sage.

Nazroo, J. (ed.) 2006 *Health and Social Research in Multiethnic Societies.* London: Routledge.

Norfolk, Suffolk and Cambridgeshire Strategic Health Authority 2003 *Independent Inquiry into the Death of David Bennett.* Report of an inquiry set up under HSG (94) 27 Chaired by Sir John Blofeld, Cambridge HSCSHA.

Nursing and Midwifery Council 2015 *The Code. Professional Standards of Practice and Behaviour for Nurses and Midwives.* London: NMC.

Office for National Statistics 2011a *Ethnicity and National Identity in England and Wales 2011.* At: <http://www.ons.gov.uk>.

Office for National Statistics 2011b *Trends in General Health and Unpaid Care Provision between Ethnic Groups, 2011* At: <http://www.ons.gov.uk>.

Office for National Statistics 2014 *Migration Statistics Quarterly Report,* November 2014. At: <http://www.ons.gov.uk>.

Office of Minority Ethnic Health 2014 *National Standards for Culturally and Linguistically Appropriate Services in Health and Health Care (The National CLAS Standards).* At: <http://minorityhealth.hhs.gov/omh>.

Papadopoulos, I. 2006 *Transcultural Health and Social Care. Development of Culturally Competent Practitioners.* Edinburgh: Churchill Livingstone.

Papadopoulos, I., Tilki, M. and Taylor, G. 1998 *Transcultural Care: A Guide for Health Care Professionals.* Dinton: Quay Publishers.

Platt, L. 2011 *Understanding Inequalities.* Cambridge: Polity.

12

Row, M., Nevill, A., Bellingham-Young, D. and Adamson-Macedo, E. 2013 Promoting positive postpartum mental health through exercise in ethnically diverse priority groups. *Diversity and Equality in Health and Care* 10/3: 185–95.

Sainsbury Centre for Mental Health, The 2002 *Breaking the Circles of Fear. A Review of the Relationship Between Mental Health Services and African and Caribbean Communities.* London: The Sainsbury Centre for Mental Health.

Scally, G. 2004 The very pests of society: the Irish and 150 years of public health in England. *Clinical Medicine* 4/1: 77–81.

World Health Organization 2011 *Mental Health Atlas.* Geneva: WHO. At: <http://www.who.int>.

World Health Organization 2015 *Diabetes.* At: <http://www.who.int>.

Zeh, P., Sandhu, H., Cannaby, A. and Sturt, J. 2014 Cultural barriers impeding ethnic minority groups from accessing effective diabetes care services: a systematic review. *Diversity and Equality in Health and Care* 11/1: 9–33.

Part III
Policy Influences on Health and Health Care

The purpose of this section is to examine the importance of policy in shaping the way health care is delivered and to consider some of the wider influences on health and health care. It is made up of four chapters which address a number of the key issues. The first, Chapter 13, discusses the policy process and relates it to health care, particularly in the UK, and emphasizes the importance of policy in this area for nursing and the provision of care. The second, Chapter 14, explores this in more detail with regard to the management of nursing in the acute/hospital sector, with reference to relevant sociological theory. The third, Chapter 15, takes a similar approach to a discussion of the organization of care provision in the community. Using theories and concepts from sociology, the aim is to demonstrate how the delivery of care is policy driven and to highlight the implications this has for nursing. Finally, Chapter 16 explores some of the wider influences on health and health care by focusing on health and disease across the world and the influence of globalization.

Health policy is a complex process, and in Chapter 13 the policy context of UK health care is examined to demonstrate how and why policy changes take place, and some key themes within contemporary health policy are introduced. It starts with an overview of what constitutes policy in health and health care, and an introduction to ways of understanding the policy process. The impact of devolution, as a wider policy trend, on the direction of health policy in the constituent parts of the UK is explored to illustrate how differences in the organization of the NHS in the home nations are policy driven. A number of key policy themes are analysed, including: structures for planning and delivering care; the role of competition; performance management; and funding care – because these are areas where there has been some divergence between the four nations. Several broader issues, such as the concept of 'choice' in health care and policy responses to obesity, are also examined. Finally, the chapter turns to the impact of policy on nursing, and the potential influence that nurses can have on the planning of care and future policy directions.

National policy sets the context for how health care is organized, and it also has an impact on how it is managed. In Chapter 14, a brief history of the approaches that have been taken to management in the NHS is included as a basis for summarizing the current position. Also examined are the developments in health-care organization, which have culminated in the more recent emphasis on culture management and leadership as being crucial to the delivery of effective services and care. This is necessary because there is no single 'answer' to the management 'problem' of health care; rather, it is important to consider a range of perspectives critically. Sociology is particularly helpful in this respect as it provides useful insights regarding the social organization of services. The policy drive for leadership and cultural change is explored and the implications for nursing discussed. Key sociological concepts, including bureaucracy, negotiated order and translational mobilization, are used to examine health-care organization and management. All nurses have some element of management in their clinical role and many have more formal organizational management responsibilities, so it is important to recognize that managing health care is part of nursing, and the more this is understood, the more likely it is that care can be better organized.

In Chapter 15, the boundaries between health and social care services, which are notoriously blurred, are explored. This is important because the implications for patients of being on either side of that boundary can have a profound effect on the level of care they receive. A number of important issues at the interface of health and social care of concern for patients and nurses are examined. These include the funding context of social care and the implications of this for the NHS and nursing staff. The extension of personal budgets from social care into Continuing Healthcare as personal health budgets, together with the challenges this presents for professional practice, are also examined. Drawing on key concepts, including social capital, personalization and the social model of disability, consideration is given to the issues that need to be addressed if 'whole person' approaches to care, which integrate health and social care services, are to be achieved. Once again, the crucial role of policy in shaping how services are delivered is evident in social care.

In Chapter 16, the final chapter of this section, attention turns to the global context. The emphasis here is to explore how individual choices can be influenced by a wide range of factors, including what is happening on a global scale. The chapter begins by exploring the global burden of disease, focusing on differences between parts of the world and the relationship between health and inequality. Then the chapter turns to a discussion of globalization and to the concept of 'acting locally' and how this is important for nursing practice. Particular attention is paid to the issue of reproductive and sexual health within a global context, exploring, in particular, the significance of this for overall well-being and the relationship between this and gender inequalities. Finally, the chapter explores the issue of nursing work at a global scale, considering, in particular, the effects of nurse migration.

Kate Thomson

> **KEY ISSUES IN THIS CHAPTER:**
> ▶ Health policy and the nurse.
> ▶ The NHS.
> ▶ Influences on health policy.
> ▶ Policy and the organization of health care.
>
> **BY THE END OF THIS CHAPTER YOU SHOULD BE ABLE TO:**
> ▶ Understand how political decisions affect the organization and management of the health system, as well as approaches to care.
> ▶ Identify the main differences between the health systems in England, Wales, Scotland and Northern Ireland.
> ▶ Appreciate how nursing practice is affected by policy changes.

1 Introduction

Have you seen the news lately? You may think that 'politics' are not interesting to you. However, political debates and decisions directly influence the health services you work in as a nurse. Having a grasp of the policy context within which changes or problems are happening in your workplace will help you to understand 'what's going on' and see the bigger picture.

Headlines at the time of writing this chapter include:

Nurses threaten strike action over '7-day NHS' plan
Cuts in acute psychiatric care may have gone too far
25 cancer drugs to be denied on NHS
Thousands of patients left waiting in ambulances outside hospital
UK government commits to £8bn NHS boost

These issues of finance, staffing, quality of and access to care are the key concerns of health policy. This chapter will help you to think about these issues in a sociological way. It starts by placing the UK's health system in a historical and social context. It then discusses what is meant by 'policy' and gives example ways of thinking about policy using a sociological perspective. How and why are policy decisions made, and whose views and interests are taken into account? The final sections of the chapter return to discuss the National Health Service in the UK in more detail, examining the different directions that health policy has taken in England, Scotland, Wales and Northern Ireland, with a particular emphasis on cost, quality and access to care.

Activity 13.1 In the news

Test it out: commit to a 'media watch' for health-related news for one week.

(a) Over your chosen week, try to listen to/watch one news radio/TV broadcast each day, and monitor one newspaper (many have excellent websites – see the end of this chapter for a few examples). Check out the lead stories; search for 'health' or 'NHS' or go to the relevant section of the site.

(b) Listen/look out for health-care or NHS-related issues in the news. Whose voices are heard (who is asked to comment on/debate the issues?)?

(c) What implications do the issues have for individual nurses, and for the nursing profession as a whole?

(d) What is the balance of stories in relation to hospital (adult acute care), community services, mental health, child health or learning-disability care?

Your 'news watch' should have indicated to you how health policy is an area of political and public debate. This is the case in most countries that have an established system of health care that necessitates making decisions about public spending and the organization of services. However, in the UK, the National Health Service (NHS) has become a potent cultural and political symbol. One example of this is the way the NHS became the focus of a whole section of the opening ceremony of the London Olympic Games in 2012 (view a video of the NHS segment at <http://www.bbc.co.uk/programmes/p01b7461>). Olympic opening ceremonies are usually designed to show the world what is unique and special about the host country – placing the NHS at the heart of this was in itself a political statement.

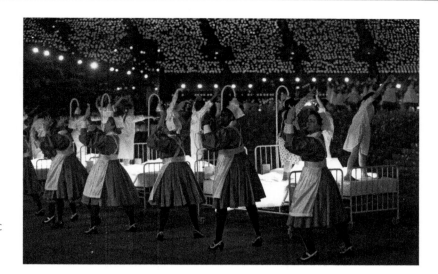

Figure 13.1 A homage to the NHS from the 2012 Olympic Games opening ceremony

2 Brief history: principles

To understand what the NHS means to UK citizens, we have to look to its origins. The National Health Service was born out of the immediate aftermath of the Second World War. It was part of a radical attempt to rebuild and improve British society after the war through creating the **'welfare state'**. The NHS was launched in July 1948 and for the first time made the full range of health-care services available to all, based on clinical need rather than ability to pay. The fact that it was paid for through general taxation meant that all contributed and helped to create a feeling of collective ownership of the system. In 2018, the NHS will have been in existence for seventy years. The majority of the UK population will only remember a time when the NHS existed.

welfare state:
state provision of services and benefits to improve citizens' well-being

> **Box 13.1 NHS history – further reading**
>
> For more on the origins of the NHS, try the following:
>
> NHS England website 'NHS History' section. At: <http://www.nhs.uk/NHSEngland/thenhs/nhshistory/Pages/the-nhs%20history.aspx>.
>
> Rudolf Klein's *New Politics of the NHS Oxford*: Radcliffe Publishing (various editions).
>
> For an account of life before the NHS, see Harry Leslie Smith, *Harry's Last Stand* (London: Icon Books, 2014). An extract was published in the *Guardian* newspaper, 4 June 2014. At: <http://www.theguardian.com/society/2014/jun/04/coalition-attacks-nhs-return-britain-age-workhouse>.

13

3 What is health policy?

Health policy is any decision that is made by the government or its representatives about how health services should be funded, provided and delivered. When we think about 'policy' we go further than just looking at laws that have been passed (legislation), although these are important. We also look at pronouncements, papers and plans produced by or on behalf of those in charge. 'Policy' may not always result in action. One example might be a political party that is not currently in power announcing its key policies relating to the NHS – they are suggesting what they would do (as part of their **manifesto**), should they be elected to government.

manifesto:
a public declaration of policies

Within the health system, policy decisions are made about a wide range of issues, including:

- How to structure the system.
- What organizations provide services within it.
- How much money the system receives.
- How the money flows through the system.
- What the money is spent on, and how other resources (staff, medications, equipment, buildings and so on) are distributed.

Many of the financial and organizational challenges facing the UK health system are not unique; they affect health systems all over the world, due to social change. These act as pressures on policy, sometimes called 'drivers'. Examples include growing and ageing populations, the rise of long-term conditions, and the possibilities offered by technological innovations such as cutting-edge drugs, prosthetics and equipment, which are often very expensive (see Mahon et al. 2009: xv). Decisions about how to meet these challenges are political ones.

4 The policy process

There are different ways of thinking about policy. One way is to view the policy process as a series of stages, as outlined in Figure 13.2 (see Hill 2012). These stages of the policy process will be traced in the response to obesity in the following case study.

Agenda setting → **Formulation** → **Implementation** 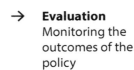 **Evaluation**
An issue comes to be seen as a policy problem   Deciding how to tackle the issue; writing policy   Putting the policy into action   Monitoring the outcomes of the policy

Figure 13.2 Stages of the policy process

Case Study: Obesity and health policy in England

In 2011, the policy document *Healthy Lives, Healthy People: A Call to Action on Obesity in England* was published (Department of Health 2011). This section uses the document to encourage you to think about the stages of the policy process.

Agenda setting: There had been growing professional, public, government and media concern about the growth in obesity rates. This is sometimes referred to as the 'obesity epidemic'. The *Foresight Report* (Government Office for Science 2007) was influential in identifying the potential social, economic and health impact for the UK of rising obesity levels. The government of the time produced a response that emphasized preventive strategies (Department of Health 2008). In 2010, the new coalition government signalled a change in approach to health policy, including, in England, moving many public-health responsibilities from the NHS to local authorities.

Formulation: The new government produced *Healthy Lives, Healthy People* (Department of Health 2011). This placed more emphasis on individual behaviour change – for example, treatment of obese adults – than the previous government's strategy. It encouraged local action rather than national directives. This mirrored the coalition government's wider ideological and political stance in health, welfare and economic policy: an emphasis on individual responsibility and a shift to more local decision-making structures in England's NHS and local government.

Implementation: Much of the implementation was expected to be tailored locally, for example by Clinical Commissioning Groups and local authorities, supported by national guidance from NICE on obesity interventions (see <http://pathways.nice.org.uk/pathways/obesity>). Change4Life, a national programme targeting children and families to promote healthier eating and more active lifestyles, was continued. There was an expectation of 'partnership' with businesses to bring about change (the Public Health 'Responsibility Deal'). For example, the food and drink industry was asked to make pledges on portion size, sugar and fat content and on calorie-labelling for take-away and restaurant foods (see <https://responsibilitydeal.dh.gov.uk/pledges/>).

Evaluation: Two long-term targets, or 'ambitions', were set:

- A sustained downward trend in the level of excess weight in children by 2020.
- A downward trend in the level of excess weight averaged across all adults by 2020.

Obesity rates are monitored locally and nationally, and there have been a number of evaluations of the impact of specific interventions. Many programmes have shown good outcomes in raising public awareness, but less clear results in relation to weight reduction (Jebb et al. 2013). Overall data indicate that the rate of increase in numbers of overweight or obese people has slowed down recently, although there is not yet a downward

13

trend (*Health Survey for England* 2013). Obesity is a very complex issue, and it is difficult to attribute overall trends to specific policy interventions.

For an in-depth discussion of obesity-related policy in England, see Jebb et al. 2013.

Activity 13.2 Discussion of strategies to prevent obesity

* What do you think about the idea of inviting the food and drink industry to get involved with implementing obesity policy? What pros and cons are there in asking for voluntary pledges (e.g., on fat, salt and sugar content)?
* This policy encourages strategies and interventions to be developed at a local level rather than imposed nationally. What benefits and disadvantages are there to this approach?
* Between 2010 and 2012, each of the devolved UK nations produced an obesity strategy or policy document. Identify a strategy/policy document on obesity for Wales, Scotland or Northern Ireland (search the Welsh government, Scottish government or DHSSPSNI websites). What similarities and differences are there between that, and England's strategy, *Healthy Lives, Healthy People*?

Influences on health policy

When we think about the policy process we should not think of it as being just about politicians (what the government says) or about the leaders of the health service. Many other factors influence policy, including professional groups, businesses, charities and the media. This section examines some of these influences.

The health-care unions and professional bodies, for example, the Royal College of Nursing (RCN), UNISON, the British Medical Association (BMA) and the Nursing and Midwifery Council (NMC), seek to influence policy on behalf of their members and patients, although they are not always successful. One illustration is the NHS reforms introduced in England after the coalition government came to power, enshrined in the Health and Social Care Act (2012). Many professional groups (including the RCN and BMA) opposed the proposed changes, partly because they were seen as enabling more **privatization** of NHS services. They involved major restructuring, for example, abolishing Primary Care Trusts and creating new bodies led by GPs, which the professional groups regarded as disruptive and expensive. After a 'listening exercise' to take account of the concerns of NHS employees, experts and members of the public, some adjustments were made to the legislation, but the key elements remained. Some questioned the extent to which the government was being led by political ideology rather than expert views about what works for a health system (Smith 2011; Pollock et al. 2012).

Businesses actively seek to influence policy through **lobbying**. Major international corporations such as pharmaceutical companies, food and drink manufacturers and private health-care providers have

privatization: public-sector services being transferred to the private sector

lobbying: influencing policymakers to benefit a particular cause, organization or business

considerable influence. Governments have to balance requirements for economic openness and free trade with their position on public policy. One example that affected public health-related policy was when the European Parliament voted on enforcing a food-labelling system across Europe in 2010. Professional and health-interest groups, including the BMA and British Heart Foundation, backed the introduction of a 'traffic lights' scheme that would label foodstuffs high in fat, sugar and salt as 'red'. However, food and drink corporations (sometimes known as 'Big Food') campaigned against this, in favour of showing Guideline Daily Amount (GDA) percentages. They produced briefings and contacted Members of the European Parliament (MEPs) directly, to persuade them that the traffic-light scheme would be unacceptable and even harmful to consumers. Their lobbying was effective and the Parliament voted against the introduction of the traffic-lights format of labelling (Hickman 2010).

Other groups actively seek to 'push' issues on to the policy agenda. Charities and organizations that represent the interests of particular patient groups or specific health conditions can be influential; for example, Cancer Research, Mencap and Mind (see an example in Box 13.2). The media can also play a role in creating momentum for policy change, by identifying something as a 'problem', generating public concern and therefore establishing it as something that politicians want to show they are acting on. (For a good discussion of influences on health policy, see Alaszewski and Brown 2012).

Box 13.2 Pressure groups and health policy process: mental health

The mental health charity, Mind, is an example of a pressure group that campaigns to raise public awareness and to change health policy. Mind produced a manifesto ahead of the 2015 General Election, and a policy briefing for a debate on mental health provision in the House of Lords in January 2015 (Mind 2014, 2015; see Hansard 2015 for a full transcript of the debate). The organization was also one of six mental health charities and professional groups (including the Royal College of Psychiatrists and the NHS Confederation's Mental Health Network) that collaborated to produce *A Manifesto for Better Mental Health* (The Mental Health Policy Group 2014). This document called upon all of the political parties to make mental health policy commitments, including increased funding, improved child and adolescent services and better access to talking therapies. Liberal Democrat leader and Deputy Prime Minister, Nick Clegg, and the leader of the Labour Party, Ed Miliband, both made statements about improving mental health policy and services in January 2015 (Meikle and Wintour 2015).

13

Those who are really implementing policy changes in public services are those on the frontline, such as nurses. In this way, people at all levels of the health service shape policy, knowingly or not. How a policy is interpreted and put into practice is often different from the way that it was envisioned by those who designed it (Harrison and McDonald 2008: 132–4). The difference between the policy intention or vision, and what happens on the ground, is sometimes known as the 'implementation gap'. Governments may introduce targets and timelines in order to enforce the implementation of a policy change, to hold local organizations to account and to monitor its impact (Buse et al. 2012: 130). In UK health policy we can see this in the waiting-time targets that were introduced from the early 2000s, in a bid to reduce waiting lists for specialist referrals and treatments (discussed later in the chapter).

Health policy in the UK: devolution

An interesting development at the beginning of this century is that health policy diverged in the individual nations that make up the United Kingdom, as a result of devolution. While the overall budget allocation comes from central government, the Scottish Parliament, Welsh and Northern Ireland Assemblies decide how to organize health services within their nations, and how to use the allocated resources. There are clear differences in how provision is organized and managed. Regional and local structures have distinct names and roles – for example, there are Clinical Commissioning Groups (CCGs) in England, Health Boards in Scotland and Wales and integrated Health and Social Care Trusts in Northern Ireland. The health system in each nation is funded centrally through taxation: decisions about spending on the NHS are made by the devolved governments, and, in England, by the Treasury.

Key differences in health policy in the four nations of the UK are summarized in Table 13.1. These differences point to key issues for health policy that are discussed in more depth in the following sections: the role of the market in health care (competition and choice), cost and quality.

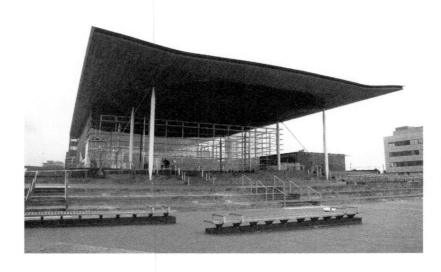

Figure 13.3 The Welsh Assembly Building (Senedd); health care in Wales is devolved to the Assembly

Table 13.1 Key differences in health policy in the four nations of the UK				
	England	**Scotland**	**Wales**	**Northern Ireland**
Prescription charges	✓	x	x	x
Free social care for over-65s	x	✓	x	x
Provider competition & patient choice	✓	x	x	x
Quality-performance targets	✓	✓	Some	Some

(Adapted from Bevan et al. 2014)

5 The role of the market in health care

One important area for discussion about health policy in the UK has been what role the market should play within the health system. In other words, should there be one main provider of health-care services, or many independent organizations? For patients, the difference might depend on whether they have a choice about where they go for treatment (there is a market), or whether they are always referred to the nearest NHS hospital that provides the service they need. For health-service providers, the key difference is in how they are structured and managed. In what is sometimes called a 'monopoly' or planned model, all the main providers basically belong to one overall organization that oversees their management and budgeting processes and decides which services will be provided where. With a market type of model, the providers (e.g., hospitals) will – in theory – be independent organizations, like businesses, which have their own management structures and ways of budgeting, are in competition with others and have to 'balance their books'. This does not necessarily mean that they are profit-making organizations.

The following sections give an overview of how market-organization principles have been introduced to the NHS in the UK, and how this has changed since devolution. They highlight the benefits and disadvantages of market ideas in health care.

Internal markets and beyond in the NHS

During the 1990s, the so-called 'purchaser–provider split' was introduced to the UK health system (with the exception of Northern Ireland). Regional bodies planned and purchased health services on behalf of their populations – a role that is now called 'commissioning'. The services were delivered by provider organizations, for example by hospitals. This organizational model is sometimes referred to as the 'internal market'. It operates rather like a marketplace, with the provider organizations competing (in theory at least) with one another to provide the best services and value for money (Harrison and McDonald 2008; Klein 2010).

There are a number of reasons why governments view an internal market as preferable to a planned system. These relate to wider

13

Table 13.2 Arguments for and against 'market' approaches in health care

	For markets	Against markets
Quality	Providers are motivated to provide satisfaction to service users (patients/ customers) and respond positively to feedback about quality to improve. Providing a better-quality service is good for business as it can increase the market share ('customer' base). Poor-quality providers may not survive.	Those buying the service on the public's behalf (commissioners) may encourage service users/ patients to access the cheapest rather than the highest-quality providers.
Value	Providers are motivated to keep costs down and work as efficiently as possible. They can focus on what is really required/demanded by service users and will not provide services that few want to use.	There are hidden costs to operating in a market. For example, the provider may need to promote itself to maintain consumer awareness and demand; or focus on bidding for contracts. There are wider costs to the system as a whole, of administering contracts and monitoring activity of a wide range of providers.
Choice	Service users can choose the location, type of service, duration or timing of the service/treatment. Having choice can increase satisfaction. Likewise, commissioners can choose to offer contracts to the best available provider (based on relevance and quality of service offered, cost, etc.)	Health-service users are less likely to be able to exercise fully informed choice, because information about medical procedures and service quality is complex. By the nature of their health problems, they may not have the capacity – or the time – to make choices. If unpopular or poor-quality services are forced out of business entirely, this may actually reduce choice.

(*Crinson 2005; Fotaki 2014; Sturgeon 2014*)

ideas about market economics, and in particular those of quality, value and choice. Table 13.2 summarizes these ideas alongside some counter-arguments.

After devolution, from 1999 onwards, Scotland and Wales abandoned the 'internal market' model in favour of regional health authorities, or boards, that plan, oversee and deliver care. Northern Ireland had always had this sort of structure. The reason for change in Wales was explained as follows:

> With simpler management structures, more money can be channelled to frontline services. The LHBs (Local Health Boards) will improve patient care by removing artificial boundaries that existed between the commissioners and the providers of services. (NHS Wales 2009)

This document also states that collaboration between NHS providers is more important than competition. In other words, the Welsh government decided that quality and value were best guaranteed by a planned system, led by government rather than the market.

The major NHS restructuring for England introduced by the 2012 Health and Social Care Act retained the purchaser–provider split and took the market principles further, with new bodies – Clinical Commissioning Groups (CCGs) – in the main 'purchaser' role. In reality, elements of a planned system remain in England's NHS. The overall organizational structure, and many processes and outcomes, remain under central control. Performance is closely monitored by the Department of Health, NHS England, Care Quality Commission, and Monitor, which oversees Foundation Trusts. This creates a potentially confusing tension between local and central priorities. Can trusts really be 'autonomous' organizations able to determine their own direction, when they are under huge pressure to adhere to central policy directives and targets (discussed in Section 7 on Quality, below)?

Activity 13.3 NHS providers and purchasers

Use an Internet search engine to find the website of a health service organization (e.g., a Health Board or Clinical Commissioning Group) that is local to you.

(a) How easy is it to find information about what the organization does, and how it works?

(b) Is the organization mainly a 'purchaser' (commissioner), planner or provider of health services? Does it combine some of these functions?

Choice

One of the differences identified in Table 13.1 was about patient choice. This is closely related to policy decisions about the market. Recent governments have expressed a commitment to choice in health care, particularly in England, where it has been built into some of the systems. For example, since the mid-2000s, patients who are referred by their GP for tests or specialist consultations can select when and where they want to have their first appointment. In theory, they have a free choice of any provider in the country, including private providers, as long as they have agreed to work with the NHS and provide services for the same price (the 'tariff').

Activity 13.4 Choice of provider

In England's NHS, patient choice of provider has been an important part of health policy since the mid-2000s. In the other nations of the UK, patient choice has not been a big part of the agenda.

Here are some questions to consider:

(a) How important do you think it is to patients to be able to choose a provider for their treatment (e.g., a hospital for their out-patient referral)?

(b) If you were a patient, what factors would you weigh up to decide whether to have your treatment at an NHS hospital or a private facility; at your local hospital or one further away?

(c) As a nurse, what factors would you recommend your patients consider when faced with a choice of provider?

13

(d) What sources of information should patients use to make such decisions?

(e) Can you think of groups of patients who would be more or less likely to exercise choice in this way? Are there groups of patients who might find it difficult?

Further reading: View the results of research on how patients make choices in Dixon et al. (2010).

The principle of patient choice of provider raises questions about equality of experience for patients. Proponents of choice argue that it creates more equality, opening up options to everybody, which were formerly only accessible to wealthier or better-connected patients. Others argue that differences in level of education, knowledge of the NHS, the nature of their condition, and their wider life circumstances, make it more or less easy for patients to exercise choice (Fotaki 2014). A wealth of evidence demonstrates the impact of social and economic conditions on health status – leading to health inequalities. Certain social groups are more likely to have greater health needs and worse experiences of the health system than others (e.g., older people, especially those from lower socioeconomic groups; people whose first language is not English; people with learning disabilities) (Mencap 2007; Marmot 2010; Lyratzopoulos et al. 2012).

There are also geographical issues and inequalities: for example, patients living in rural or sparsely populated areas will not have a realistic range of provider 'choices', unless they are willing to travel long distances for treatment. Many patients want to defer to the health-care provider's view about what is best. Finally, there will be some types of condition or treatments that are only catered for in a small number of specialist facilities. These capacity constraints mean that, even in areas with a wide range of health-care providers, some patients may have no real 'choice'.

In a health system that is organized like a market patients can become a type of customer. Having choice is meant to promote empowerment, enhance patients' commitment to the treatment process and produce greater patient satisfaction with the experience. This reflects a move to a more **consumer-oriented** approach to public services like health care. While opening up choices to health-service users can be empowering, it also marks a shift of responsibility from professional to patient: 'What happens to those individuals who do not make appropriate choices about their health needs; does this represent a system failure or an individual one?' (Crinson 2005: 510).

consumer oriented/ consumerism: people (e.g., patients) being regarded like customers

6 Cost and funding

One of the differences within the UK that was indicated in Table 13.1 is whether there are prescription charges. This is one example of a decision being made about how the system is funded and whether there are direct costs to the patient.

Wales, Scotland and Northern Ireland all removed prescription charges entirely (in 2007, 2011 and 2010 respectively). England's prescription charge is a 'flat rate', which means patients pay the same price, whatever the actual cost of the medication. At the time of writing, this is £8.05. There is a complicated system of exemptions from prescription charges, and about 90 per cent of prescriptions in England are actually dispensed free of charge (HSCIC 2013). However, the prescription charge is seen as a way of keeping costs down. For example, it encourages direct purchasing of lower-cost items that can be bought without a prescription (such as some painkillers), at no cost to the NHS.

Those who argue against prescription charges point out that they affect people on low incomes disproportionately. For example, patients may choose not to get all of their prescribed drugs because of cost concerns. Ultimately, this can contribute to worsening health and potentially to additional costs to the system. Northern Ireland's Health Minister, Michael McGimpsey, summed up some of these points in his announcement that prescription charges were to be abolished:

> It is simply unacceptable that people who have to cope with the burden of ill health should have the additional anxiety of trying to find the money to pay for much-needed medication which they cannot afford. This is totally against the principles of the NHS which promises free health services to all. (Northern Ireland Executive 2008)

Activity 13.5 Paying for services

Prescription charges are an example of what is known as a 'co-payment' in some health-care systems. Other co-payment ideas that are sometimes debated in the UK include charging people to visit their GP, for inappropriate A & E visits or missed appointments.

Think about the questions and discuss with a fellow student or colleague:

(a) Do you think that charges to patients (for example, the prescription charge) are a good way to balance the costs of the health system?

(b) Should other charges be introduced (e.g., a small charge for GP visits; payment for 'hotel' costs in hospital, e.g., food and laundry services)?

(c) What disadvantages are there? (think about equality of access; administrative costs)

13

7 Quality

What is most important to society and politicians: the cost of the health system; the quality of care provided; or the ability of all to access care? These three aspects have been called the 'eternal triangle' in relation to discussions about health-care policy (Friedman 1991). Is it possible to find the optimum balance between all three: the highest quality of care, to all who need it, for a reasonable expenditure? It does not seem controversial to say that 'quality' in health care is important to all. Who would not want to give, or receive, good-quality care? But this is another area where policy can be influential, and where the nations of the UK have diverged since devolution – this section uses the specific examples of using targets and measuring patient satisfaction to monitor and improve quality.

Targets

The NHS in England has many performance targets and performance management strategies for the providers of care (NHS Trusts, private providers and so on). The other UK nations have fewer, with Scotland the closest to England in having a system of performance measurement and indicators.

Examples of targets in England are:

- Waiting times: eighteen-week maximum time between GP referral and starting specialist treatment;
- Accident and Emergency (A & E) departments: four-hour maximum time from arrival to admission, discharge or transfer.
- Readmissions: if patients are readmitted as an emergency with a related problem, within thirty days of being discharged, the hospital will not be paid for the patients' care
- Hospital-acquired infections: Clostridium difficile (C-diff) infection rates have to be within a specific range.

NHS trusts that fail to meet these targets can have financial penalties imposed through fines or withholding payments. These penalties can run to many thousands, even millions, of pounds (Pulse 2012).

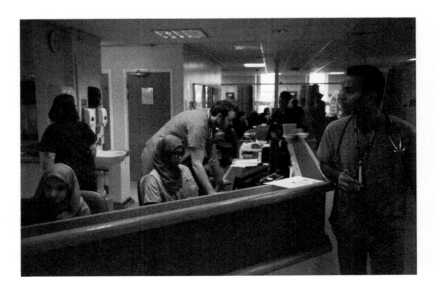

Figure 13.4 Waiting times in A & E departments have been the focus of targets

Introduction of targets changed the way that hospital departments worked – how they prioritized patients and managed their 'flow' through the system. However, there is evidence that they distorted hospitals' priorities and did not always improve patients' experiences of care; for example, generating a flurry of activity to treat, admit or discharge A & E patients in the final twenty minutes of the four-hour period (Weber et al. 2012). Efforts to meet targets also resulted in 'gaming', that is, management strategies to document that the targets had been met but in the letter rather than in the spirit (Bevan and Hood 2006). One example might be ambulances having to wait outside busy A & E departments. The clock does not start on the official four-hour wait until the patient is inside the department. Therefore the hospital may ensure it makes the target even though the patient has experienced a longer total wait. In the meantime, there is a negative impact on the wider system while the ambulance is out of action.

The Francis Report into poor care and higher than expected death rates at Mid Staffordshire NHS Foundation Trust has been used as an example of how performance targets do not necessarily improve actual care standards. The hospital met all its targets and had been praised by the inspectorate, the Care Quality Commission. However, the inquiry found that, to quote one headline, 'a hospital is able to tick all the boxes, yet still utterly fail patients' (Edemariam 2009).

It is difficult to make direct comparisons about which of the four nations is doing 'better' in relation, for example, to waiting times, because of differences in how they are calculated. It seems that people in Wales have longer waits for operations such as hip replacement than in the other nations, although it is unclear what has caused this (Bevan et al. 2014). It is even harder to use the comparisons to assess whether more targets really improve care. Overall it seems that targets may be important to maintain and improve performance in areas such as waiting times and infection rates, but that an over-reliance on them as a way of managing provision can have a negative impact; for example, on organizational cultures, management willingness to innovate, and sometimes on patient experience (Ham 2014). This reminds us that quality is made up of many elements, and time-related targets can address only one of these (see the 'eternal triangle' discussed earlier).

Patient satisfaction

Patient feedback is another mechanism for judging the quality of services, which has become increasingly important. One example is NHS England's 'Friends and Family Test', which was introduced as a key evaluator for health services (NHS England 2013). It involves users answering a single question: 'How likely are you to recommend our service to friends and family if they needed similar care or treatment?' At the time of writing, the question is asked following acute inpatient stays, visits to A & E and use of maternity services. Staff members are

13

also asked whether they would recommend their service to friends or family who required treatment; and if they would recommend it as a workplace. Results are updated regularly and can be viewed and compared on NHS England/NHS Choices websites. Although this is a simple test that can highlight quality and safety issues, its usefulness to compare care quality between different hospitals may be questionable because of differences in test administration and patient populations (Dixon-Woods et al. 2014; Sizmur et al. 2014).

Activity 13.6 Targets and patient views on quality

Consider the following questions. Discuss in a group:

(a) Do you know of any targets that apply in your field of nursing? Are they less appropriate for use in children's, mental health and learning-disability services than in adult acute services? Give reasons for your answer.

(b) Some writers such as Greener (2009) argue that the use of targets can be demoralizing for health professionals, as it calls into question their integrity. Do you agree? Why may targets have this effect?

(c) What do you think about the 'Friends and Family Test'? Does it capture the essential information that people need in order to judge how good health services are? Are there fields or areas of nursing where it would be less effective?

---

8 Health policy and nursing

Why is it relevant for you, as a nurse, to take an interest in policy? Whether you are aware of it or not, policy shapes a lot of your experience both as a student and as a qualified nurse. The curriculum you study has been planned and adjusted to reflect changing policy concerns. An example is the impact of the Francis Inquiry (Mid Staffordshire NHS Foundation Trust Public Inquiry 2013). Its investigation of care failures in a Midlands hospital fed directly into the way that care, caring and nurses' responsibilities are taught in universities, requiring a greater emphasis on compassionate care and the 'six Cs'(see p. 35), for example (Willis Commission 2012; NHS Careers 2014).

Policy also shapes the organizations you will work in as a nurse, where you will work and what tasks are expected of you. For example, since England's implementation of the Health and Social Care Act (2012), many nurses in public-health related roles, including many health visitors and school nurses, are now employed by Local Authorities (councils) rather than the NHS (Seccombe 2014). The Disability Discrimination Act (2005), Equality Act (2010) and Mental Capacity Act (2005) introduced new duties and expectations for learning-disability nurses (Moulster et al. 2012). Finally, the roles and career pathways open to you as a nurse change over time as a result of policy developments. In recent years, opportunities that have expanded for nurses in the UK, supported by policy, include acting as a case manager in the community (Drennan et al. 2011) or nurse practitioner in primary care (Hoare et al. 2011), and in commissioning and evaluating health-care services (Jerram and Fox 2014).

Nurses influencing policy

As qualified practitioners working on the 'front line' of health care, nurses are experts in the reality of health practice, with a particular insight into the impact of services (and policy changes) on patients, service users and carers. Nurse voices are essential in influencing future policy decisions and should be helpful to governments in determining cost-effective and rational approaches to policy issues (International Council of Nurses 2005). Even though nurses are the largest professional group in the NHS, they have been under-represented at decision-making levels and should be recognized as 'experts' in the policy process (Greener 2009: 243).

Conclusion

This chapter has demonstrated how health services, and the work of nurses, are shaped by health policy that is made by governments. Policy can change frequently, and is influenced by many factors. These include political ideology (of the government in power), public concern, campaigns by professional groups or charities, business interests and international pressures. A sociological perspective on policy can help us to better appreciate these influences and to understand where policy changes come from and what their impact might be.

Summary and Resources

Summary

▷ The way that the health service is organized and delivered results from political decision-making.
▷ Nurses' work is affected both directly and indirectly by policy decisions.
▷ Nurses can make a contribution to debates about policy.
▷ The four nations of the UK have been developing health policy in different directions.
▷ Questions to do with equality of access, the quality of patient experience, and cost, are central within health policy discussions.

13

Questions for Discussion

1 What do you think the role of the private sector should be in formulating policy and delivering health services?
2 How important is having a choice of service provider, for patients or service users in your field of nursing?
3 What do you think about the individual nations of the UK being able to make their own decisions on health policy and structuring the health service? Are the differences beneficial?
4 What is the best way to measure the quality of health services – is it possible to strike a balance between clinical outcomes, targets such as waiting times and patient experiences?

Glossary

consumer oriented/
consumerism:
a 'consumer' society is one where people are encouraged to find value in getting more and more things; consumption of products and services takes on central importance in people's lives, and in how they view each other; people start to be viewed as active consumers (customers), rather than just recipients, of products and services, including health care

lobbying:
trying to influence policymakers to make decisions that are beneficial to a particular cause, organization or business

manifesto:
a public declaration of policies, positions and intentions; in the UK, the major political parties usually publish a manifesto in the months preceding a General Election, which provides the voting public with an indication of the actions that party would take, should they be voted into government

privatization:
transferring services from the public sector (i.e., being run and owned by government) to the private sector; privatized services may be run and owned by profit-making companies

welfare state:
state provision of services and benefits to improve citizens' well-being; in Britain this usually refers to services and structures brought in after the Second World War to address health, education, social security, housing and care needs

Further Reading

K. Buse, N. Mays and G. Walt: *Making Health Policy*, 2nd edn. Maidenhead: Open University Press, 2012.
Provides good detail on ways of understanding health-policy processes. International rather than UK focus.

A. Fatchett: *Social Policy for Nurses*. Cambridge: Polity, 2012.
More detail on specific aspects of policy that affect the contexts within which nurses work – not just 'health-care' policy.

C. Ham: *Health Policy in Britain*, 6th edn. Basingstoke: Palgrave, 2009.
Excellent overview that provides rich background information about debates and changes to health policy in Britain, by a leading expert.

G. Taylor: *Using Health Policy in Nursing Practice*. London: Learning Matters, 2013.
Focuses on the policy context for specific issues in nursing practice, with an emphasis on how policy and practice influence one another.

Also useful are the following online resources:

BBC News <http://www.bbc.co.uk/news/health/News>
A site with good coverage of health and NHS issues. You can also find items specific to Wales, Scotland, Northern Ireland and England or to your local area.

The *Guardian* <http://www.theguardian.com/society/health>
National newspaper with good coverage of health and social policy issues.

King's Fund <www.kingsfund.org.uk>
A health policy research think tank. Produces regular research reports, blogs, information and opinion pieces on health and social care policy issues.

Nuffield Trust <www.nuffieldtrust.org.uk/our-work>
A health and care policy research think tank. Produces regular reports on a range of key health policy topics.

References

Alaszewski, A. and Brown, P. 2012 *Making Health Policy: A Critical Introduction*. Cambridge: Polity.

Bevan, G. and Hood, C. 2006 What's measured is what matters: targets and gaming in the English public health care system. *Public Administration* 84/3: 517–38.

Bevan, G., Karinakolos, M., Exley, J., Nolte, E., Connolly, S. and Mays, N. 2014 The four health systems of the United Kingdom: how do they compare? London: Nuffield Trust and Health Foundation. At: <http://www.nuffieldtrust.org.uk/compare-UK-health>.

Buse, K., Mays, N. and Walt, G. 2012 *Making Health Policy*, 2nd edn. Maidenhead: Open University Press/McGraw-Hill Education.

Crinson, I. 2005 The direction of health policy in New Labour's third term. *Critical Social Policy* 25/4: 507–16.

Department of Health 2008 *Healthy Weight, Healthy Lives*. London: Department of Health.

13

Department of Health 2011 *Healthy Lives, Healthy People: A Call to Action.* London: Department of Health.

Dixon, A., Appleby, J., Robertson, R., Burge, P., Devlin, N. and Magee, H. 2010 *Patient Choice: How Patients Choose and How Providers Respond.* London: King's Fund. At: <http://www.kingsfund.org.uk/publications/patient_choice.html>.

Dixon-Woods, M., Minion, J. T., Mckee, L., Willars, J. and Martin, G. 2014 The friends and family test: a qualitative study of concerns that influence the willingness of English National Health Service staff to recommend their organization. *Journal of the Royal Society of Medicine* 107/8: 318–25.

Drennan, V., Goodman, C., Manthorpe, J., Davies, S., Scott, C., Gage, H. and Iliffe, S. 2011 Establishing new nursing roles: a case study of the English community matron initiative. *Journal of Clinical Nursing* 20: 2948–57.

Edemariam, A. 2009 A hospital is able to tick all the boxes yet still utterly fail patients. *Guardian*, 19 March 2009. Available at: <http://www.theguardian.com>.

Fotaki, M. 2014 *What Market-based Choice Can't Do for the NHS: The Theory and Evidence of How Choice Works in Health Care.* London: Centre for Health and the Public Interest. At: <http://chpi.org.uk/wp-content/uploads/2014/03/What-market-based-patient-choice-cant-do-for-the-NHS-CHPI.pdf>.

Friedman, E. 1991 The eternal triangle: cost, access, and quality. *Physician Executive* 17/4: 3–9.

Government Office for Science 2007 *Tackling Obesities: Future Choices-Project Report* ['Foresight Report']. London: Office for Science.

Greener, I. 2009 *Healthcare in the UK: Understanding Continuity and Change.* Bristol: Policy Press.

Ham, C. 2014 *Reforming the NHS from Within: Beyond Hierarchy, Inspection and Markets.* London: King's Fund.

Hansard 2015 House of Lords Debate (Mental Health), 15 January 2015, Columns 948–80. At: <http://www.publications.parliament.uk/pa/ld201415/ldhansrd/text/150115-0002.htm>.

Harrison, S. and McDonald, R. 2008 *The Politics of Healthcare in Britain.* London: Sage.

Health and Social Care Information Centre 2013a *Health Survey for England 2013.* Available at: <http://www.hscic.gov.uk/catalogue/PUB16076>.

Health and Social Care Information Centre 2013b *Prescriptions Dispensed in the Community, Statistics for England – 2002–12.* Leeds: HSCIC. At: <http://www.hscic.gov.uk/catalogue/PUB11291>.

Hickman, M. 2010 Laid bare, the lobbying campaign that won the food labelling battle. *Independent*, 18 June 2010. At: <http://www.independent.co.uk/life-style/food-and-drink/news/laid-bare-the-lobbying-campaign-that-won-the-food-labelling-battle-2003686.html>.

Hill, M. 2012 *The Public Policy Process*, 6th edn. London: Routledge.

Hoare, K. J., Mills, J. and Francis, K. 2011 The role of government policy in supporting nurse-led care in general practice in the United Kingdom, New Zealand and Australia: an adapted realist review. *Journal of Advanced Nursing* 68/5: 963–80.

International Council of Nurses 2005 *Guidelines on Shaping Effective Health Policy.* Geneva: ICN.

Jebb, S. A., Aveyard, P. N. and Hawkes, C. 2013 The evolution of policy and actions to tackle obesity in England. *Obesity Reviews* 14/S2: 42–59.

Jerram, S. and Fox, A. 2014 New responsibilities in purchasing and developing services. *Nursing Older People* 26/5: 24–5.

Klein, R. 2010 *The New Politics of the NHS*, 6th edn. Oxford: Radcliffe Publishing.

Lyratzopoulos, G., Elliott, M., Barbiere, J. M., Henderson, A., Staetsky, L., Paddison, C., Campbell, J. and Roland, M. 2011 Understanding ethnic and other socio-demographic differences in patient experience of primary care: evidence from the English General Practice Patient Survey. *BMJ Quality & Safety* 21/1: 21–9.

Lyratzopoulos, G., Neal, R. D., Barbiere, J. M., Rubin, G. P. and Abel, G. A. 2012 Variation in number of general practitioner consultations before hospital referral for cancer: findings from the 2010 National Cancer Patient Experience Survey in England. *The Lancet oncology* 13/4: 353–65.

Mahon, A., Walshe, K. and Chambers, N. 2009 Introduction. In A. Mahon, K. Walshe and N. Chambers (eds), *A Reader in Health Policy and Management*. Maidenhead: Open University Press.

Marmot, M. 2010 *Strategic Review of Health Inequalities in England post-2010*. London: Marmot Review.

Mason, S., Weber, E. J., Coster, J., Freeman, J. and Locker, T. 2012 Time patients spend in the emergency department: England's 4-hour rule – a case of hitting the target but missing the point? *Annals of Emergency Medicine* 59/5: 341–9.

Meikle, J. and Wintour, P. 2015 Lib Dems announce campaign for NHS to set 'zero suicide' goal. *Guardian*, 19 January 2015. At: <http://www.theguardian.com/society/2015/jan/18/lib-dems-zero-suicides-nhs-blue-monday-labour-children-mental-health>.

Mencap 2007 *Death by Indifference*. London: Mencap.

Mental Health Policy Group, The 2014 *A Manifesto for Better Mental Health*. Published online 22 August 2014. At: <http://www.mind.org.uk/media/1113989/a-manifesto-for-better-mental-health.pdf>.

The Mid Staffordshire NHS Foundation Trust Public Inquiry 2013 *Report of the Mid Staffordshire NHS Foundation Trust Public Inquiry: Executive Summary*. London: Stationery Office (Chair: R Francis). At: <www.midstaffspublicinquiry.com/report>.

Mind 2014 *Take Action for Better Mental Health: Our Manifesto for the General Election, 2015*. London: Mind. At: <http://www.mind.org.uk/media/1081517/Mind-Manifesto-Jun14.pdf>.

Mind 2015 *Parliamentary Briefing from Mind: House of Lords Debate – Mental Health Care Provision*, 15 January 2015. London: Mind. At: <http://www.mind.org.uk/media/1775204/lords-debate-on-mental-health.pdf>.

Moulster, G., Ames, S. and Griffiths, T. 2012 A new learning disability nursing framework. *Learning Disability Practice* 15/6: 14–18.

NHS Careers 2014 *Implications of the Francis Report* (online). At: <http://www.nhscareers.nhs.uk/promotions/implications-of-the-francis-report/>.

NHS England 2013 *Putting Patients First: The NHS England Business Plan for 2013/14–2015/16*. London: NHS England.

13

NHS England 2014 *Patient Friends and Family Test Infographics – November 2014*. London: NHS England. At: <http://www.england.nhs.uk/statistics/wp-content/uploads/sites/2/2013/07/Nov-14-Patient-FFT.pdf>.

NHS Wales 2009 *NHS in Wales: Why We are Changing the Structure*. Cardiff: Welsh Assembly Government. At: <http://www.wales.nhs.uk/documents/NHS%20Reform%20leaflet_October%202009.pdf>.

Northern Ireland Executive 2008 *Free Prescriptions Gets Green Light* (press release) 20 November 2008. At: <http://www.northernireland.gov.uk/news/news-dhssps/news-dhssps-201108-free_prescriptions_gets.htm>.

Pollock, A., Price, D., Roderick, P., Treuherz, T., Mccoy, D., Mckee, M. and Reynolds, L. 2012 How the Health and Social Care Bill 2011 would end entitlement to comprehensive health care in England. *Lancet* 379/9814: 387–9.

PULSE 2012 GPs fine hospitals over failure to meet A&E waiting time targets. *Pulse*, 13 February 2012. At: <http://www.pulsetoday.co.uk/gps-fine-hospitals-over-failure-to-meet-ae-waiting-time-targets/13423958.article>.

Seccombe, I. 2014 *New Responsibilities, New Opportunities for Local Government and Health Partners*. Viv Bennett (blog), Department of Health. At: <https://vivbennett.blog.gov.uk/2014/11/21/new-responsibilities-new-opportunities-for-local-government-and-health-partners-by-izzi-seccombe/>.

Sizmur, S., Graham, C. and Walsh, J. 2014 Influence of patients' age and sex and the mode of administration on results from the NHS Friends and Family Test of patient experience. *Journal of Health Services Research and Policy* 20/1: 5–10.

Smith, J. 2011 NHS Future Forum: is anyone listening? *British Journal of Nursing* 20/16: 963.

Sturgeon, D. 2014 The business of the NHS: The rise and rise of consumer culture and commodification in the provision of health services. *Critical Social Policy* 34/3: 405–16.

Weber, E. J., Mason, S., Freeman, J. V. and Coster, J. 2012. Implications of England's four-hour target for quality of care and resource use in the emergency department. *Annals of Emergency Medicine* 60/6: 699–706.

Willis Commission 2012 *Quality with Compassion: The Future of Nursing Education*. Report of the Willis Commission on Nursing Education. London: Royal College of Nursing.

Alistair Hewison

> **KEY ISSUES IN THIS CHAPTER:**
> ▶ What is management?
> ▶ The contribution of sociology to our understanding of the management and organization of health care.
> ▶ The importance of management in the role of the nurse.
> ▶ The involvement of nurses in the organization and management of health care.
>
> **BY THE END OF THIS CHAPTER YOU SHOULD BE ABLE TO:**
> ▶ Summarize the main phases in the development of the organization of the National Health Service.
> ▶ Describe the features of hospital organization that characterize it as a bureaucracy.
> ▶ Examine critically the negotiated order of health-care organization.
> ▶ Discuss the challenges of health-care organization.
> ▶ Evaluate critically the role of the nurse as a manager.

1 Introduction

The National Health Service (NHS) deals with over 1 million patients every thirty-six hours (NHS Choices 2015) and in 2011 there were 15 million in-patient admissions to NHS hospitals in England (Health and Social Care Information Centre undated). It is a vast organization employing more than 1.7 million people (NHS Choices 2015), making it the fourth-largest organization in the world after the Chinese Red Army, the Walmart conglomerate, and the Indian State Railways (NHS Choices 2015; Trefgarne 2005). In March 2014 there were 315,000 nurses, midwives and health visitors working in the NHS (King's Fund

2014). However, while the NHS embodies the social conscience of the country, positively transforms the lives of millions of people, and is a source of pride, there are times when it fails (Keogh 2013). This was demonstrated very starkly in the events that occurred at the Mid Staffordshire NHS Foundation Trust, reported in the Public Inquiry Chaired by Sir Robert Francis (Francis 2013). The three-volume, 1,782-page report presents a detailed analysis of the factors contributing to the poor standards of care at the hospital. For example, as a result of poor leadership and staffing policies, unsatisfactory nursing care was provided on some wards, there was a decline in professionalism and a tolerance of poor standards (Francis 2013). The findings of the inquiry (Francis 2013) and the subsequent Berwick Review (2013) highlighted the need for a fundamental change in culture and improved leadership if such failures in care were to be avoided in the future. This demonstrates the importance of considering the management of care. The NHS is a large and complex organization, and if patients are to receive good-quality care it needs to be well managed.

The purpose of this chapter is to discuss how this has been approached in the past, to examine the current focus on organizational culture and leadership as key elements in health-service organization, and to draw out the implications for nursing of these developments. In order to do this, the chapter is organized into three main sections. First, a history of the management and organization of the NHS is presented to provide some context; this is followed by a discussion of organizational culture and leadership, because attention to these areas has been advocated as a means of ensuring that services are managed in the best interests of patients. Finally, the role of the nurse as a manager and organizer of care is explored, and it is argued that further development of this element of the role in an appropriately supportive structure could help ensure care is managed with the patient at its heart.

2 Management

The term 'manage' derives from the Italian word *maneggiare*, which means to control or to train, and was originally applied to the management of horses (Grint 1995). One of the foremost writers on management summarizes a view that many share: 'Management is a curious phenomenon. It is generously paid, enormously influential, and significantly devoid of common sense' (Mintzberg 1996: 61). For the purposes of this chapter, management is regarded as an expression of human **agency**. Management has been characterized as consisting of five elements:

agency:
the capacity of individuals to shape their social world

1 deciding/planning what is to be done, and how;
2 allocating time and effort to what is to be done;
3 motivating or generating the effort to do it;

4   co-ordinating and combining disparate efforts;
5   controlling what is to be done to ensure that it conforms with
    what was intended. (Hales 1993: 2)

However, if these five elements of management are to be achieved, a
complex blend of knowledge and action is required. Mintzberg argues
that managing is learned primarily through experience, and rooted in
context. It involves a combination of craft and art alongside some use
of science, resulting in an activity that is above all a practice (Mintzberg
2011). This is relevant for people working in all organizations, including health care. As Iles (2005: 5) observes: 'As soon as we ask someone
else to do something, rather than undertaking it ourselves, we become
managers. We rely on someone else to perform that task in the way
we would do it.' Nurses soon find they have to ask others, including
health-care assistants, parents, carers, and members of the multidisciplinary team, to undertake a range of tasks, and so are involved in
management as part of their practice from an early stage in their career.

The contribution of sociology

Given that the NHS is a vast and complex organization, it can be difficult to appreciate how it all fits together. Figure 14.1 to illustrate this.
Yet this only conveys one 'picture' of the NHS as an organization.
Sociologists have been interested in organizations since the days of
Marx, Weber and Durkheim (Lammers 1978), and bring particular
perspectives and concepts that provide useful approaches for explanation and analysis. These are summarized in Table 14.1, and examples
of studies that have used some of these approaches are discussed
below.

Management and organization of the National Health Service

The famous US industrialist Henry Ford is credited with declaring that
'history is bunk' (Lockerby 2011), and in a fast-moving, constantly
changing health-care environment consideration of what has happened in the past may seem to be of little value. Indeed, statements
such as 'the NHS must change if it is to survive and remain sustainable',
and 'the old ways will not sustain it and we will only see a managed
decline' (Nicholson 2014), suggest that what has gone before is now
irrelevant and new solutions are needed. However, the past informs
and re-informs the present, in shaping the structure and management of organizations (Bedeian 1998; Pollitt 2008). Without some
knowledge of how the organization has developed, structures can be
difficult to understand and earlier management mistakes repeated
(Timmins 2008). This indicates why it is helpful to examine some key
phases in the development of health-care provision, before moving

14

The health & care system from April 2013

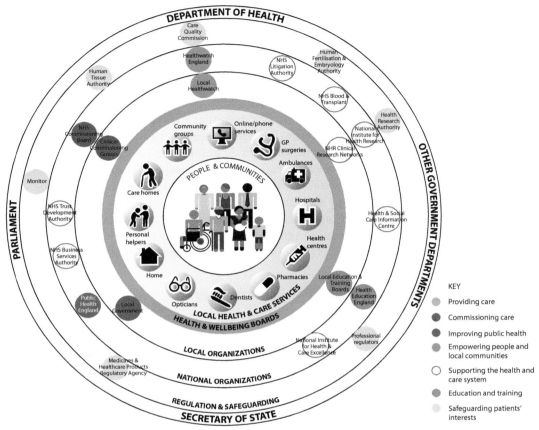

Figure 14.1 The health and care system (*Department of Health 2014*)

Table 14.1 Six theoretical strands in the sociology of organizations	
Theoretical strand	**Application and developments**
Managerial-psychologistic	Scientific management
	Democratic humanism
Durkheim-systems	Human relations
	Systems thinking in organizational analysis
Interactionist	Occupations and professions in society
	Organizations as negotiated orders
	Ethnomethodology
Weberian-social action	Social action perspective on organizations
	Bureaucratic principles of work organization
	Orientations to work
Marxian	Individual experiences and capitalist labour processes
	Structural contradictions in society and economy
Post-modern	Discourse and human subjectivity
	Post-modern organizations

(*Adapted from Watson 1995*)

on to consider more contemporary concerns. Mannion et al. (2010) identified four main phases in the organization of the NHS, which are summarized here to provide the context for the studies which demonstrate the contribution sociology has made to our understanding of health-care organization.

From the beginning: 1948–1983

The NHS was established following a period of significant upheaval and unrest, particularly in Europe (see Chapter 13 for more detail). This influenced the thinking of the politicians, and the foundations of the health service were laid in a series of landmark reports expressing commitment to the development of the welfare state. One of these, a report on Social Insurance and Allied Services, or the Beveridge Report as it was generally referred to, was published in 1942 as the 'blueprint' for welfare reform in the UK. As part of this programme of reform, the National Health Service Act came into force in July 1948, resulting in the establishment of a universal state health service, providing diagnosis and treatment of illnesses at home or in hospital for the first time in Britain. This embodied the principle of the NHS providing care and treatment for citizens 'from cradle to grave', which was free at the point of delivery, which remains a central tenet of NHS organization (DH 2013). The founding principle of NHS organization still affects current approaches.

In its early days, the service was run on the basis of supporting the health professionals to deliver care and treatment through effective administration of the service (Webster 1988, 1998; Rivett 1998; Harrison 1988). In the following twenty years, there were two major reforms undertaken in an effort to organize and manage the service more effectively. The Salmon Report (Ministry of Health 1966) encouraged the development of a senior nursing staff structure and was influenced by principles derived from scientific management approaches (Taylor 1947). For example, the different elements of the nursing role were subdivided, in accordance with the scientific management approach of breaking work down into its component parts, resulting in a more layered hierarchy of roles. In this way, it was hoped that the management of the service would improve. The 1974 reorganization (DHSS 1974) was characterized by its emphasis on the management structures and organizational control inherent in systems theory (Burns and Stalker 1961). The dominant organizational form during this phase of NHS management was **bureaucracy**. This term is often used to describe rule-bound organizations where it is difficult to get any explanation or response because of 'red tape'. If a process or person is referred to as being 'bureaucratic', it generally indicates that this is negative and unhelpful. In an extreme form, bureaucratic organizations fail to do what they are supposed to do because rules and regulations are applied so rigidly that employees lose sight of

bureaucracy: structure in organizations, with specialization of tasks, rules and regulations, systems and authority

14

what their job is. Bureaucracy, as a sociological concept, was originally developed by Max Weber, one of the first sociologists to consider the role of individuals in relation to the structural determinants of social action. Much of his work was concerned with the notion of 'rationality', which he used to explain the development of Western society, which was increasingly based on science and calculation (Jary and Jary 1991). This, combined with the growth of large organizations throughout the nineteenth century, led Weber to conclude that the decisive reason for the advance of bureaucratic organization was its purely technical superiority over any other form of organization (Weber 1947: 214). In short, it was a description of an **ideal type** of organization – not ideal in the sense that it was perfect or one that should be aimed for, rather that its structure contained specific elements that characterized it as a bureaucracy and that were necessary to manage the organizations of the day (see Box 14.1). Bureaucracy can be observed in the barriers that sometimes exist between different wards and departments and the lack of cooperation that ensues. At a more basic level, nurses can become so concerned with all of the forms that need to be completed when a patient is admitted, either on paper or increasingly using hand-held computers, that they have less time to spend delivering direct care. This is not a criticism of the individual nurse who is trying to balance these aspects of her work; rather, it is an indication of how an understanding of the concept of bureaucracy can help explain some of the more puzzling aspects of nursing practice. Activity 14.1 further illustrates how it can be applied to make sense of the organization as a whole. The bureaucratic nature of health-care organizations persists (Schofield 2001) and application of the concept from sociology continues to provide useful insights. For example, it has been found that, despite widespread criticisms of bureaucracy for its negative elements, its rules concerning equity and fairness can have benefits (Du Gay 2000).

ideal type: model of a phenomenon which identifies its essential elements

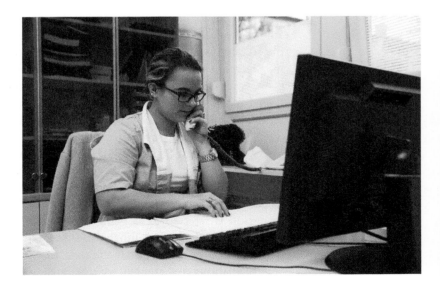

Figure 14.2
Bureaucracy is evident in most large organizations

relationship to the reality of the situation people working in health care face (Howieson and Thigarajah 2011; Hewison and Morrell 2013).

Activity 14.3 Leadership and nursing

Complete the NHS Leadership Academy self assessment tool at: <http:// www.leadershipacademy.nhs.uk/wp-content/uploads/2012/11/ NHSLeadership -Framework-LeadershipFrameworkSelfAssessmentTool.pdf>.

(a) What are your strengths as a leader?
(b) What areas do you need to develop?
(c) To what extent do you think that leaders as individuals can have an impact on care?
(d) Do you think nurses should be leaders?

---

negotiated order:
network and norms of behaviour developed outside the organizational structure by people working together

social interactionist:
theories that social reality is created through social interaction

Much thinking about leadership incorporates notions of **negotiated order** which, in contrast to the ideal type of bureaucracy, emphasizes the importance of negotiation between individuals. Bond and Bond (1986) locate the concept of negotiated order within a broad **social interactionist** tradition. This theorizes that social phenomena, particularly organizational arrangements, emerge from the ongoing interaction among people. It involves negotiation and renegotiation over actions and decisions, and stresses the fluidity and uncertainty of social arrangements. As long ago as 1963 Strauss et al. (1963) concluded that the hospital is a locale where staff are enmeshed in a complex negotiative process in order to accomplish their individual and organizational objectives. The dynamics of how this is accomplished on a day-to-day basis are illustrated in the work of Stein (1967), who characterized it as the 'doctor–nurse game'. This involves subtle and nuanced communication on the part of the nurse to ensure that doctors adhere to nurses' requests without the nurse seeming to give direction. In playing the game, the intention is that the work can be done without creating too much friction. The role of the nurse has developed considerably since 1967, and in 1990 Stein et al. noted that, in an increasing number of hospital settings, nurses feel free to confront and even challenge physicians more directly on issues of patient care. However, elements of negotiated order can still be discerned in models of leadership. For example, the NHS Leadership Framework includes statements that reflect a recognition of the need to take account of the negotiated order approach: 'Leaders are sensitive to the concerns and needs of different individuals, groups and organizations, and use this to build networks of influence and plan how to reach agreement about priorities, allocation of resources or approaches to service delivery' (NHS Leadership Academy 2013).

This is intended to contrast interactions of this nature with 'transactional leadership' whereby leaders use rewards and 'trade-offs' when interacting with staff (Barr and Dowding 2008). It also reflects the importance of engaging staff more directly in the organization of care (Ham 2014). This demonstrates how sociological perspectives can

14

uncover some of the complexities behind seemingly straightforward managerial prescriptions. Another useful concept in this respect is the informal organization.

Case Study: Leadership and diabetes

In 2012, it was estimated that worldwide there were 382 million adults aged between twenty and seventy-nine years with diabetes. It was predicted this figure will rise to 592 million by 2035. There are 3.2 million people with diabetes in the UK, and by 2025 it is estimated that there will be 5 million (Diabetes UK 2014).

A National Service Framework (Department of Health 2001), setting out what needed to be done, was produced. This was later reviewed by the House of Commons Public Accounts Committee (HCCPA 2012), which concluded that although there is consensus about what needs to be done for people with diabetes, progress in delivering the recommended standards of care and in achieving treatment targets has been depressingly poor. There is no strong national leadership, no effective accountability arrangements for commissioners and no appropriate performance incentives for providers. We have seen no evidence that the department will ensure that these issues are addressed effectively in the new NHS structure. Failure on the part of the department to do so will lead to higher costs to the NHS, as well as less than adequate support for people with diabetes (HCCPA 2012: 3).

In response to this criticism, NHS England published *Action for Diabetes* (2014), presented as a 'one-stop shop', bringing all the strands of work together in one place, for anyone interested in what NHS England is doing now and over the next few years in this important area.

Consider the two extracts below.

a) *In the future, we would want to see personalised and integrated care, designed in partnership with people with diabetes, and delivered by a competent workforce in specialist and non-specialist settings (p. 11)*

b) *We are here also to provide leadership and support to Clinical Commissioning Groups as commissioners of secondary and community healthcare services. Improving outcomes for people with or at risk of diabetes will be achieved through actions in each of these roles. (p. 13)*

- How might you help manage achievement of (a)?
- What sort of leadership is required if outcomes are to be improved for people with diabetes (b)?
- What leadership skills do you think you need to develop to make an impact on this aspect of care?

Activity 14.4 Negotiating care

The next time you are involved in a handover report or case conference concerning a patient you are caring for on one of your clinical placements, think about the way decisions are being made about patient/client care.

(a) To what extent are decisions the outcome of a formal process and based on 'objective' clinical evidence, and to what extent are they the outcome of informal discussion?
(b) Whose views prevail and why?
(c) How does the ward/department leader take account of staff views when organizing care?

Organizational culture

informal organization: norms of behaviour that develop outside formal organizational structure

The **informal organization** is the network of relationships that spontaneously establish themselves among members of an organization on the basis of their common interests and friendships (Huczynski and Buchanan 2007). The importance of this can be demonstrated through consideration of the concept of organizational culture in health care, which incorporates the informal organization. The Francis Report (Francis 2013) and the Berwick Review (Berwick 2013) both called for a fundamental change in the culture of health care. However, this is a far from straightforward process because arriving at a precise and agreed definition of organizational culture is problematic. The term '**organizational culture**' refers to the pattern of beliefs, values and learned way of coping with experiences which have developed during the course of an organization's history, and which tend to be manifested in its material arrangements and the behaviours of its members (Brown 1995). Much of this is an outcome of the informal organization. Although others contend that things are more complex, with Pacanowsky and O'Donnell-Trujillo (1982) arguing that organizational culture is not just another piece of the puzzle, it *is* the puzzle. They maintain that culture is not something an organization has; it is something an organization *is*. Similarly, Davies and Mannion (2013) refer to a 'cultural mosaic' where organizations are constituted of multiple subcultures of ward teams, services and occupational groups, operating within a hierarchy, and argue that it is necessary to understand this if the concept is to be of benefit. One way of dealing with these contrasting perspectives is to view organizational culture as being like an 'iceberg' (see Figure 14.3).

organizational culture: basic assumptions developed by a group to cope with external adaptation/internal integration problems

Three levels of organizational culture can be identified and these are:

Level 1: Artefacts – the visible manifestations of organizational culture; for example, uniforms, job titles, logos, layout of buildings, routines and the language of health care. These are the 'tip of the iceberg' and visible to all.
Level 2: Expressed beliefs and values about the organization. These arise from what organizational members believe to be important. They are used to justify actions and behaviours; for example, professional values in health care. They are buried deep in the iceberg.

14

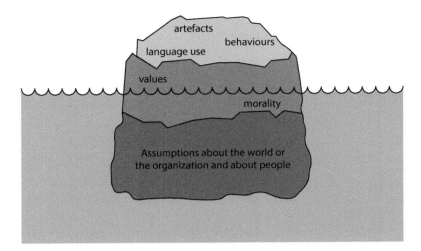

Figure 14.3 The
Iceberg model of
culture

Level 3: Basic underlying assumptions. These are the implicit
assumptions that guide behaviour and shape how members of
the organization think and feel about things. For example, health
care is viewed as a public service that has distinct qualities, but is
it an organization like any other? These assumptions are deeply
embedded, below the waterline. This is why culture can be so
difficult to change because such assumptions are often hidden, yet
very powerful.

Activity 14.5 Organizational culture

Consider the three levels of culture in organizations:

(a) Identify some artefacts; for example, what message is conveyed by the
range of uniforms people wear?
(b) What do people say about the hospital/service? Is it mainly positive or
negative? Are there specific issues of concern?
(c) What is the 'feel' of a place of work you have worked in or visited
recently? How did you come to this conclusion?

However, managing and changing organizational culture is seen as
an essential element of system reform, which can take many years to
bring about (Scott et al. 2003). It is recognized as being important by
patients and professionals (Konteh et al. 2010), yet there is no evidence
to demonstrate that effective strategies to bring about cultural change
that can be widely applied exist (Parmelli et al. 2011). This suggests that
this will be a continuing challenge for all those working in health care
for the foreseeable future.

4 Actor network theory

actor network theory:
that social phenomena are created by people through interaction with the social and material world

translational mobilization:
involves the synthesis of knowledge necessary to bring about action

ethnographic research:
direct observation of activity of members of a group or organization

holism:
a person is considered as a functioning whole rather than separate systems

The final contribution of sociology to understanding contemporary management challenges to be considered here can be found in the work of Davina Allen (2015, 2014). Using **actor network theory**, she has conducted a programme of research which recasts the nature of nursing work and raises some important implications for the future of health-care organization. Central to her account of nursing work is the concept of **translational mobilization**. In a study of front-line nursing activity in forty UK hospitals, using **ethnographic** methods, she found that through their organizing work, nurses were the network builders, system enablers and principal mediators through which the diverse elements of care were coordinated and managed (Allen 2014). Nurses were the 'glue' that ensured care was planned and delivered (Allen 2015). This involved interacting with a vast array of personnel to ensure the needs of patients and the organization were met. As she observes: 'There is very little that moves in health care without passing through the hands of a nurse' (Allen 2015: 136). She argues that traditional conceptualizations of nursing, which have emphasized 'holistic' care and **holism** as the professional ideal, and involve nurses caring for patients on a one-to-one basis to meet their individual needs, do not accurately reflect much of what happens in practice (Allen 2014). The picture of individual qualified nurses providing direct care was not borne out by her data; rather, they have the central role in coordinating diverse lines of action that contribute to the care of patients, while coping with the overall work of the ward or department (Allen 2015). Nurses are the organizers and coordinators of care. She concludes that 'holism' should be reformulated to incorporate the organizing work that nurses do because this would be more accurate, their contribution

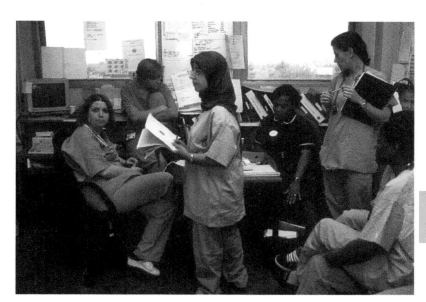

Figure 14.4 Handover reports are crucial in the organization of patient care

14

to health care would be more visible and it may reduce disillusionment as expectations of practice would be more realistic (Allen 2014). In this way, the application of a sociological approach demonstrates how seemingly familiar roles and activities can be explained in different ways that shed light on the reality of practice. This has implications for the future organization of nursing work and health care more widely. If nurses are the de-facto managers of health care in hospitals, structures and processes may need to be reviewed to capitalize on this in order to improve patient care.

Summary and Resources

Summary

▶ Health-care organizations are large and complex and will not function unless they are managed.

▶ Key concepts and theories from the study of sociology, such as bureaucracy, negotiated order, the informal organization and actor network theory, can provide useful insights into the way health-care organizations operate. Similarly, research methods developed in the discipline of sociology have been used to shed light on important aspects of health-care organizations.

▶ Nurses are increasingly involved in management from an early stage in their careers, and so an understanding of how organizations work is important. The study of sociology is helpful in developing the composite knowledge base all nurses need.

▶ Management is a prominent feature of the government's plans for health care over the next few years. Health policy is predicated on notions of the NHS being effectively managed and organized. Sociology provides a means of studying this development.

Questions for Discussion

1 Why is it important for health-care organizations to be managed effectively?
2 What are the advantages and disadvantages of nurses being managers of care?
3 Are leaders born or made?
4 Is the NHS too big to be managed?
5 Should the role of the nurse be refocused on the management of care rather than its delivery?

Glossary

actor network theory: is based on the premise of human agency, and that social phenomena are

agency:
the capacity to actively shape and direct the world, rather than simply to react to external events and forces

bureaucracy:
a structure found in large organizations, based on the specialization of tasks, rules and regulations, systems and authority

ethnographic research:
a research approach which involves the direct observation of the activity of members of a group or organization

holism:
an approach or philosophy in which the person is considered as a functioning whole rather than as a composite of different separate systems

ideologies:
bodies of beliefs organized around sets of central values

ideal type:
a model of a phenomenon which identifies its essential elements

informal organization:
the relationships, networks and norms of behaviour that people who work together develop outside the formal organizational structure and processes

organizational culture:
the pattern of basic assumptions that a given group has invented, discovered or developed in learning to cope with its problems of external adaptation and internal integration, and that have worked well enough to be considered valid and, therefore, to be taught to new members as the correct way to perceive, think and feel in relation to these problems (Schein 1984)

negotiated order:
the relationships, networks and norms of behaviour that people who work together develop outside the formal organizational structure and processes; it is characterized by fluid and uncertain social arrangements

New Public Management:
the application of a wide range of management theories and approaches to the organization of public services

14

The first entry continues from a previous page:

created by people through interaction with the social and material world; application of the theory involves the study of what people do, the tools they use and the practices they engage in

| social interactionist: | a theoretical tradition in which it is argued that social reality is created through social interaction |
| translational mobilization: | involves the synthesis of knowledge necessary to bring about action |

Further Reading

A. A. Huczynski and D. A. Buchanan: *Organizational Behaviour*, 8th edn. London: Financial Times Prentice Hall, 2013.
A comprehensive and accessible textbook which examines organizational behaviour and management.

J. Hewitt-Taylor: *Understanding and Managing Change in Health Care*. Houndmills: Palgrave Macmillan, 2013.
A useful primer on the main areas of managing change in health-care organizations.

K. Walshe and J. Smith: *Healthcare Management*, 2nd edn. Maidenhead: Open University Press, 2011.
An edited book, which includes a wide range of detailed material examining a number of health management issues.

Also useful are the following online resources:

<www.leadershipacademy.nhs.uk>
Useful source of information and resources regarding current approaches to leadership in the English NHS.

<http://www.nhsiq.nhs.uk/capacity-capability/nhs-change-model.aspx>
This is a useful source of information about organizational change. Given the constant drive to bring about change in health care, consideration of the NHS Change Model would be helpful.

<http://www.kingsfund.org.uk/>
The King's Fund is a health and social care 'think tank'. It is a useful source of up-to-date commentary and analysis on a range of health issues including management.

<http://www.reallylearning.com/>
The website of health commentator Valerie Iles. It includes useful free resources and independent comment on health management.

References

Allen, D. 2014 Re-conceptualizing holism in the contemporary nursing mandate: from individual to organizational relationships. *Social Science & Medicine* 119: 131–8.

Allen, D. 2015 *The Invisible Work of Nurses: Hospitals, Organization and Healthcare*. London: Routledge.

Ansof, H. I. 1980 Strategic issue management. *Strategic Management Journal* 1/2: 131–48.

Appleby, J. 1994 The reformed National Health Service: a commentary. *Social Policy & Administration* 28/4: 345–58.

Barr, J. and Dowding, L. 2008 *Leadership in Health Care*. London: Sage.

Bedeian, A. G. 1998 Exploring the past. *Journal of Management History* 4/1: 4–15.

Berwick, D. 2013. *A Promise to Learn, a Commitment to Act: Improving the Safety of Patients in England*. National Advisory Group on the Safety of Patients in England. At: <https://www.gov.uk/government/uploads/system/uploads/ attachment_data/file/226703/Berwick_Report.pdf>.

Beveridge, W. 1942 *Social Insurance and Allied Services*. Cmnd 6404. London: HMSO.

Blundell, B. and Murdock, A. 1997 *Managing in the Public Sector*. London: Butterworth Heinemann.

Bond, J. and Bond, S. 1986 *Sociology and Health Care*. Edinburgh: Churchill Livingstone.

Brown, A. D. 1992 Managing change in the NHS: the Resource Management Initiative. *Leadership and Organization Development Journal* 13/6: 13–17.

Brown, A. 1995 *Organizational Culture*. London: Pitman Publishing.

Burns, T. and Stalker, G. M. 1961 *The Management of Innovation*. Oxford: Oxford University Press.

Chote, R. 2007 Health and the public spending squeeze: funding prospects for the NHS. In J. Appleby (ed.), *Funding Health Care 2008 and Beyond. Report from the Leeds Castle Summit*. London: King's Fund, pp. 35–42.

Davies, H. T. O. and Mannion, R. 2013 Will prescriptions for cultural change improve the NHS? *British Medical Journal* 346: 1–4.

Dawson, S., Garside, P., Hudson, R. and Bicknell, C. 2009 *The Design and Establishment of the Leadership Council*. NHS Leadership Council. At: <http://www.dh.gov.uk/prod_consum_dh/groups/dh_digitalassets/documents/digitalasset/dh_093388.pdf>.

Department of Health (DH) 1989 *Working for Patients*. London: Department of Health.

Department of Health (DH) 1998 *A First Class Service: Quality in the New NHS*. London: Department of Health.

Department of Health (DH) 2000 *The NHS Plan: A Plan for Investment a Plan for Reform*. London: Department of Health.

Department of Health (DH) 2001 *National Service Framework for Diabetes: Standards*. London: Department of Health.

Department of Health (DH) 2007 *The Modernization Agency*. At: <http://www.dh.gov.uk/en/Publicationsandstatistics/Publications/AnnualReports/Browsable/DH_4937234>.

Department of Health (DH) 2008a *High Quality Care For All: NHS Next Stage Review Final Report (The Darzi Review)*. London: Department of Health.

Department of Health (DH) 2008b *A High Quality Workforce: NHS Next Stage Review*. London: Department of Health.

Department of Health (DH) 2009 *Inspiring Leaders: Leadership for Quality*. London: Department of Health.

Department of Health (DH) 2012 *The Operating Framework for the NHS in England 2012/13*. London: Department of Health.

Department of Health (DH) 2013 *The NHS Constitution*. London: Department of Health.

14

Department of Health (DH) 2014 *The Health and Care System Explained*. At: https://www.gov.uk/government/publications/the-health-and-care-system-explained>..

Department of Health and Social Security 1974 *Management Arrangements for the Reorganized National Health Service*. London: HMSO.

Department of Health and Social Security 1983 *The NHS Management Enquiry (The Griffiths Report) DA(83)38*. London: DHSS.

Diabetes UK 2014 *Diabetes: Facts and Stats – Version 3*. London: Diabetes UK. At: <www.U:\SociologyBook\Diabetes-key-stats-guidelines-April2014.pdf>.

Dixon, J. 1998 The context. In J. Le Grand, N. Mays and J. Mulligan (eds), *Learning from the Internal Market*. London: King's Fund, pp. 1–14.

Dopson, S. and Waddington, I. 1996 Managing social change: a process-sociological approach to understanding organisational change in the NHS. *Sociology of Health & Illness* 18/4: 525–50.

Du Gay, P. 2000 *In Praise of Bureaucracy*. London: Sage Publications.

Dutton, J. and Ashford, S. 1993 Selling issues to top management. *Academy of Management Review* 18/30: 397–428.

Ferlie, E. 2010 Public management 'reform' narratives and the changing organization of primary care. *London Journal of Primary Care* 3: 76–80.

Ferlie, E., Ashburner, L., Fitzgerald, L. and Pettigrew, A. 1996 *The New Public Management in Action*. Oxford: Oxford University Press.

Ford, J. 2005 Examining leadership through critical feminist readings. *Journal of Health Organization and Management* 19/3: 236–51.

Francis, R. 2013 *Report of the Mid-Staffordshire NHS Foundation Trust Public Inquiry*. London: HMSO.

Giddens, A. 1998 *The Third Way – The Renewal of Social Democracy*. Bristol: Policy Press.

Gorsky, M. (ed.) 2010 *The Griffiths NHS Management Inquiry: Its Origins, Nature and Impact*. Held 11 November 2008, Centre for History in Public Health, London School of Hygiene and Tropical Medicine, January 2010. Available at: <http://history.lshtm.ac.uk.witness-seminars.html>.

Grint, K. 1995 *Management: A Sociological Introduction*. Cambridge: Polity.

Hales, C. P. 1993 *Managing through Organization*. London: Routledge.

Ham, C. 2014 *Staff Engagement and Empowerment in the NHS*. London: King's Fund.

Harrison, S. 1988 *Managing the NHS – Shifting the Frontier*. London: Chapman and Hall.

Health and Social Care Information Centre (undated) *Hospital Care*. At: <http://www.hscic.gov.uk/hospital-care>.

Hewison, A. and Morrell, K. 2013 Leadership development in healthcare: a counter narrative to inform policy. *International Journal of Nursing Studies* 51/4: 677–88.

Hood, C. 1991 A public management for all seasons. *Public Administration* 69: 3–19.

House of Commons (HCCPA) 2012 *Department of Health: The Management of Adult Diabetes Services in the NHS Seventeenth Report of Session 2012–13 HC 289*. London: House of Commons, HMSO.

Howieson, B. and Thigarajah, T. 2011 What is clinical leadership? A journal-based metareview. *International Journal of Clinical Leadership* 17/1: 7–18.

Huczynski, A. A. and Buchanan, D. 2007 *Organizational Behaviour: An Introductory Text*, 6th edn. Harlow: Pearson Education.

Hunter, D. J. 2005 The National Health Service 1980–2005. *Public Money & Management* 25/4: 209–12.

Jary, D. and Jary, J. 1991 *Collins Dictionary of Sociology*. Glasgow: HarperCollins.

Keogh, B. 2013 *Review into the Quality of Care provided by 14 Hospital Trusts in England*. Overview Report. At: <http://www.nhs.uk/NHSEngland/bruce-keogh-review/Documents/outcomes/keogh-review-final-report.pdf>.

King's Fund 2011 *The Future of Leadership and Management in the NHS – No More Heroes* (Report from the King's Fund Commission on Leadership and Management in the NHS). London: King's Fund.

King's Fund 2014 *Quarterly Monitoring Report* 12. At: <http://qmr.kingsfund.org.uk/2014/12/>.

Klein, R. 1995 *The New Politics of the NHS*, 3rd edn. London: Longman.

Konteh, F. H., Mannion, R. and Davies H. T. O. 2010 Understanding culture and culture management in the English NHS: a comparison of professional and patient perspectives. *Journal of Evaluation in Clinical Practice* 17: 111–17.

Lammers, C. J. 1978 The comparative sociology of organizations. *Annual Review of Sociology* 4: 485–510.

Lockerby, P. 2011 *Henry Ford – Quote: 'History Is Bunk'*. At: <http://www.science20.com/chatter_box/henry_ford_quote_history_bunk-79505>.

Mannion, R., Davies, H. and Harrison, S. et al. 2010 *Changing Management Cultures and Organizational Performance in the NHS (OC2)*. National Institute for Health Research Service Delivery and Organization Programme. London: HMSO.

Ministry of Health (MOH) 1966 *Report of the Committee on Senior Nursing Staff (Salmon Report)*. London: HMSO.

Mintzberg, H. 1996 Musings on management. *Harvard Business Review* (July–August) 74: 61–7.

Mintzberg, H. 2011 *Managing*. Harlow: Prentice Hall.

National Leadership Centre 2004 *NHS Leadership Qualities Framework – A Good Practice Guide*. London: NHS Leadership Centre (Modernization Agency).

NHS Choices 2015 *The NHS in England*. At: <http://www.nhs.uk/NHSEngland/thenhs/about/Pages/overview.aspx>.

NHS England 2014 *Action for Diabetes*. At https://www.england.nhs.uk/ourwork/qual-clin-lead/diabetes-prevention/action-for-diabetes/

NHS Leadership Academy 2013 *Healthcare Leadership Model – The Nine Dimensions of Leadership Behaviour*. At: <www.leadershipacademy.nhs.uk>.

Nicholson, D. 2014 *Change is the Key to NHS Survival. National Health Service England*. At: <http://www.england.nhs.uk/2014/03/03/nhs-survival/>.

Owens, P. and Glennerster, H. 1990 *Nursing in Conflict*. Basingstoke: Macmillan Educational.

Pacanowsky, M. E. and O'Donnell-Trujillo, N. 1982. Communication and organizational cultures. *Western Journal of Speech Communication* 46: 115–30.

14

Packwood, T., Kerrison, S. and Buxton, M. 1992 The audit process and medical organization. *Quality in Health Care* 1: 192–6.

Parmelli, E., Flodgren, G., Beyer F., Baillie, N., Schaafsma M. E. and Eccles, M. P. 2011 The effectiveness of strategies to change organizational culture to improve healthcare performance: a systematic review. *Implementation Science* 6: 33.

Pollitt, C. 2007 New Labour's re-disorganization. *Public Management Review* 9/4: 529–43.

Pollitt, C. 2008 *Time, Policy, Management – Governing with the Past*. Oxford: Oxford University Press.

Rea, D. M. 1994 Better informed judgements: Resource Management in the NHS. Accounting. *Auditing and Accountability Journal* 7/1: 86–110.

Rivett, G. C. 1998 *From Cradle to Grave, the First 50 Years of the NHS*. London: King's Fund.

Schein, E. 1984 Coming to a new awareness of organizational culture. *Sloan Management Review* (winter) 22/2: 3–6.

Schein, E. 1985 *Organizational Culture and Leadership*. San Francisco: Jossey-Bass.

Schofield, J. 2001 The old ways are the best? The durability and usefulness of bureaucracy in public sector management. *Organization* 8/1: 77–96.

Scott, T., Mannion, R., Davies, H. T. O. and Marshall, M. N. 2003 Implementing culture change in health care: theory and practice. *International Journal for Quality in Health Care* 15/2: 111–18.

Stein, L. I. 1967 The doctor–nurse game. *Archives of General Psychiatry* 16: 699–703.

Stein, L. I., Watts, D. T. and Howell, T. 1990 The doctor–nurse game revisited. *New England Journal of Medicine* 322/8: 546–9.

Stevens, S. 2014 *Five Year Forward View*. London: Department of Health.

Storey, J. and Holti, R. 2013 The contribution of clinical leadership to service redesign: a naturalistic inquiry. *Health Services Management Research* 25/3: 144–51.

Strauss, A., Schatzman, L., Ehrlich, D., Bucher, R. and Sabshin, M. 1963 The hospital and its negotiated order. In E. Freidson (ed.), *The Hospital in Modern Society*. Basingstoke: Macmillan, pp. 147–69.

Taylor, F. W. 1947 *Scientific Management*. London: Harper and Row.

Timmins, N. 2008 History matters. *Nursing Standard* 22/17: 22–4.

Trefgarne, G. 2005 *Chinese Army, Indian Railway . . . Then Comes the NHS*. At: <http://www.telegraph.co.uk/finance/2907780/Chinese-army-Indian-railways. . .-then-comes-the-NHS.html>.

Watson, T. J. 1995 *Sociology Work and Industry*, 3rd edn. London: Routledge.

Weber, M. 1947 *The Theory of Social and Economic Organization*. New York: Free Press.

Webster, C. 1988 *The National Health Service Since the War: Volume 1 Problems of Health Care – The National Health Service before 1957*. London: HMSO.

Webster, C. 1998 *The National Health Service: A Political History*. Oxford: Oxford University Press.

criticized for creating local monopolies which limited the range of social care services available and minimized choice for service users (Baxter et al. 2011).

The limits of community

The second strand of the 1990 Community Care legislation – the commitment to keep people in their own homes or other community settings – was largely welcomed. However, by linking it with the commitment to the outsourcing of care services, there was concern that this was largely about cost savings (Lewis and Glennerster, 1996). More people with long-term care needs – particularly older people who might have been looked after in hospital geriatric wards in the past – were to be shifted to the social care side of the divide, and therefore liable to contribute towards their care costs if they had the means. NHS Continuing Health Care (CHC) was available for some patients who were deemed to have both health and care needs, but was tightly rationed, with demand far outstripping supply. The criteria demanded a 'primary health need' which was subject to different thresholds in different parts of the country, and often left patients and families bewildered and upset if they had to foot the bill for meeting what they saw as health conditions.

Activity 15.1 Means-testing

(a) Is the concept of means-testing consistent with an NHS free at the point of delivery?

(b) Should people be forced to sell their houses to fund their own care?

Is it fair that someone who has been frugal and saved all of their life has to pay for their care, when someone with no savings will have their care paid for?

(c) Should people be forced to give up work to care for their relatives?

(d) These are the sorts of issues that policymakers have to consider when deciding how to fund care. Discuss these with a group of your colleagues and gauge the different views. What other approaches to social care might there be?

The community care element of the 1990 legislation was also controversial because it was never clear that adequate investment had been made in what was to be the alternative to institutional life. As Roulstone and Prideaux put it, 'The decanting of ex-asylum patients into unwelcoming and unprepared communities and the sense that informal care actually meant greater reliance on family made some commentators question whether the "community" aspect of community care actually had any meaning' (2012: 15). It intensified the pressure on unpaid family carers who were expected to be able to sustain their family members in a domestic setting. Such informal care remains a core element of the social care system, with twice as

15

many unpaid carers – nearly 6.4 million – as there are paid staff in the health and social care systems combined (House of Lords 2013; 59).

The shift away from institutional settings has also changed the pattern of residential care use for older people, with more older people opting for support in their own home. Residential homes now tend to be the destination only for the very frail, many of whom will have a cognitive impairment. For people staying at home, there has been a move away from the low-level cleaning and home-help services that local authorities used to provide, with support more narrowly focused on **personal care** (help with washing and dressing) (Lloyd 2014: 60). With an emphasis on efficiency and task-based care, local authorities purchase this personal care in fifteen- or thirty-minute 'slots' from mostly private providers.

It has been argued that domiciliary care is a 'sector in crisis' due to the poor quality of care that is often provided and the difficulties it faces in recruiting and retaining workers. A report into social care by the Equality and Human Rights Commission (EHRC) found 'serious, systemic threats to the basic human rights of older people who are getting home care services' (EHRC 2011: 7). Leece (2010) lists a number of difficulties facing the domiciliary care sector, which include low pay and status, financial constraints on local authorities, poor working conditions (unsociable hours, poor job security), requirements for high standards of care and staff qualifications and competition with other employers, including supermarkets and residential homes. Bolton and Wibberley (2013) suggest that, despite the popular belief that care work is unskilled, domiciliary care work now requires higher levels of skill than in the past, including performing health-care tasks such as changing dressings or offering physiotherapy.

personal care:
care at home or in residential setting which includes washing and dressing

---

Activity 15.2 The health and social care divide

Research and read some news items regarding health and social care. There are many of these online – see one example on the BBC News website at: <http://www.bbc.co.uk/news/health-29047190>.

(a) Why do you think politicians are reluctant to address this issue?

(b) What are the implications of this divide for patients and their carers?

(c) What advice would you give to a relative who asks you about how best to organize continuing care of her mother who needs help with washing and using the toilet?

---

3 Personalization

personalization:
approach enabling people using care services to have choice and control over their support

If community was the dominant policy theme of care in the 1980s and 1990s, social care in the twenty-first century has been dominated by the theme of **personalization**. A reform agenda which covers adult and children's care services (and is increasingly stretching into health), personalization is a way of thinking about public services and those who use them, rather than being a worked-out set of policy prescriptions. As Carr puts it, personalization involves 'thinking about public services ... in an entirely different way – starting with the person rather than the service' (Carr 2010: 67). This guide to action makes personalization highly flexible when translated into specific policy agendas, being applicable to a range of different ways of reforming the welfare state.

The care management reforms of the early 1990s had promised to 'promot[e] individual choice and self-determination' (Department of Health 1989). However, local authorities tended to focus on the administrative aspects of the reforms rather than their scope for empowering users, as social workers found more of their time taken up with filling in forms (Lewis and Glennerster 1996: 104). Momentum for more personalized approaches to care and support continued to gather during the 1990s, fuelled by the disappointing experience of care management.

Although personalized social care is about more than devolved budgets for service users, it was the introduction of **direct payments** legislation in 1996, following years of campaigning by disability organizations, which marked a key policy change. It allowed service users with disabilities to receive a budget to manage their own care needs and purchase services which contribute to an agreed outcome. The legislation was later extended to include older people, disabled children, mental health service users and carers. In 2005, the Department of Health piloted devolved budgets in thirteen councils. Evaluation of the pilots found that the initiative was generally welcomed by participants, who reported feeling they had more control over their daily lives (Glendinning et al. 2008). Mental health service users, physically disabled adults and people with learning disabilities were more positive about the scheme than older participants. **Personal budgets** have since become the main vehicle through which people receive their care spend. They can be taken as a direct payment where the money goes to the service user or their family, or can be a managed personal budget, looked after by a local authority or agreed third party.

In 2007, the Putting People First concordat, signed by central government, local government and the social care sector, widened the agenda, emphasizing that personalization should not just be seen as personal budgets or direct payments (HM Government 2007). Personalization was to be about choice and control for the individual, with a number of strands, including early intervention and prevention, **social capital**, and improved access to universal services. Personalization was also expected to facilitate a more positive account of risk to overcome a culture in which safeguarding could be used excessively to limit people's choice and control.

direct payments: cash allocation enabling people or their families using care services to purchase their own care support

personal budgets: allocation of money for people using care services

social capital: theory explaining and measuring extent to which people are connected to others in their locality

15

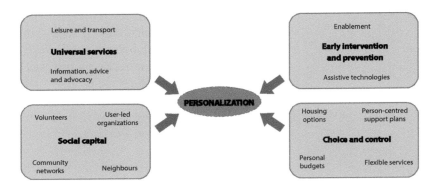

Figure 15.2 Key themes in personalization

The progress, following a decade of personalization-oriented reforms, has varied, by locality and by user group. Numerical targets for the take-up of personal budgets were initially used but later abandoned, amid a fear that some councils were taking a tick-box approach to meeting the targets, ostensibly moving people on to a managed personal budget while leaving the services unchanged. There is now an expectation that direct payments should be the default offer for all eligible social care service users, with other options, such as third-party or council management of a budget, to be a fallback option when people don't want the responsibility of looking after a budget themselves.

Personalization and older people

Take-up rates of personal budgets are at around three-quarters of eligible people (Samuel 2013). There has been much optimism about the scope for personal budgets to have a transformative impact on people's lives, and the evaluation data suggest that many people are able to rethink their care and support in ways that meet their needs much more fully (Waters and Hatton 2014). However, much of this transformation has been for younger people with learning and/or physical disabilities, who have been able to employ a personal assistant to give them more tailored support. It does not appear to be as appropriate for older people (the largest group of adult social care users), where take-up of personal budgets is lower than for people with learning disabilities (45 per cent of older people compared to 59 per cent of people with a learning disability (Age UK 2013)). The difference is particularly stark for direct payments, which are associated with the most transformative outcomes for people: only 7 per cent of older people are in receipt of a direct payment, compared to 25 per cent of people with learning disabilities (Age UK 2013).

There are likely to be a number of reasons for this. Older people or their family carers may not want the complexity of managing a budget and employing a personal assistant. The tendency to provide smaller packages of care to older people rather than younger also means that the money may only be enough to cover personal care. For many older people, the reality of social care continues to be limited to domiciliary care in the home – provided by minimum-wage care staff with high turnover rates – or residential care. Although the Social Care Institute for Excellence (SCIE 2009) has developed guidance on how to make the experience of being in residential care more personalized, such institutional settings can struggle to offer tailored support.

Children's services

Personalization in children's services has proceeded in a less focused and more ad hoc way than for those of adults, even though some of the early pioneering work on personal care planning and budgets was done with disabled children and their families. The social innovation network In Control has worked with local authorities and central government to develop more personalized approaches for children, young people and families (Crosby 2010). In 2007, the then Department for Education and Skills (DfES) announced pilots to provide individual budgets for disabled children and their families through the Aiming High programme and, building on the success of these pilots, local authorities now offer personal budgets to families with disabled children. The government has been exploring the scope to extend this to families where children have Special Educational Needs and to adoptive families. In all cases, the principle is that people will get better outcomes if they have the choice and flexibility to purchase the services that fit their needs, rather than relying on existing statutory provision.

Has personalization improved social care?

For all the optimism about personalization, and the vignettes about transformational change that some people have experienced through having a personal budget, its impact on care outcomes remains highly contested. The attempt to bring in more personalized care services at a time of austerity has proved very challenging for local authorities, and has made it difficult to achieve the transformational outcomes that its advocates envisaged. Social workers have expressed grave concerns about the problems of overlaying personalization on top of austerity – with additional bureaucracy and time spent on brokerage or support planning limiting the scope to review and support people once they are in the system (Hart 2014).

One of the originators of the idea of personalized public services, Charles Leadbeater, suggested that personalization is a continuum. At the 'shallow' end it involves 'modest modification of mass-produced, standardized services to partially adapt them to user needs' (2004: 20). He favours an approach called 'deep personalization', or 'personalization through participation', at the other end of the continuum, in which people 'devise their own bottom-up solutions, which create the public

15

good' (2004: 26). There is a danger that the personalization on offer in social care services gets stuck at the shallow end of this continuum.

Activity 15.3 Personalization

Personalization is an approach to the delivery of care services which aims to give as much choice and control as possible to the person using services.

(a) Think of a patient you have cared for recently. What support, advice and guidance would he or she have needed to take the lead in the organization and funding of their care?

(b) Is personalization 'practical' in your field of nursing?

Box 15.1 Personal health budgets

Drawing inspiration from the perceived success of personal budgets in social care, in 2007, the then Labour government proposed the introduction of personal health budgets in the NHS. In a pilot study, involving people with long-term health conditions such as diabetes and chronic pulmonary heart disease, patients were able to gain access to some of the money that would be spent on treating them. This could be taken as a direct payment or a managed personal budget, and patients worked with clinicians to agree how the money would be spent. According to the Department of Health, such budgets 'could support innovative services, potentially including those currently outside the scope of traditional NHS commissioning practice' (Department of Health 2009a: 45).

A national evaluation of the pilots found that use of personal health budgets was associated with a significant improvement in the care-related quality of life and psychological well-being of patients receiving the budgets, although there was not a significant impact on health-related quality of life (Forder et al. 2012). The evaluation team concluded: 'The findings suggest that the benefits of personal health budgets stemmed from the value that people placed on having increased choice and control in their lives, and the capacity this gave them to improve the more complex or higher-order aspects of their quality of life' (Forder et al. 2012: 131). Following the pilot, personal health budgets are now in place for people using NHS Continuing Healthcare, with some local discretion about their use for people with other health conditions. Nurses are likely to need a working knowledge of personal health budgets to advise patients on whether or not they might be eligible, and what some of the risks and opportunities of controlling their own care spend might be.

---

4 Integrating health and care

If the first phase of the post-war welfare state set up a health and care divide in which people falling on the care side of the border found themselves in hostile and abusive institutions, the de-institutionalization phase from the 1980s did little to reduce the divide between health and social care. However, the twin imperatives of personalization and austerity in recent years have seen sustained efforts to bring health and care services together in ways which recognize the need to treat the 'whole person'. The benefits of more collaboration, summarized by Gray and Birrell (2013), are well known:

1 People's needs do not neatly fit into the two categories of health or care, leading to confusion and to a tendency to treat different parts of a person's needs in different systems. This is becoming particularly pronounced as more people have long-term conditions and multiple morbidities.

2 Institutional separation leads to boundary clashes and funding disputes, as well as perpetuating cultural differences in attitudes and work practices between workforces.

3 An integrated system is likely to enable people to stay independent for longer, keeping them out of over-stretched A & E wards. Intermediate care and reablement packages allow people to receive support outside of hospital settings as part of a transition back towards independent living.

4 Multidisciplinary working is increasingly recognized to bring benefits in terms of developing long-term and sustainable support for patients.

There is no shortage of political commitment to integration. The incoming New Labour government in 1997 insisted it would tackle the 'Berlin Wall' between health and social care by stimulating loose forms of partnership working. The Health Act 1999 allowed funds to be transferred between local authorities and the NHS to finance joint working. The NHS Plan 2000 permitted the creation of Care Trusts, which were NHS bodies with social care responsibilities delegated to them. The coalition government from 2010 made an early commitment to 'break down barriers between health and social care funding to incentivize preventative action' (Department of Health 2010). However, there has been remarkably little progress on making integration a reality, and in some ways the system has been getting more fragmented. For example, the Health and Social Care Act 2012 reinforced the split between primary and secondary care as GPs became commissioners through Clinical Commissioning Groups.

Activity 15.4 Personal choice vs universal provision

(a) To what extent is variability in provision of services acceptable?

(b) Is there a need for agreed standards of care for all?

(c) How can individual needs be balanced with universal care for all?

Barriers to integration

Reflecting the lack of progress on integration, Glasby notes, 'Arising out of these separate categories of health and social care are different organizations with different budgets, different catchment areas,

15

different legal frameworks, different cultures, different IT systems and different ways of training and educating professionals' (2013). Gray and Birrell (2013: ch.6) argue that various attempts at different kinds of integrated working (structural integration, pooled budgets, co-location and joint management posts) have often failed to produce the benefits that were promised. They highlight four particular barriers to effective joint working:

- Professional differences, which may be linked to modes of practice or to cultural differences. It has often been found that health professionals – who are usually considered to occupy a higher social status than social workers and care staff – come to dominate partnerships.
- Human resource issues, relating to differences in contracts, pensions and terms and conditions.
- Funding difficulties, for example in relation to what is and is not included in a pooled funding arrangement. The intense financial pressures facing local government in particular are leading to a fraught environment in which to attempt the sharing of funds.
- Lack of coterminous boundaries, particularly given the abolition of Primary Care Trusts following the Health and Social Care Act 2012. Clinical Commissioning Groups rarely cover the same patch as local authorities.

A Better Care Fund, to encourage a greater pooling of health and social care resources, has been announced and £3.8 billion was earmarked in the 2014 Spending Review settlement to bring together health and social care budgets. However, there has been criticism from health service leaders about the extent to which they are being asked to use their funds to prop up creaking social services. Social care leaders for their part have suggested that the relatively small amount of money available for the Better Care Fund risks being swallowed without trace into massive NHS institutions. Whatever the merits of these claims, they further affirm the extent to which low trust relationships between the health and social care community impede effective integrated working.

Activity 15.5 Integrated working

On the next clinical placement where you are caring for elderly people with complex needs, try and find out:

(a) The number of staff involved in making the arrangements for the discharge/transfer of a patient with 'social care' needs.
(b) The details of the planned care package.
(c) The time it takes to organize this.
(d) The extent to which it is patient led.

How effective is partnership working between health and social care?

5 The Care Act 2014

The passing of the Care Act in 2014 was described by government as 'the most significant reform of care and support in more than 60 years' (HM Government 2014). The Act, which came into force in April 2015, looks likely to set the agenda for future decades in the way that the Community Care Act did from the early 1990s. The key points from the Act are summarized in Box 15.2.

Box 15.2 Key points from the Care Act 2014

1 The law surrounding care has been simplified and updated.
2 Councils now have a duty to think about the physical, mental and emotional well-being of people who need care, and to invest in prevention and early intervention.
3 Service users and carers are given parity of entitlement.
4 From 2020 care spending for older people is capped at £72,000, and will be adjusted each year.
5 The eligibility threshold for care is to be set nationally rather than locally.
6 Councils must assist people in accessing independent financial advice.
7 Self-funders are to be given more support in their care.
8 Personal budgets are embedded in law as the default for all eligible care service users.

One of the most significant changes in the Act is that from 2020 the amount people spend on social care will be subject to a cap. People who do not currently meet the means-testing threshold for local authority funded care will pay for their own care only until they reach the threshold of £72,000. This means that local authorities need to keep track of these people and how much they are spending, in order to have a record of when the cap has been reached. There are significant administrative complexities here: local authorities have to account for not how much people have actually spent but how much the local authority would have spent if it had been purchasing the care, which is likely to be a somewhat lower figure given bulk buying by local authorities. The so-called hotel costs of residential care – accommodation and food – are not covered by the cap. Henwood (2014) argues that the proposals are likely to be of marginal benefit given the small number of people who will qualify for support. She points out: 'Moreover, in reality most people needing care and paying for it themselves will never reach the cap' (Henwood 2014). A House of Lords report on ageing also criticized the new funding proposals:

> [I]n our view [this] will not be sufficient because it will largely benefit higher income groups by protecting them from depleting their housing assets . . . It does not bring extra funding into the system to tackle the current funding crisis or address the problem of expanding need in the coming decades. (2013: 12)

15

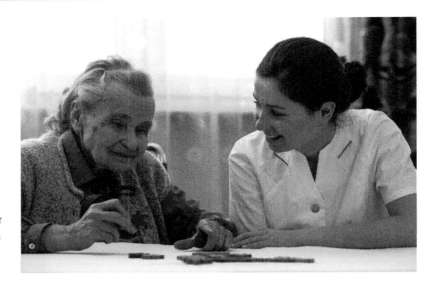

Figure 15.3 Caring for patients with dementia involves both social and medical aspects

Case Study: Dementia

It is estimated by the Alzheimer's Society that 800,000 people in the UK have dementia, affecting one in six people over eighty. Over 17,000 people under the age of sixty-five have early onset dementia (Alzheimer's Society 2014a). It is the leading cause of death for women in England and Wales. By 2038, the number of people with dementia is predicted to rise to 1.4 million people, costing over £50 billion in care (Department of Health 2009b). Two-thirds of people with dementia live in the community in their own homes and are supported by a range of professionals.

Diagnosing dementia can be difficult, with the Alzheimer's Society estimating that half of people with the condition do not have a formal diagnosis, despite the known benefits of early diagnosis. An announcement that GPs would have a financial incentive of £55 per patient to increase diagnosis rates created controversy, with the Patients' Association suggesting that it put a 'bounty on the head' of some patients (BBC 2014).

Dementia is an example of a condition that spans the divide between health and social care services. Some of the support needed will be medical, for example drugs and NHS services such as memory clinics, but many people with the condition will also need personal care at home or in residential care to assist with washing, dressing and preparing food, which will fall under social care eligibility criteria. The Alzheimer's Society has been highly critical of the impact of the health and social care divide on people living with dementia, and the burden that this places on unpaid family carers: 'If you have cancer or heart disease you can quite rightly expect that the care you need will be free. That is just not the case for people with dementia. Families are forced to break the bank to pay for basic care for a loved one' (Alzheimer's Society 2014b).

Efforts have been made to ensure that people with dementia are not left out of the personalization agenda. The Think Local Act Personal (TLAP) team, which promotes personalization and is funded by the Department of Health, has produced a number of guides that show how personalization can work for people with dementia (e.g., TLAP 2013). The emphasis is on a range of person-centred approaches, recognizing that personal budgets may not be as appropriate for dementia as for other conditions. For people eligible for NHS funding, there is some evidence that personal health budgets can be beneficial, as Colin Royle's account of supporting his father's dementia demonstrates:

> [W]e were approached by our social worker about the prospect of having a personal health budget (PHB). It was explained that the idea behind a PHB was to allow more choice and control over the care that we received. The budget was to be set at the cost equivalent as if my dad had gone into a care home, as anticipated some months earlier . . . By receiving his care in this manner, his entire care package could be tailored around his own needs, and not designed to fit in with the needs of other service users . . . My dad was thriving under his new package of care. Within 18 months of receiving a personal health budget, his medication had reduced by two-thirds and any need for input from care managers or consultants had dissipated . . . Unfortunately, dementia is a degenerative disease and my dad's condition will continue to get worse. What a personal health budget has allowed him to do however is get the most out of the life that he has left and live it in the dignified way that he deserves. (Royle 2014: 122–3)

However, not everyone with dementia will have a family member who is willing to play an active role in managing a personal budget. And for those people who are not eligible for NHS funding, the lack of resources within social care will be a major limiting factor. A former social worker has written of the difficulties that she faced in trying to reconcile the claims of personalization advocates with the reality of a cash-strapped service for people with advanced dementia:

> While the shiny policy brochures look at the different day opportunities for people and choices about going to local leisure centres rather than day centres, the realities, in my experience, due to the levels of funding we had to "play" with was more like a choice between one shower a day or two baths a week. (Hart 2014: 117)

Conclusion

Social care services for older people, people with disabilities and people with mental health problems have undergone substantial change during the era of the welfare state. Care has moved out of large-scale institutions and is primarily located in community and home settings. The state is no longer the provider of much social care provision. A commitment to person-centred care, embodying choice and control, is the organizing principle for care services. Integration and prevention are core principles of future planning in local authorities and health services.

What has not changed since 1945 is that social care continues to be the poor relation of the National Health Service. While political parties

15

fall over themselves to announce the protection of NHS budgets, social care budgets have borne a disproportionate amount of the funding cuts since 2010. The high political profile of the NHS is in sharp contrast to the relatively low profile of social care, which is surprising given that an estimated three-quarters of us will need formal care and support in later life (Lloyd 2014). Campaigners have hailed the Care Act 2014 a great step forward in embedding in law a commitment to capping care costs, investing in prevention, facilitating integration and supporting carers. But it is no substitute for public debate about ensuring that there is sufficient money available for vulnerable people to be supported in a safe, caring and dignified environment.

Summary and Resources

Summary

▶ Social care since 1948 has been separated from health, even though it can be difficult to identify whether someone has a health or a social care need. Health services are free at the point of use whereas social care services are means-tested.

▶ Reforms in the early 1990s privatized much of social care provision, and made it a policy goal to look after people in communities and homes rather than in large institutions.

▶ These reforms appeared to exacerbate rather than improve many of the failings of care quality. Increasingly campaigns focused on the need to make services more personalized to the individual to give them as much choice and control as possible.

▶ The personalization reform agenda has been very effective for some people – particularly younger disabled people who have taken up a direct payment – but its effects have been variable, by geography and by type of user group. Older people in particular have not yet experienced many of its benefits.

▶ Campaigns to make services more integrated have a high profile in health and social care sectors, but achieving progress on these goals remains slow. There is hope that the Care Act 2014 will be a focal point for a renewed push on integration and prevention.

▶ The rising incidence of dementia is putting a strain on health and social care services, and drawing attention to the problem of services which assume that health and care can be treated separately.

Questions for Discussion

1 What approaches might make it easier to integrate health and social care services?

2 What impact might a different professional background (nursing or social work, for example) have on how you assessed someone with a long-term health condition?

3 What are some of the advantages and disadvantages of broadening the use of personal budgets?

Glossary

care management: this dated from the NHS and Community Care Act 1990 and was a government policy designed to involve people using services more fully in the assessment and planning of care, but it is largely considered to have failed to achieve this due to an overemphasis on cost-containment, which prevented social workers from undertaking assessments that were person-centred; the policy of personalization from 2007 was developed in response to the perceived failings of the care management approach

community care: this approach stemmed from the NHS and Community Care Act 1990 and aimed to ensure that people using social care services could do so in their own homes or close to their families rather than in large institutions, but it drew criticism because of a perceived failure of supply of adequate types of support housing within communities; sections of the media were also critical of the perceived risks of putting people with mental health problems and learning disabilities into communities rather than containing them within isolated institutional settings

direct payments: these were legalized in 1996 following pressure from disability rights organizations to allow people with disabilities to have direct financial control over their support; this commitment to 'independent living' was originally pioneered by people with physical disabilities, but the legislation has been extended so that now anyone with an assessed social care need is eligible for a direct payment; the government wants to move as many people as possible on to this form of funding as it is associated with better outcomes for people than when their care money is managed by the local authority

personalization: this became a mainstream social care policy objective following the Putting People First concordat signed by government and social care

15

stakeholder organizations in 2007, which has cross-party support and has continued as a national policy despite the changes in government; personalization has four aspects – early intervention and prevention, increased choice and control, enhanced social capital, and better access to universal services; of these, it has been choice and control – and particularly personal budgets – which fall within this quadrant, which has become the most high-profile aspect of personalization

personal budgets: these refer to the allocation of money which is granted to people using social care services; the money can be received as cash (a direct payment) or managed on their behalf by the local authority or a third party (then called a managed personal budget)

personal care: refers to a set of highly personal practices – primarily washing and dressing – which people may be supported to do because of their social care need; providers of this type of service must be registered with the sector regulator, the Care Quality Commission

social capital: an academic theory which helps to measure and explain the connections that people have within their communities (bonding social capital) and across different communities (bridging social capital); people with higher levels of social capital are considered likely to have higher levels of well-being and to be able to access more informal community support than people with lower levels who may be reliant on statutory services

Further Reading

A. M. Gray and D. Birrell: *Transforming Adult Social Care*. Bristol: Policy Press, 2013.
This book provides an introduction to social care issues.

C. Needham and J. Glasby (eds): *Debates in Personalisation*. Bristol: Policy Press, 2014.
This books gives discussion of the advantages and disadvantages of personalization and direct payments.

A. Cameron, R. Lart, L. Bostock and C. Coomber (2012): *Factors that Promote and Hinder Joint and Integrated Working across the Health and Social Care Interface*. London: Social Care Institute for Excellence.

This book provides an overview of research findings on factors which promote and inhibit integrated working between health and social care.

SCIE: *Research Briefing 4*. London: Social Care Institute for Excellence, 2004. This report gives a discussion of factors that promote and hinder joint and integrated working between health and social care services.

M. Barnes: *Care in Everyday Life*. Bristol: Policy Press, 2012. This book gives a discussion of the practices of care, and some of the ethical issues of delivering social care.

J. Lewis and A. West: Re-shaping social care services for older people in England: policy development and the problem of achieving 'good care', *Journal of Social Policy* 43 (2014): 1–18. This article focuses on some of the issues involved in providing 'good care' for older people.

Also useful are the following online resources:

The Social Care Institute for Excellence (<www.scie.org.uk/>) A very comprehensive range of care resources, including videos and easy-read versions of reports.

Age UK (<www.ageuk.org.uk/>) Information about older people's services.

In Control (<http://www.in-control.org.uk/>) Personalization in social care services has been promoted by the social innovation network. See their website for reports on the progress of personalization and information about the ideas behind the personalization reforms.

The Alzheimer's Society (<www.alzheimers.org.uk>) This is a good place to find information and resources about dementia.

References

Age UK 2013 *Making Managed Personal Budgets Work for Older People*. London: Age UK. At: <http://www.ageuk.org.uk/professional-resources-home/services-and-practice/care-and-support/personalisation-hub/making-personal-budgets-work-for-older-people/>.

Alzheimer's Society 2014a *Alzheimer's Society Calls for Action as Scale and Cost of Dementia Soars*. At: <http://www.alzheimers.org.uk/site/scripts/news_article.php?newsID=2168>.

Alzheimer's Society 2014b *The Dementia Guide: Living Well after Diagnosis*. London: Alzheimer's Society.

Baxter K., Wilberforce, M. and Glendinning, C. 2011 Personal budgets and the workforce implications for social care providers. *Social Policy and Society* 10/1: 55–65.

BBC 2014 *GPs To Be Paid £55 for Each Dementia Diagnosis*, 22 October. At: <http://www.bbc.co.uk/news/health-29718618>.

Bolton, S. C. and Wibberley, G. 2013 Domiciliary care: the formal and informal labour process. *Sociology* 48/4: 682–97.

Cameron, A. M., Lart, R. A., Bostock, L. and Coomber, C. 2012 *Factors that Promote and Hinder Joint and Integrated Working across the Health and Social Care Interface*. London: Social Care Institute for Excellence.

15

Carr, S. 2010 *Personalization: A Rough Guide* (revised edn). London: Social Care Institute for Excellence.

Crosby, N. 2010 *Personalization: Children, Young People and Families*. Wythall: In Control.

Department of Health 1989 *Caring for People: Community Care in the Next Decade and Beyond*. London: HMSO.

Department of Health 2001 *Valuing People: A New Strategy for Learning Disability for the Twenty-first Century*. London: Department of Health.

Department of Health 2009a *Personal Health Budgets: First Steps*. London: Department of Health.

Department of Health 2009b *Living Well with Dementia: A National Dementia Strategy*. London: Department of Health.

Department of Health 2010 *A Vision for Adult Social Care: Capable Communities and Active Citizens*. London: Department of Health.

EHRC (Equalities and Human Rights Commission) 2011 *Close to Home: An Inquiry into Older People and Human Rights in Home Care*. London: Equalities and Human Rights Commission.

Forder, J., Jones, K., Glendinning, C., Caiels, J., Welch, E., Baxter, K., Davidson, J., Windle, K., Irvine, A., King, D. and Dolan, P. 2012 *Evaluation of the Personal Health Budget Pilot Programme*. London: Department of Health.

Glasby, J. 2005 The integration dilemma: how deep and how broad to go? *Journal of Integrated Care* 13/5: 27–30.

Glasby, J. 2007 *Understanding Health and Social Care*. Bristol: Policy Press.

Glasby, J. 2013 Distinction between sick, frail and disabled has to go. *The Conversation*, 3 July. At: <http://theconversation.com/distinction-between-sick-frail-and-disabled-has-to-go-15735>.

Glendinning, C., Halliwell, S., Jacobs, S. et al. 2008 *Evaluation of the Individual Budgets Pilot Programme*. York: Social Policy Research Unit.

Gray, A. M. and Birrell, D. 2013 *Transforming Adult Social Care*. Bristol: Policy Press.

Hart, V. 2014 A view from social work practice. In C. Needham and J. Glasby (eds), *Debates in Personalisation*. Bristol: Policy Press, pp. 113–18.

Henwood, M. 2014 Self-funders: the road from perdition? In C. Needham and J. Glasby (eds), *Debates in Personalisation*. Bristol: Policy Press, pp. 77–85.

HM Government 2007 *Putting People First*. London: HM Government.

HM Government 2014 *Care and Support Minister Norman Lamb Talks about the Biggest Reforms to the Social Care System in more than 60 Years*. At: <https://www.gov.uk/government/speeches/care-bill-becomes-care-act-2014>.

House of Lords 2013 *Ready for Ageing: Report from the Select Committee on Public Service and Demographic Change*. London: The Stationery Office.

Leadbeater, C. 2004 *Personalization through Participation: A New Script for Public Services*. London: Demos.

Leece, J. 2010 Paying the piper and calling the tune: Power and the direct payment relationship. *British Journal of Social Work* 40/1: 188–206.

Lewis, J. and Glennerster, H. 1996 *Implementing the New Community Care*. Buckingham: Open University Press.

Lewis, J. and West, A. 2014 Re-shaping social care services for older people in England: policy development and the problem of achieving 'good care'. *Journal of Social Policy* 43: 1–18.

Lloyd, L. 2014 Can personalization work for older people? In C. Needham and J. Glasby (eds), *Debates in Personalization*. Bristol: Policy Press, pp. 57–66.

Means, R., Richards, S. and Smith, R. 2008 *Community Care*, 4th edn. Basingstoke: Palgrave.

Nuffield Trust 2012 *A Decade of Austerity?* London: Nuffield Trust.

O'Brien, J. and Tyne, A. 1981 *The Principle of Normalization: A Foundation for Effective Services*. London: Campaign for Mentally Handicapped People.

Oliver, M. 1990 *The Politics of Disablement*. Basingstoke: Macmillan.

Roulstone, A. and Prideaux, S. 2012 *Understanding Disability Policy*. Bristol: Policy Press.

Royle, C. 2014 Managing a personal health budget: Malcolm's story(book). In C. Needham and J. Glasby (eds), *Debates in Personalization*. Bristol: Policy Press, pp. 119–23.

Samuel, M. 2013 Most councils met 70 percent personal budgets target, say directors. *Community Care*, 9 September. Available at: <http://www.communitycare.co.uk/2013/09/10/most-councils-met-70-personal-budgets-target-say-directors/http://www.communitycare.co.uk/2013/09/10/most-councils-met-70-personal-budgets-target-say-directors/>.

SCIE (Social Care Institute for Excellence) 2009 *At a Glance 17: Personalization Briefing, Implications for Residential Care Homes*. London: SCIE.

SCIE (Social Care Institute for Excellence) 2013 *Fair Access to Care Services: Prioritizing Eligibility for Care and Support*. London: SCIE. Available at: <http://www.scie.org.uk/publications/guides/guide33/>.

Scourfield, P. 2006 'What matters is what works'? How discourses of modernization have both silenced and limited debate on domiciliary care for older people. *Critical Social Policy* 26/1: 5–30.

Skills for Care 2013 *The Size and Structure of the Adult Social Care Sector and Workforce in England*. Leeds: Skills for Care.

Stanley, N., Manthorpe, J. and Penhale, B. (eds) 1999 *Institutional Abuse: Perspectives across the Life Course*. London: Psychology Press.

Think Local, Act Personal (TLAP) 2013 *Making it Real for People with Dementia*. London: Think Local, Act Personal.

Waters, J. and Hatton, C. 2014 *The Third National Personal Budgets Survey*. London: In Control.

15

Global Health

Sarah Earle

KEY ISSUES IN THIS CHAPTER:
- ▶ Global patterns of health and disease.
- ▶ Globalization, nursing and health.
- ▶ Reproductive and sexual health in a global context.
- ▶ Nursing and migration.

BY THE END OF THIS CHAPTER YOU SHOULD BE ABLE TO:
- ▶ Explain general patterns of health and disease across the world.
- ▶ Define and understand the concept of globalization as it applies to health and nursing.
- ▶ Discuss why reproduction and sexuality are important to global health.
- ▶ Discuss the significance of the global context for the nursing workforce.

1 Introduction

Every day, individuals make choices that influence their own health and that of those around them. Individual choices can have far-reaching consequences, but these choices are shaped, influenced and sometimes even determined by local, national and international events. Sociology is significant because it can throw light on the relationship between the individual and the wider society. In recent years, events such as the ebola crisis, the 9/11 terrorist attacks, the impact of global warming and the financial crisis of 2008 demonstrate the global consequences of individual actions and the impact of global events on individual health and well-being. This chapter is organized into four sections. The first section begins by outlining global patterns of health and disease.

The next section defines and explores globalization and considers the impact of this for health and well-being. Next, and in order to explore globalization and well-being in more detail, the focus turns to the issue of reproductive and sexual health. The final section of this chapter examines the phenomenon of international nurse migration within the context of a global health workforce crisis.

16

2 Global patterns of health and disease

child mortality: child death under the age of five

Globally, health is improving. Over the last fifty years, global life expectancy has increased by twenty years and **child mortalit**y (which is an excellent indicator of a nation's present and future health) has decreased by approximately 7 million (WHO 2003). However, good health is not shared by all and it is not equally distributed. For example, according to the World Health Organization (WHO 2005), more than half of all child deaths across the world occur in just six countries (China, the Democratic Republic of the Congo, Ethiopia, India, Nigeria and Pakistan). Children, especially those under the age of five, are particularly at risk from inequalities in health, facing the acute dangers of birth injury, infectious diseases, malnutrition and pollution. Maternal health and child health are strongly intertwined and the need for improved reproductive and sexual health across the world is widely recognized (Section 4 in this chapter explores this topic). Read Box 16.1 which tells you more about global health inequalities.

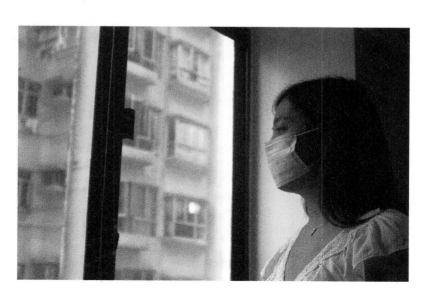

Figure 16.1 Diseases such as SARS and swine flu can affect people around the whole world

> ### Box 16.1 Global health inequalities
>
> - About 4 million children die each year before one month of age and an additional 3.3 million are stillborn. Of all these child deaths, 99 per cent occur in low- and middle-income countries.
> - Approximately a quarter of all children in developing countries are underweight and at risk of the longer-term effects of undernourishment.
> - More than 500,000 women in developing countries die each year in childbirth or of complications from pregnancy.
> - In low- and middle-income countries, 30 per cent of all deaths occur at ages fifteen to fifty-nine, compared with 15 per cent in high-income countries.
> - Virtually all deaths from communicable diseases, maternal and perinatal conditions, and nutritional deficiencies occur in low- and middle-income countries.
> - In sub-Saharan Africa, two thirds of all deaths can be attributed to communicable diseases (including HIV/AIDS), perinatal conditions and nutritional deficiencies; these causes were responsible for a third of all deaths in South Asia.
>
> *(Lopez, Begg and Bos 2006; UNDESA 2008)*

More recently, the global burden of neuropsychiatric disorders, which had previously been largely ignored, has come to the attention of policymakers. While mortality is undoubtedly an important measure of health and disease, it is accepted that disability and ill health caused by disease, injury, war and disasters can play an important role in determining the overall health of populations across the world (see Box 16.2).

> ### Box 16.2 Global mental health issues
>
> - Approximately 20 per cent of the world's children and young people have mental disorders or problems.
> - Mental disorders are important risk factors for other diseases, as well as unintentional and intentional injury.
> - Mental and substance-use disorders are the leading cause of disability worldwide.
> - Around 800,000 people commit suicide every year.
> - War and disasters have a big impact on mental health and psychosocial well-being.
> - Discrimination and stigma against patients and families prevent people from seeking mental health care.
>
> *(WHO 2015)*

Globally, neuropsychiatric conditions are the most important cause of disability, affecting both men and women equally. Depression is the leading cause of disability for men and women, but women have higher burdens from anxiety disorders, migraine and dementia. In contrast, the global burden for alcohol and drug-use disorders is six times higher for men than for women. Children who survive malnutrition,

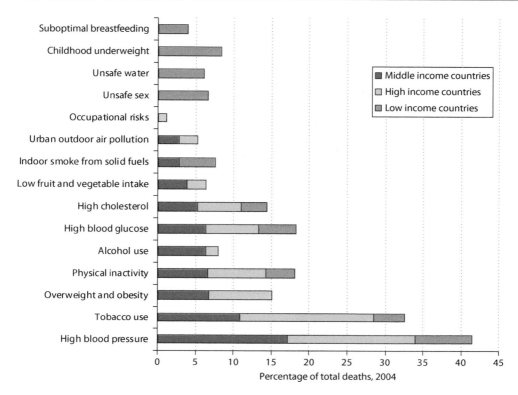

Figure 16.2 Deaths attributed to ten leading risk factors, by country income level, 2004

infectious diseases and other childhood threats are also likely to suffer from physical and learning disabilities into adult life. For example, children who have survived cerebral malaria can experience severe anaemia and neurological complications that can irreversibly impair cognitive function (Global Health Council, online).

Activity 16.1 The global burden of disease

Study the information provided in Figure 16.2 and then answer the questions below.

(a) Describe the main differences in global patterns of disease between low- and middle-income countries compared to high-income countries.

(b) What is the leading cause of death in low- and middle-income countries?

(c) What is the leading cause of death in high-income countries?

(d) What does this graph tell you about the comparative global burden of non-fatal illnesses?

The measurement of global patterns of disease and mortality is not an easy task. Data are drawn from a variety of sources that are not always comparable. For example, death registration systems are not universally implemented and, even when implemented, are not always complete. Cause of death is also not always recorded accurately and,

epidemiological:
branch of medicine that studies causes, distribution, and control of disease in populations

for deaths from causes such as HIV/AIDS, malaria and tuberculosis (TB), **epidemiological** estimates are used (Mathers, Lopez and Murray 2006). However, in general, people living in developing countries have shorter life expectancies than those in developed countries and they tend to live a higher proportion of their lives in poorer health.

Demographic changes to the world's population also have a profound impact on the global burden of disease and on patterns of health and illness; two global demographic changes are particularly significant.

First, the world population has increased exponentially since the beginning of the twentieth century and it continues to rise. In 2008, the world population was approximately 6.7 billion (IPC online) and it is expected to continue to rise to over 9 billion by 2050, with population growth at its highest in developing countries (UNDESA 2007). However, the countries with the largest populations are also often the ones with the least resources available to support this growth. Over 60 per cent of the global population will most likely live in Africa and Asia by 2050, and 70 per cent of this growth will take place in the world's poorest countries (Oxford Martin Commission 2013).

ageing population:
increase in number of older people coupled with reduced amount of children and persons of working age

Second, the population is also **ageing**. A report on world population ageing, published by the United Nations Department of Economic and Social Affairs (UNDESA 2007), has shown that the ageing population is an unprecedented process without parallel in the history of humanity (see Box 16.3). The report of the Oxford Martin Commission for Future Generations (2013) describes this phenomenon as a **megatrend**.

megatrend:
important shift in the evolution of society

Box 16.3 Global population ageing

Globally, the number of older people in the population is expected to exceed the number of children for the first time in 2047. In developed countries, the number of older people exceeded the number of children in 1998.

* Population ageing affects nearly all the countries of the world.
* Population ageing results mainly from reductions of fertility. Fertility is unlikely to increase substantially to reverse this trend.
* Population ageing has major consequences for all aspects of human life. At an economic level it affects: economic growth, savings, investment, consumption, labour markets, pensions and taxation. In the social sphere it affects: family composition and living arrangements, housing demand, migration trends, epidemiology and the demand for health and social care services.

(Source: UNDESA 2007)

Demographic changes across the world can have enormous consequences for health and well-being, and can place different and competing demands on health-care services. Good health is not enjoyed equally by all and there are considerable inequalities in health across the globe. The next section in this chapter further examines global change by exploring the concept and process of globalization.

3 Globalization, nursing and health

Globalization is much discussed and debated. It has been described as a concept, a process, a project and even a revolution. However it is described or defined, though, it is associated with some of the most important changes in the late twentieth and early twenty-first centuries, and cannot be ignored (Scriven 2005).

Attempting to critically theorize the concept of globalization, Kellner argues:

> [T]he key to understanding globalization is theorizing it as at once a product of technological revolution and the global restructuring of capitalism in which economic, technological, political, and cultural features are inter-twined. From this perspective, one should avoid both technological and economic determinism and all one-sided optics of globalization in favour of a view that theorizes globalization as a highly complex, contradictory, and thus ambiguous set of institutions and social relations, as well as one involving flows of goods, services, ideas, technologies, cultural forms, and people. (Kellner 2002: 285)

In a nutshell, globalization refers to the expansion of capitalism and is an economic phenomenon (Geertz 1998). However, as Kellner suggests, globalization is also much more than this. For example, changes in information and communications technologies (ICTs) are also part of globalization. Mobile phones and the increasing availability of broadband Internet facilitate commerce and communication across international borders in a way never seen before.

There is considerable debate between globalization scholars, including sociologists, as to the nature of globalization, how and why it has come about and even if it really exists! (For example, see Castells 1996.)

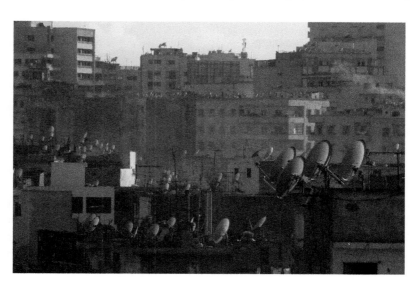

Figure 16.3
Globalization means that people all over the world are becoming interconnected in unprecedented ways, spreading messages and ideas around the globe

Leaving that debate aside, there is also extensive discussion on whether globalization is a force for good, or a negative influence on society. Many sociologists believe that globalization is 'Janus-faced' (Guillén 2001); that is, they believe that globalization is simultaneously positive and negative. Pro-globalization groups (for example, the International Policy Network or World Growth) argue that free trade, in the form of goods, services, ideas and technologies, creates global wealth which, in turn, creates peaceful, prosperous and healthy societies. In contrast, anti-globalization groups (such as Consumers International or Friends of the Earth International) argue that free trade is not fair trade and that globalization destroys traditional cultures, communities and local economies, leading to poverty and inequalities in health.

Referring specifically to the impact of globalization on health, McMichael and Beaglehole (2000) describe it as a 'mixed blessing'. On the one hand, they highlight how rapid economic growth and the availability of new technologies have led to a welcome global increase in life expectancy and indeed dramatically enhanced health and well-being for some. On the other hand, they suggest that globalization – including the flow of goods, services, ideas, technologies, cultural forms and people – poses a serious health risk across the world (McMichael and Beaglehole 2000, 2009; see Box 16.4).

Box 16.4 Globalization and potential health risks

- Marginalization and poverty, which develop and maintain higher morbidity and mortality rates.
- Global environmental degradation such as the spread of invasive species, the dispersal of organic pollutants and atmospheric changes.
- Increased power of global capital, together with fragmentation of labour markets, leading to lower standards of occupational health and safety.
- The expansion of the international drug trade.
- The expansion of trafficking in people.
- Increased international travel, leading to the faster spread of toxins and infectious diseases.
- Increased refugee populations and rapid population growth, leading to greater chance of ethnic and civil conflict.
- Increased consumerism and the global marketing of harmful commodities such as tobacco.

(Yach and Bettcher, 1998: 737; McMichael and Beaglehole 2009: 12)

The 2007 World Health Report (WHO 2007), which focused on global public health security, noted some of these concerns and stated:

Today's highly mobile, interdependent and interconnected world provides myriad opportunities for the rapid spread of infectious diseases, and radionuclear and toxic threats.... Infectious diseases are now spreading geographically much faster than at any time in history. It is estimated that 2.1 billion airline passengers travelled in 2006; an outbreak or epidemic in any one part of the world is only a few hours away from becoming an imminent threat somewhere else. (WHO 2007: 6)

The UK government strategy *Health is Global* (Department of Health 2008) was the first cross-government strategy to tackle the issues connected to global health. This strategy outlined a set of principles and actions for the UK government, which set out to improve the health of people across the world, including those living in the UK. *Health is Global* outlined five specific areas for action and commits billion of pounds to the project of global health security. Most recently, Public Health England's *Global Health Strategy* (TSO 2014) outlines a set of strategic areas and actions that the English government will focus on between 2014 and 2019 to improve the health of people across the world, including those living in the UK (see Box 16.5).

> **Box 16.5 England's global health strategy: five priority areas**
> 1. Improving global health security
> 2. Responding to outbreaks and incidents of international concern, and supporting humanitarian disasters
> 3. Building public health capacity, particularly in low- and middle-income countries
> 4. Developing capacity for engagement on international aspects of health and well-being
> 5. Strengthening UK partnerships for global health activity
>
> *(TSO 2014: 5)*

In relation to the impact of globalization on nursing, Grootjans and Newman (2012) suggest that there are three essential issues that nurses should grasp in order to respond to the challenge of nursing within a globalized world.

- Nurses should acknowledge that absence of disease is not their primary goal; it is well-being.

human ecology:
relationship between individuals and natural, social and built environments

- Nurses should move away from human biology to **human ecology**, recognizing the importance of social and structural determinants of health.
- Nurses should look beyond local influences on well-being and towards national and global events and how these impact on everyday life.

In essence, Grootjans and Newman (2012: 83) argue that responding to globalization is about 'what each of us does locally but now also includes a broader context for nurses who now need to reflect on the idea that to act locally is to have a global impact'.

So far, this chapter has demonstrated that globalization is a process with far-reaching consequences for the health of people and populations. Globalization also impacts on nursing work and nursing knowledge. The next section focuses specifically on reproductive and sexual health within a global context and on the role of nurses in realizing this important aspect of health.

4 Reproductive and sexual health in a global context

Achieving reproductive and sexual health for all is a vital part of a healthy world. It is an important goal in itself because it is a human right and people should be able to make their own choices. It is also important because it is essential to human development and to the achievement and maintenance of a good level of health. In addition to this, reproductive and sexual health is inextricably linked to the achievement of other important aims, such as those set out in the United Nations Millennium Development Goals (see Box 16.6). For example, making progress on sexual and reproductive health is thought to impact on better child health as well as on the wider goals of eradicating extreme poverty, promoting gender equality and achieving universal primary education. The UK Department for International Development (2004) argues that even a small investment in improving reproductive and sexual health can have a massive impact on the health of individuals and populations at local and global levels.

Box 16.6 United Nations Millennium Development Goals
1. Eradicate extreme poverty and hunger
2. Achieve universal primary education
3. Promote gender equality and empower women
4. Reduce child mortality
5. Improve maternal health
6. Combat HIV/AIDS, malaria and other diseases
7. Ensure environmental sustainability
8. Develop a global partnership for development
(UNDP 2008: online)

The joint declaration of the 1994 International Conference on Population and Development (ICPD) held in Cairo defined reproductive health as:

> a state of complete physical, mental and social well-being and not merely the absence of disease or infirmity, in all matters relating to the reproductive systems and to its functions and processes. Men and women should be able to enjoy a satisfying and safe sex life, have the capability to reproduce and the freedom to decide if, when and how often to do so. This requires informed choice and access to safe, effective affordable and acceptable health-care services. (ICPD 1994: online)

16

Arguably, realizing reproductive and sexual health requires an acknowledgement of women's sexual rights and the need for gender equality. Some of the key elements of providing reproductive and sexual health care can be found in Box 16.7.

Box 16.7 The key elements of reproductive and sexual health care

(a) Family planning.
(b) Antenatal, safe delivery and post-natal care.
(c) Prevention and appropriate treatment of infertility.
(d) Prevention of abortion and management of the consequences of abortion.
(e) Treatment of reproductive tract infections.
(f) Prevention, care and treatment of STIs and HIV/AIDS.
(g) Information, education and counselling, as appropriate, on human sexuality and reproductive health.
(h) Prevention and surveillance of violence against women, care for survivors of violence and other actions to eliminate traditional harmful practices, such as Female genital mutilation/circumcision.

(UNFPA 2008)

While there have been some improvements in the global experience of reproductive and sexual health, in many parts of the world access to health care falls considerably short of what would be required to achieve good health for all. Sexual and reproductive health problems account for a third of health issues for women of reproductive age. Many of these health problems are preventable.

Unsafe sex is a particular risk factor in developing countries. Sexual behaviour varies a lot across the world, but in Africa unsafe sex – associated with non-use or ineffective use of barrier methods of contraception – accounts for nearly 100 per cent of HIV infection.

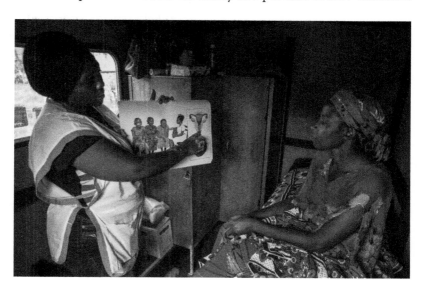

Figure 16.4 Mobile sexual health clinics play a vital role in ensuring access to reproductive health care

Young women and girls are especially at risk, also leaving themselves vulnerable to tuberculosis, which is a leading cause of death. Globally 222 million women do not have access to the contraceptive services they need. This means that many people are also at increased risk of other sexually acquired infections such as gonorrhoea, chlamydia and syphilis. Syphilis alone accounts for 20,000 stillbirths each year and 90,000 neonatal deaths globally.

A lack of contraception and the risk of unintended pregnancy is also very significant, as is the risk of unsafe abortions and the complications that arise from these. It is thought that in Africa only 14 per cent of women use modern contraception (which includes the pill, condoms, sterilization or an intrauterine device). According to WHO (2009), if all of the women who wanted to use contraception were able to do so the usage figure would probably be 46 per cent. WHO (2015) have set out a framework to ensure human rights within contraceptive service delivery. As part of this, the framework focuses on providing quality care that is comprehensive and promotes privacy, confidentiality and informed decision-making. However, it is not always easy to realize these goals in practice. A global report on the right to decide for people with learning disabilities, *Independent but not Alone* (Inclusion International 2014), reveals that people with intellectual disabilities are often denied the basic right to control what happens to their own bodies. In relation to their reproductive and sexual rights – and in general – particular issues were highlighted:

- They are often excluded from participation in health-care education and programmes.
- When they are included in health-care programmes the information is not always easy to understand.
- Because information is not always understood, it is difficult to make informed decisions.
- They are not always invited to consent to treatment and decisions are often made on their behalf by relatives or carers.
- Their views are sometimes discounted and not taken seriously.

Appropriate reproductive and sexual health services are the cornerstone of improving health and well-being. However, this means that services should be responsive, appropriate to local needs, high quality, affordable, accessible and non-discriminatory (DFID 2004). There can be many barriers to the provision of high-quality services in the area of reproductive and sexual health. At a most basic level these include issues relating to economic and health infrastructures, including the availability of health-care workers and services, but other issues are also impactful. For example, in times of war and disaster, reproductive and sexual health is often neglected, and indeed women are often at a higher risk of sexual and physical violence and sexually acquired infection (Health Poverty Action 2015: online).

Fundamentalist and religious views can also make a difference to whether contraception and abortion are available and in what circumstances. For example, writing specifically about Pentecostalism in Brazil, Ogland and Verona (2011) suggest that commitment to religious attendance and participation, together with a conservative moral orientation and pro-family discourse, has served to politicize the abortion debate.

However, there are many individuals and organizations who work towards challenging the cultural norms which impact negatively on women's health and well-being, and on the well-being of their children and communities. In Box 16.8 the NGO Health Poverty Action reports on a life-changing initiative in Ethiopia that questions the traditional practice of female genital cutting:

Box 16.8 Islamic religious leader challenges cultural norms in Ethiopia

As an Islamic religious leader, Sheik Tesfaye Abate is a well-respected and influential member of his community in the Bale Lowlands, Ethiopia. We have trained him to lead open discussions about sensitive health issues and move his community towards a consensus.

In these meetings, he challenges the community to rethink the cultural norms that they have been practising for decades, like female genital cutting. He also takes other opportunities to broach difficult topics. 'I have been using every opportunity to discuss health issues, and in my role as a religious leader I also start discussions after worship. People often come to me for advice, and I talk with them.'

Before the project trained him and provided him with reading materials on sexual and reproductive health issues, Sheik Abate had very little knowledge of the issues himself. Gesturing to the dusty surroundings of his home, he says, 'Before, we didn't know about HIV testing and that harmful traditional practices were so prevalent here.'

Sheik Abate feels that the project has really helped his community. 'It should continue and grow. We are working for the sake of the community. If the project ended tomorrow, we would still continue. The community is happy to have learnt about harmful traditional practices. Some still want to have many wives and to practise female genital cutting, but we are challenging each other on these issues now. People are changing.'

(Health Poverty Action 2015: online)

It is increasingly recognized that reproductive and sexual health is not simply a women's issue and that it is vital to engage boys and men in this area, as well as in the promotion of gender equality more generally. The example above illustrates how community leaders – often men – can influence change and improve health. There are many initiatives globally that seek to involve boys and men in one of three areas: (a) as clients; (b) as supportive partners; and (c) as agents of change (WHO 2015). You can read about one such example of a community-based programme specifically focused on engaging boys and men in Activity 16.2.

Activity 16.2 Community-based reproductive health services in Uganda: the Family Life Education Program

Read about the Family Life Education Program in Uganda and then answer the questions below:

> The Family Life Education Program (FLEP), through its Community-Based Reproductive Health Services (CBRHS), implemented strategies to engage men and male adolescents and improve access to family planning and reproductive health services in order to remedy Uganda's high maternal mortality rate, poor antenatal care, low contraceptive use and increasing cases of STIs, including HIV. FLEP collaborates with the Church of Uganda through the Parish Development Committee on programme implementation and monitoring. Community-based drug agents (CBDAs) are trained to deliver health education, group discussions and couple counselling on family planning, STIs, HIV and other reproductive health issues. FLEP recruited male CBDAs to work along with female CBDAs and strengthened men's involvement in pregnancy and women's reproductive health. The programme operates from stationary and mobile clinics. Additionally, youth centres were established to develop youth peer educators (YPEs) who provide counselling, information sharing and basic health care services to young people. A radio teen show, drama skits and sports are also used to reach teens. (UNFPA 2011: 57)

(a) How are boys and men being involved in this case study? As clients, supportive partners or agents of change?

(b) Do you agree that reproductive and sexual health is not just a women's issue? Do you agree that boys and men should be more engaged?

(c) If you were involved in planning and delivering nurse-led sexual health services, how would you go about encouraging and including boys and men to make better use of services or to support their partners?

---

5 Nursing work: a global view

Globally, there is a health workforce crisis (WHO 2006). That is, there is a serious shortage of health-care workers across the world, and this is seen as a crucial factor in the achievement of health and development goals, such as the United Nation's Millennium Development Goals. Overall, there is a critical shortage of nurses, midwives and doctors equivalent to 2.4 billion workers worldwide. According to the World Health Report 2006 (WHO 2006), there are fifty-seven countries (mostly in Africa, Asia and South America) that face a particularly acute crisis. There is considerable inequity between countries, with those that have the greatest need for quality health care experiencing the greatest threat to their workforce. There is also inequity between urban populations – where there are sometimes high concentrations of health workers – and rural populations, where there is often scarcity at unsafe levels, especially in the least developed countries. Organizations such as the Global Health Workforce Alliance, which is an alliance hosted and administered by the World Health Organization, work in partnership with governments, civil society, finance institutions, international agencies, professional associations and others to identify and implement solutions to the global health workforce crisis.

The global health workforce is large and diverse. It consists of a range of individuals employed in a variety of occupations working with individuals, groups and communities at local, regional, national and international levels. In all countries, a well-educated and flexible health workforce is essential to the delivery of health-care services, as well as to the performance of health systems in more general terms. Beaglehole and Bonita (2001) argue that most governments have neglected public-health workforce development and that, in some developing countries, the situation is especially acute.

In a globalized world the migration of people across borders is not uncommon. Nurse migration happens for a variety of reasons; economists describe this as the 'push' and the 'pull'. **Push** factors might include low wages, job insecurity, poor prospects and discrimination. **Pull** factors include higher salaries, safe work environments, job security and better training and education opportunities.

While low-income countries often rely on NGOs for health service delivery, high-income countries such as the UK, the United States, New Zealand and Australia often recruit nurses from other countries; indeed, industrialized countries such as these have a long history of welcoming health-care workers from overseas. However, when nurses and other health-care workers migrate from poorer to richer economies, this instability can have a very negative impact on the health-care workforce and, in turn, on health and health-care provision. A recent review suggests that mass migration can have a negative impact on nurse education (Hancock 2008) and that migrant nurses are socially devalued (Allan, Tschudin and Horton 2008). 'NHS bosses have been accused of adding to a developing world "skills drain" in nursing,' reports the UK national news (BBC 2000: online). Writing specifically about African countries, other commentators (Sanders et al. 2009) suggest that the 'brain drain' from Africa to the developed world is one of the most serious problems facing African countries. Furthermore, they argue that high levels of expatriation means that health-care workers who stay have increased workloads, which leads to low productivity, poorer service delivery and, thus, the conditions that push further migration.

However, the movement of health workers can have advantages for all concerned, and what is seen as a 'brain drain' can actually become a 'brain gain'. For example, recipient countries are helped to resolve worker shortages or skill-mix gaps. Migrants, who migrate for many different reasons, often learn new skills and – if they return home – bring back with them a wealth of experience and expertise. Additionally, remittances (money sent back home by migrants) are thought to reduce poverty in their country of origin. Some countries, such as the

push:
push factors refer to conditions or circumstances that encourage nurses to leave their country

pull:
pull factors refer to conditions in the destination country which attract movement into that country

Philippines, have traditionally seen large numbers of nurses migrating to work in other parts of the world (see Box 16.9). But the Philippine Overseas Employment Administration has developed an incentive programme, including tax-free shopping, subsidized business loans and scholarships, to encourage migrants to return home (WHO 2006). In an article reported in the *Nursing Times*, one British nurse acknowledges her gain in having worked with migrant nurses during her career:

> I feel very privileged to work with such compassionate and knowledgeable people, and to be given the chance to learn about life and attitudes in different parts of the world. Without foreign nurses, some of our hospitals would not be able to cope with the demands made on them, and people would not receive the care they need. The burden on existing nurses such as myself would be intolerable, and any joy or satisfaction from nursing would disappear under an increasing mountain of work. (Crampton 2003: 13)

However, not everybody paints such a rosy picture of nurse migration. Drawing on a study designed to examine why Nepali nurses migrate to the UK, Adhikari and Melia (2013) argue that Nepali nurses – who are highly qualified and specialized – have been wrongly placed in the health-care system and that their qualifications, experience and knowledge are largely ignored. Instead of working in their specialist fields of critical care, education or management, migrant Nepali nurses end up working in the care sector, often providing personal care for elderly people; this is something that migrant nurses sometimes refer to as BBC, or British Bottom Care.

Box 16.9 Providing nurses for the world? The Philippines

An estimated 150,000 Filipino nurses – 85 per cent of employed Filipino nurses – work abroad. The combination of degree-prepared nurses mostly with a good standard of English, and a Filipino government-approved programme of producing nurses for export, has resulted in thousands of nurses working overseas. Remittance income from nurses is a major source of hard currency for developing countries and has been a major motivator for the Philippines to train nurses for overseas.

Research in 1993 estimated that Filipinos working abroad sent home more than US$800 million in remittance income. The exodus of nurses from the Philippines prompted a warning from the Philippine Nurses' Association in 2003 that if the exodus continued, it would prompt a serious public health crisis by 2006. There are an estimated 30,000 nursing vacancies in the Philippines and government agencies and the Department of Health have noted that inexperienced health workers were the ones remaining in the Philippines (O'Connor 2005: online).

National policies and incentive programmes which encourage the return of emigrant workers are beneficial. However, given the huge global crisis, organizations such as the World Health Organization suggest that global solidarity is needed to resolve this problem. In particular, the World Health

16

Organisation argues that three specific actions should be taken to respond to the global health workforce crisis:

1. Catalysing knowledge and learning to include the pooling of experience and expertise to help countries tap into the best talent and practices, including identification and support for priority research issues.

2. Striking cooperative agreements to protect the health and safety of global migrants, relief workers and volunteers, the adoption of ethical recruitment practices and a willingness to commit human resources to assist in humanitarian emergencies.

3. Responding to workforce crises in the poorest developing countries to include both the immediate and long-term financing of the health care workforce. (Source: WHO 2006)

Activity 16.3 Globalization, migration and nursing work

Read the case study and then answer the questions below.

Fatima Ansari*. . . is a trim, well-dressed woman in her mid-thirties with dark eyes that communicate calm and strength. She was born in the Middle East, and is a member of an ethnic community representing only 7 per cent of the national population. Life was difficult but she grew up in a happy home, sheltered by her immediate and extended family. Ansari dreamed of being a nurse, but making the wish a reality was a continuing challenge. Women were expected to marry young, care for their husbands, and immediately build families. In spite of the powerful social pressures, Ansari persevered and with the support of her parents finished nursing school. What a momentous occasion, the day she received her diploma! It came with the promise of a wonderful future.

In her first job Ansari faced what would become an insurmountable obstacle. The fact that she belonged to an ethnic minority made her the butt off intolerable discrimination. In the eleven years Ansari worked as a nurse in her home country, she was never given a permanent position and was daily victimized by the harmful and unfair practices of her colleagues and employers. Eager to pursue her nursing education, she made countless unsuccessful attempts to enrol in continuing education courses and advanced university programmes. Despite her qualifications and willingness to learn, she was consistently refused admittance. Earning very little money and only offered sporadic temporary work contracts, she often had to work more than one job to make ends meet. Despite all her efforts, a permanent position, professional fulfilment, and career advancement became an illusion. Every day she felt more insecure and unsafe . . .

Ansari knew that in her country there was a serious nursing shortage. Seeing the desperate need for nurses made her job insecurities and poor working conditions that much more stressful and difficult to bear. Given no hope for a better future in her home country, Ansari finally decided to join her sister and brother in Sweden. (Kingma 2006: 9–10)

*This is a pseudonym.

(a) Why did Ansari become a nurse migrant?

(b) Can you think of other reasons why nurses might migrate to work in another country? Make a list of these.

(c) What are the benefits of nurse migration and what are the costs?

The UK government strategy *Health is Global* (TSO 2008) also recognized that action needed to be taken to ensure that the global shortage of health-care workers is addressed. The strategy promised up to £6 billion for the development of health systems and services, especially in low- to middle-income countries, and effective development assistance to low-income countries to help them train and retain staff.

Summary and Resources

Summary

▶ Globally health is improving. However, there is considerable disparity in health and disease across different parts of the world.
▶ Globalization can be defined in different ways and can be described as 'Janus-faced'.
▶ Improving reproductive and sexual health is important to improving overall health and well-being.
▶ International nurse migration is influenced by both 'push' and 'pull' factors, and has been described as both a 'brain drain' and a 'brain gain'.

Questions for Discussion

1 Define globalization and describe the impact of globalization on health.
2 Why is an understanding of the global context important for nurses and nursing work?
3 Would you migrate to work as a nurse in another country? What sort of 'push' and 'pull' factors would influence your decision?

Glossary

ageing population: a population ages when an increase in the proportion of older people is coupled with a reduction in the proportion of children and persons of working age; influenced by rising life expectancy coupled with a decline in fertility rates

child mortality: child death under the age of five

epidemiological: referring to epidemiology, the branch of medicine that studies the causes, distribution and control of disease in populations; also deals with the measurement of a range of factors that determine and influence health

globalization: an economic, cultural, technological and political process involving the movement of people, goods, services, cultures, technologies and ideas across international borders

human ecology:	a theory that is concerned with the relationships between individuals and their natural, social and built environments; a branch of sociology that draws on ecology and focuses especially on environment and communities
megatrend:	an important shift in the evolution of society; global and sustained forces of development that impact on all aspects of the social world
pull:	pull factors refer to conditions in the destination country which attract movement into that country; migration into a country that offers better conditions, circumstances or opportunities
push:	push factors refer to conditions or circumstances that encourage nurses to leave their country; migration away from a country due to some problem or difficulty

Further Reading

M. Kingma: *Nurses on the Move: Migration and the Global Health Care Economy*. London: ILR Press, 2006.
This is a really comprehensive book, which explores the social, economic and political context of international nurse migration. It draws on poignant interviews with nurse migrants and offers an excellent insight into the 'real face' of nurse migration.

L. Ray: *Globalization and Everyday Life*. London: Routledge, 2006.
This provides a more detailed yet accessible sociological introduction to globalization, with a focus on understanding the process of globalization and the way that it is created and sustained by the everyday actions of individuals.

M. MacLachlan: *Culture and Health: A Critical Perspective Towards Global Health*, 2nd edn. Oxford: Wiley Blackwell, 2006.
This is a much more challenging text but one that you might want to pick up if you decide to pursue a project or dissertation on the subject of global health. The book begins with the premise that most nurses and other health-care professionals practise in a multicultural society and should, therefore, seek to understand the relationship between culture, health and health care.

Also useful is the following online resource:

Health Poverty Action 2015 At: <http://www.healthpovertyaction.org/where-we-work/spotlight-stories-2/sheik-abate/v>.

References

Adhikari, R. and Melia, K.M. 2013 The (mis)management of migrant nurses in the UK: a sociological study. *Journal of Nursing Management*, early online: DOI: 10.1111/jonm.12141.

Allan, C. L. and Clarke, J. 2005 Are HIV/AIDS services in Leeds, UK, able to meet the needs of asylum seekers? *Public Health* 119: 305–11.

Allan, H., Tschudin, V. and Horton, K. 2008 The devaluation of nursing: a position statement. *Nursing Ethics* 15/4: 549–56.

BBC News Online 2000 *UK 'Fuelling Global Nurse Shortage'*, Thursday, 21 December, 18:32 GMT. Available at: <http://news.bbc.co.uk/1/hi/health/1082120.stm>.

Beaglehole, R. and Bonita, R. 2001 Challenges for public health in the global context – prevention and surveillance. *Scandinavian Journal of Public Health* 29: 81–3.

Castells, M. 1996 *The Rise of the Network Society*. Cambridge, MA: Blackwell.

Crampton, J. 2003 Foreign nurses are highly valued members of the NHS. *Nursing Times* 99/18: 13.

DFID 2004 *Sexual and Reproductive Health and Rights: A Position Paper*. London: DFID.

Feldman, R. 2006 Primary health care for refugees and asylum seekers: a review of the literature and a framework for services. *Public Health* 120/9: 809–16.

Geertz, C. 1998 The world in pieces: culture and politics at the end of the century. *Focaal: Tijdschrift voor Antropologie* 32: 91–117.

Global Health Council 2007 *Child Development in Developing Countries*. Available at: <http://www.globalhealth.org/child_health/impact/>.

Grootjans, J. and Newman, S. 2012 The relevance of globalization to nursing: a concept analysis. *International Nursing Review* 60: 78–85.

Guillén, M. 2001 Is globalization civilizing, destructive or feeble? A critique of five key debates in the social science literature. *Annual Review of Sociology* 27: 235–60.

Hancock, P. K. 2008 Nurse migration: the effects on nursing education. *International Nursing Review* 55/3: 258–64.

Inclusion International 2014 *Independent but Not Alone: A Global Report on the Right to Decide*. London: Inclusion International.

IPC 2008 *Population Division*. US Census Bureau. Available at: <http://www.census.gov/ipc/www/>.

Kellner, D. 2002 Theorizing globalization. *Sociological Theory* 20/3: 285–305.

Kingma, M. 2006 *Nurses on the Move: Migration and the Global Health Care Economy*. London: ILR Press.

Lopez, A. D., Begg, S. and Bos, E. 2006 Demographic and epidemiological characteristics of major regions, 1990–2001. In A. D. Lopez, C. D. Mathers, M. Ezzati, D. T. Jamison and C. J. L. Murray (eds), *Global Burden of Disease and Risk Factors*. Washington, DC/New York: World Bank/Oxford University Press, pp. 17–44.

Lopez, A. D., Mathers, C. D., Ezzati, M., Jamison, D. T. and Murray, C. J. L. 2006 Measuring the global burden of disease and risk factors, 1990–2001. In A. D. Lopez, C. D. Mathers, M. Ezzati, D. T. Jamison and C. J. L. Murray (eds), *Global Burden of Disease and Risk Factors*. Washington, DC/New York: World Bank/Oxford University Press, pp. 1–14.

McMichael, A. J. and Beaglehole, R. 2000 The changing global context of public health. *The Lancet* 356/9228: 495–9.

McMichael, A. J. and Beaglehole, R. 2009 The global context for public health. In R. Beaglehole (ed.), *Global Public Health: A New Era*, 2nd edn. Oxford: Oxford University Press, pp. 1–22.

Mathers, C, D., Lopez, A. D. and Murray, C. J. L. 2006 The burden of disease and mortality by condition: data, methods, and results for 2001. In A. D. Lopez, C. D. Mathers, M. Ezzati, D. T. Jamison and C. J. L. Murray (eds), *Global Burden of Disease and Risk Factors*. Washington, DC/ New York: World Bank/Oxford University Press, pp. 45–240.

O'Connor, T. 2005 The Philippines – providing nurses for the world. *Kai Tiaki: Nursing New Zealand* (May). At: <http://findarticles.com/p/articles/ mi_hb4839/is_/ai_n29183078>.

Ogland, C. P. and Verona A. P. 2011 Religion and attitudes towards abortion policy in Brazil. *Journal for the Scientific Study of Religion* 50/4: 812–21.

Oxford Martin Commission 2013 *Now for the Long Term: The Report of the Oxford Martin Commission for Future Generations*. Oxford: Oxford Martin School.

Pfeil, M. and Howe, A. 2004 Ensuring primary care reaches the 'hard to reach'. *Quality in Primary Care* 12/3: 185–90.

Sanders, D., Dovlo, D., Wilma, M. and Lehmann, U. 2009 Public health in Africa. In R. Beaglehole (ed.), *Global Public Health: A New Era*, 2nd edn. Oxford: Oxford University Press, pp. 161–84.

Scriven, A. 2005 Promoting health: a global context and rationale. In A. Scriven and S. Garman (eds), *Promoting Health: Global Perspectives*. Houndmills: Palgrave, pp. 1–13.

TSO 2008 *Health is Global: A UK Government Strategy 2008–13*. London: TSO.

UNDESA 2007 *World Population Ageing*. New York: United Nations.

UNDESA 2008 *The Millennium Development Goals Report*. New York: United Nations.

UNDP 2008 *Millennium Development Goals*. Available at: <http://www.undp. org/mdg/basics.shtml>.

UNPFA 2008 *Making Reproductive Rights and Sexual and Reproductive Health a Reality for All: Reproductive Rights and Sexual and Reproductive Health Framework*. New York: UNPFA.

UNPFA 2011 *Engaging Men and Boys in Gender Equality: Vignettes from Asia and Africa*. New York: UNPFA.

UNPFA/WHO 2015 *Ensuring Human Rights within Contraceptive Service Delivery: Implementation Guide*. Geneva: WHO/UNPFA.

Van Cleemput, P. and Parry, G. 2001 Health status of gypsy travellers. *Journal of Public Health Medicine* 23: 129–34.

WHO 2003 *The World Health Report: Shaping the Future*. Geneva: WHO.

WHO 2005 *World Health Report 2005: Make Every Mother and Child Count*. Geneva: WHO.

WHO 2006 *World Health Report 2006: Working Together for Health*. Geneva: WHO.

WHO 2007 *World Health Report 2007. A Safer Future: Global Public Health Security in the 21st Century*. Geneva: WHO.

WHO 2009 *Global Health Risks: Mortality and Burden of Disease Attributable to Selected Major Risks*. Geneva: WHO.

WHO 2015 *10 Facts on Mental Health*. Available at: <http://www.who.int/ features/factfiles/mental_health/en/>.

Yach, D. and Bettcher, D. 1998 The globalization of public health, I: Threats and opportunities. *American Journal of Public Health* 88/5: 735–8.

Index